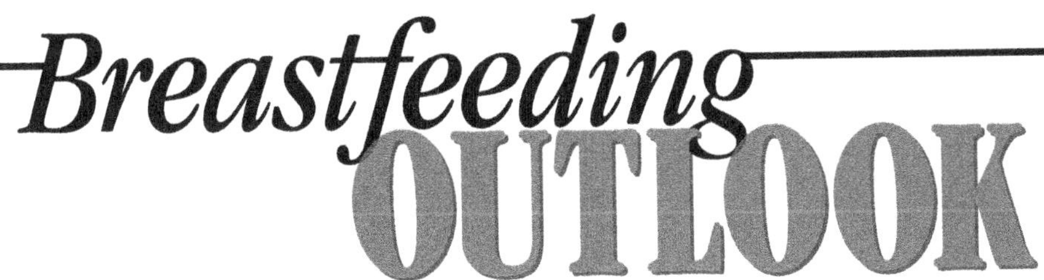

Marie Biancuzzo's
Picture Perfect Guide to Decoding Photos:
A Workbook for Passing the IBLCE Exam

Marie Biancuzzo, RN MS CCL IBCLC

Gold Standard Publishing

Graphics and Layout: *Breastfeeding Outlook*
Cover Design: *Breastfeeding Outlook*

A Note to the Reader
The author and publisher have made every attempt to check content for accuracy. Because the health care sciences are continually advancing, our knowledge base continues to expand. Therefore, we recommend that the reader check product information for changes in dosages, contraindications, and other information about any medication or intervention.

Marie Biancuzzo and Breastfeeding Outlook are not affiliated with IBLCE nor with *The Breastfeeding Atlas.*

The International Board of Lactation Consultant Examiners® (IBLCE®) owns certain names, trademarks, and logos, including IBLCE and the certification marks International Board Certified Lactation Consultant® and IBCLC® (the "Marks"). Use of these Marks in this publication does not state or imply IBLCE endorsement.

The Breastfeeding Atlas, Sixth Edition is copyrighted by Barbara Wilson-Clay and Kathleen L. Hoover, and reference to the images in that publication does not state or imply endorsement of this book by those authors.

A Request to the Reader
We invite your comments and constructive suggestions. If you find an error, please notify us at *info@breastfeedingoutlook.com.*

The most recent version of this document may always be obtained at ***breastfeedingoutlook.com***

Breastfeeding Outlook
Box 387
Herndon VA 20172-0387
breastfeedingoutlook.com

ISBN 978-1-931048-57-6

10 9 8 7 6 5 4 3

Chapter 1

Introduction

Marie Biancuzzo's Picture Perfect Guide to Decoding Photos: A Workbook for Passing the IBLCE Exam

The clock is ticking, the pressure is on. You're looking at a photo on the IBLCE exam. You see a white spot on the pictured nipple, but what does it mean? Is it yeast? Is it a sign of Raynaud's? Is it a bleb? All of those could involve a white spot! So, which is it? Will you make the right choice?

Take a deep breath. You don't need to worry anymore. Considering the many exam prep courses I've taught over the years, a good estimate is that I've taught more than 25 percent of currently-certified US IBCLCs! In other words, I've helped thousands of IBCLCs learn to distinguish between *this* and *that*. I can help you, too— on the exam, or in real life! That's why I wrote this workbook!

Maybe you've already discovered the value of viewing the photos in *The Breastfeeding Atlas*. Maybe you've flipped through the many pages of crisp, high-quality photos, but still find that conditions like "white spots" are hard to figure out. I hear this from participants in my exam prep courses often. Book in hand, they tell me: "I understand the photo when I read its caption. But I worry that if I saw a photo like it on the exam without a caption, I wouldn't be able to tell if it was *this* or *that*."

It's time to stop flipping through the photos and start developing your skills to methodically analyze them. Once you have, you'll be better prepared to care for mothers and infants in clinical practice—and also, pass the IBLCE exam!

The aim of this workbook is to help you to:

- accurately distinguish between similar but different clinical conditions shown in the photos
- use written exercises to recall and apply knowledge of typical features and their implications
- provide detailed context and clarification of terms as they may relate to items on the IBLCE exam

Focusing on the color plates found in *The Breastfeeding Atlas 6th Edition*, this workbook is chock-full of learning exercises that will help you to decode key features, confusing terminology, and more. Make the most of several different types of learning exercises—match terms to their definitions, or match photos to their clinical management. Start writing short answers for those exercises that ask you to compare and contrast key features. Respond to some provocative questions to help you identify not only what you have learned, but also what you still need to learn! Don't skip the written learning exercises, which are designed as cues to help you reflect on your learning gaps—and cement your knowledge so that you can decode the clues that—long after you pass the IBLCE exam—will help you provide top-notch, evidence-based care to breastfeeding mothers and their infants.

At the end of each chapter, you'll find a set of multiple-choice questions to help you know exactly where you stand. Although you may feel you've "got it" and want to move on to the next topic, these questions give you a much clearer understanding of your mastery before you head to the IBLCE exam.

Wilson-Clay and Hoover wrote *The Breastfeeding Atlas* as a pictorial story of individual cases; as such, the book will remain an invaluable resource throughout your lactation career. (I often tell IBLCE exam candidates they would be crazy to sit for the exam without carefully studying the *Atlas*!) In this workbook, I take a different approach. From a conceptual standpoint, I highlight relationships of photos within and between chapters. I'll help you to see features that typify common—and not-so-common—clinical conditions.

I'll help you nail the medical and lactation terminology you need to know. If you've been tripping over words like craniosynostosis, hypoplasia, nevus, hemangioma, induration or peau d'orange while reading The *Breastfeeding Atlas,* you'll be glad to find that each chapter includes a list of key terms and a vocabulary learning exercise to help you strengthen your understanding of the necessary terminology. I also provide links to YouTube videos and podcasts to help you truly master the content.

When you finish, you'll be able to recognize the characteristics that typify conditions as normal, variations of normal, or abnormal.

The first several chapters of this workbook focus on normal appearances, sleep-wake states, birth trauma and feeding issues, birthmarks and signs of abuse, stooling patterns of breastfed infants, milk color and volume in different circumstances, and positioning and latch. Later chapters address congenital and acquired breast and nipple conditions, localized infectious and breast or nipple lesions, and lactation management. The workbook also addresses data-gathering and breastfeeding management, twins and multiple births, tandem breastfeeding, supplementation, cancer, and congenital conditions such as ankyloglossia and cleft lip/palate.

In short, this workbook is an indispensable guide whether you're an experienced lactation consultant, nurse practitioner, midwife, or breastfeeding helper—or are aspiring to be one.

- *Marie Biancuzzo*

Chapter 2

Infant States and General Appearance

Parents and professionals alike know that breastfeeding is the normal method of infant feeding. They also realize that there is a range of normal breastfeeding behaviors, but they may find it difficult to distinguish between what's normal and what's abnormal. Such distinctions are key to facilitating optimal breastfeeding.

Anyone who has worked with breastfeeding families for more than a few days knows that many "breastfeeding" questions are often more about infant sleep patterns, behaviors, or skin and general appearance. Although they are not specifically "breastfeeding," those questions certainly relate to breastfeeding!

Then, there are the unasked questions that can affect the breastfeeding experience, especially those related to birth trauma. What's normal? What's a variation of normal? What's abnormal? Understanding the bigger context can very much affect the care implications for successful breastfeeding.

I promise that by the time you finish this chapter, you will be able to distinguish between normal variants (behavioral states, skin or general appearance, and birth trauma) and identify feeding implications (if any) for the breastfeeding newborn. By looking carefully and methodically at the photos in *The Breastfeeding Atlas* and doing the learning exercises here, you will soon be able to do that!

Objectives

Given a clinical photo, you will be able to:

- Recognize key features that distinguish one sleep state from another.
- Recognize newborn sleep states or behaviors that indicate feeding readiness, resistance, or satiety and their meaning for the caregiver.
- Describe newborn jaundice in terms of how to blanch for its presence, the technology to treat it, and its relationship to breastfeeding.
- Compare and contrast at least three types of skin conditions that are considered normal in newborns.
- Recognize the most common examples of birth trauma (including those related to diagnostic testing and therapeutic intervention) and their effect on feeding behavior.
- Distinguish between a caput succedaneum and a cephalohematoma in terms of their visible clues, as well as their implications for breastfeeding.
- State the definition of at least 10 terms related to newborn appearance, state, behavior, and general well-being.

Key Terms

- active alert state
- approach (engaging) behaviors
- avoidance behaviors
- blanching
- brachial plexus
- caput succedaneum
- cephalohematoma
- deep sleep
- drowsy sleep
- erythema toxicum
- forceps
- facial palsy
- Epstein's pearls
- Erb's palsy
- hematoma
- Harlequin's sign
- hypothermia
- jaundice
- light sleep
- milia
- molding
- mottling
- noxious stimuli
- phototherapy
- quiet alert state
- satiety
- subconjunctival hemorrhage
- vacuum extraction

Sleep/Wake States

Recognizing sleep/wake states is an important skill for both parents and professionals to acquire. Infants in wake states are more interested in feeding, whereas those in sleep states are not. However, sometimes the signs are subtle, causing the caregiver to try to help a hungry infant to sleep, or a sleepy infant to eat.

Newborns have six sleep-wake states, which can be described along a continuum, from the sleepiest to the most alert:

- deep sleep, with good facial muscle tone (**Figure 1**) or poor muscle tone (**Figure 2**)
- light sleep, as shown with hands-to-mouth activity (**Figure 3**)
- drowsy (note sucking on the hand, **Figure 4**)
- quiet alert (**Figure 6**)
- active alert (**Figure 7, Figure 8**)
- crying (**Figure 10**)

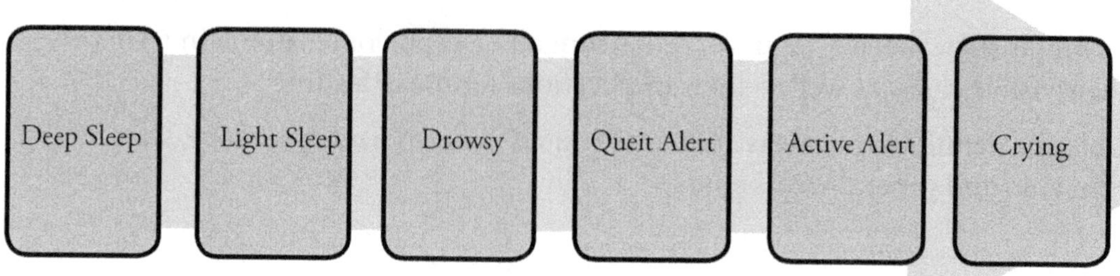

Figure 2-1. The sleep-wake continuum.

Once you know about these 6 states, you will have a better understanding of how to help with infant feeding. How can you distinguish one sleep/wake state from the other? To determine which sleep state is being shown, look for these five key features:

- bodily movement
- eye movement
- facial movements and expressions
- breathing patterns
- level of response to internal and external stimuli

Even when you are viewing a still photo, such as is used on the IBLCE exam, it is entirely possible to see moving body parts—mouth, arms, legs, and more. Eye movement, although subtle, can sometimes be seen in a photo if the infant is in a light sleep state. Facial movements and expressions are distinct in a photo. The other cues—breathing patterns and level of response to stimuli—are unlikely to be evident in a still photo.

There is more to learn on sleep-wake states. Download and study the material available from the March of Dimes, listed at the end of the chapter. Without doing so, you might miss one or more of this chapter's quiz questions!

Complete Learning Exercise 2-2 to help you recognize four big clues to infant sleep states.

Behaviors: Signs of Approach & Avoidance

Swedish physician and researcher Kerstin Uvnas-Moberg[1] describes three phases of social interaction that provide a framework for understanding behavior: approach, interaction, and satiety. Whether you're a newborn looking for food, a political candidate seeking a voter's favor, or an IBCLC candidate signing up for a course, the first step in the interactive process is *approach*! *Every* social interaction starts with an approach.

An infant in the *approach* phase (sometimes called "engagement") shows distinct signs of readiness to engage. These include signs of hunger (such as rooting, oral searching, and hands-to-mouth activity), or alertness (such as a bright-eyed look or turning towards someone who is talking). In general, infants who show signs of engagement are willing to suckle. Many of the newborns shown on page 161 of *The Breastfeeding Atlas* are showing signs of the approach phase, some more than others. It's critical to differentiate between signs of approach (often, but not always, hunger cues) and signs of *avoidance*.

An infant in the *avoidance (or "disengagement")* phase—the opposite of *approach*—may demonstrate that he finds the situation negative or intrusive. He may be grimacing or closing his eyes, having jerky movements, hiccoughing, spitting, or gagging. A newborn may respond this way due to some touch or event that is unpleasant or harmful, often referred to as *noxious stimuli* (**Figure 5**). The newborn in the photo has little desire to suckle at this time.

The second phase of social interaction is *interaction*. Whenever the infant is actively feeding, he is engaged in the process of interaction. Assuming the feeding was successful, the final phase is *satiety*, the feeling of being satisfied. This is illustrated in **Figure 11**.

Luckily, recognizing cues that the infant is in the approach, interaction, or satiety phase is relatively easy. Newborns who are awake and displaying early hunger cues are likely to be interested in suckling. Newborns who are in deep sleep are generally not interested; it is very difficult to rouse an infant from this state. Similarly, those who have already had a full feeding and are satiated are uninterested in continuing to feed (**Figure 11**).

Skin and General Appearance

Observing the skin and general appearance can give us clues about how receptive the infant will be to feeding. Our skin is our largest organ, and it reveals much about recent events. For example, experiences from childbirth can affect the infant's interest in feeding or his ability to suckle. Even mild trauma, such as molding of his head during labor, may reduce his enthusiasm for breastfeeding. He may have undergone invasive testing (e.g., **Figure 17, Figure 22 or Figure 23**), another source of noxious stimuli.

All the observations that one might make about newborn skin are well beyond the scope of this workbook. Several factors, including gestational age, affect what is "normal." However, there are several variations of normal that should be recognized as requiring little or no further action.

Jaundice

Newborn *jaundice* is a yellowing of the skin (and possibly the whites of the eyes). It occurs when the newborn has high levels of bilirubin circulating in the blood. Bilirubin is a yellow substance that is made when the body breaks down red blood cells. Because the newborn's liver is immature, it often doesn't remove bilirubin well. Bilirubin builds up, causing the yellowish discoloration of the skin which indicates an accumulation of red blood cells. Jaundice is not a medical diagnosis; it is merely a skin coloration. (Hyperbilirubinemia *is* a medical diagnosis).

Most times, jaundice is "physiologic." That is, it is a reflection of the newborn's immature liver, rather than a pathologic event. (While there are other types of jaundice in newborns, this is the most common.)

Not all newborns have jaundice. Breastfeeding does not increase the risk of jaundice. Infants with certain conditions are more at risk for jaundice, however. An excellent example is a *cephalohematoma* (**Figure 21**)—a collection of blood between the skull and the membranes covering the bones. A cephalohemotoma puts the newborn at risk for jaundice because there are more red blood cells to be broken down (compared to infants who do not have this condition).

There are certainly tests that determine the amount of bilirubin a newborn has in his blood. However, a simple way to determine the presence of jaundice is by pressing on the skin. This is called *blanching.* (**Figure 24** and **Figure 25**) After exerting pressure on the skin (the forehead, mid-sternum, or other places) the underlying color of the skin and the tissue just beneath the skin can reveal a yellow color.

Treatments: There are several types of treatments for jaundice. Many times, the best treatment is frequent feedings. If needed, jaundice is treated with a fiberoptic bili blanket (**Figure 26**) or bili lights (**Figure 27**). Note that the newborn has his eyes covered, to protect them from the lights. In many hospitals, a newborn undergoing this treatment is not in the same room with his mother throughout the day. These factors can impact the breastfeeding experience.

Implications for feeding: The best prevention for physiologic jaundice is breastfeeding—early and often! Bilirubin is excreted through the feces. Colostrum has a laxative effect on the gut, and therefore, breastfeeding can prevent, or minimize, the build-up of bilirubin. However, newborns who are jaundiced are often lethargic. Sometimes, they are not taking in enough fluid, and the physician may order supplemental donor milk or formula.

Erythema Toxicum

About half of newborns have *erythema toxicum* known to parents as newborn rash (**Figure 12** —an extreme case). Not all infants experience erythema toxicum, but it is completely normal. No one knows its exact cause. Typically, it shows up on Day 2. It is usually gone by about Day 5.

Frequently, IBLCE exam candidates ask, "How will I know if it's a normal newborn rash and not something else?" The key is to look for the clues. For this and other skin conditions, be aware of what is at the surface of the skin, what is above the surface of the skin, and what is below the surface of the skin. Also, color and locations are key to distinguishing one skin condition from another. Erythema toxicum rarely covers more than half of the skin's surface, and it is always most concentrated on the newborn's back. It consists of little bumps that are raised and arranged in a splotchy fashion above the skin's surface, and have a yellow or white center (**Figure 12**). Note how this looks different from **Figure 13** or **Figure 14**.

Other Skin Conditions

The word "rash" is an imprecise word used to describe many different skin conditions. Unless you are legally authorized to make a medical diagnosis, you may not diagnose a particular "rash." However, all healthcare team members should be able to distinguish normal skin conditions that require no further action from those that require referral.

Mottling is often referred to as a "rash" but it is not. Common in newborns, *mottling* reflects the tube-like structure of the capillaries below the surface of the skin. It is most often caused when the infant is *hypothermic* (cold). When the infant's body is cold stressed, a lacy pattern of dilated blood vessels is visible beneath the skin. The exact number that defines hypothermia depends on where the newborn's temperature is being measured (skin, rectal, or axillary temperatures) and the agency's policy. However, as a general rule it is defined as when the newborn's drops below 36.5 °C (97.7 °F).

Sometimes, as in **Figure 14**, there is a clear difference in color at the midline; this is called *Harlequin's sign.* Here, the infant is tilted onto his left side, so the "warmer" side is more pink/red; the right side is more white/blue. If the newborn were to be tilted onto his right side, the colors would spontaneously reverse with the postural change. This is common during the newborn period, but does indicate that the infant is cold stressed.

Other commonly-seen newborn skin conditions—not rashes—include newborn acne, dry peeling skin, and birth marks (birth marks will be discussed in chapter 3). *Milia* (**Figure 58**) are tiny inclusion cysts that occur on about half of all newborns. They are frequently visible on the nose, or around the eyes, cheek, chin or forehead. They disappear within a few weeks or more. *Epstein's pearls* (**Figure 59**) are also tiny cysts. These small hard, raised white nodules appear in the midline of the hard palate, mainly in the posterior section. They are very common, and they will spontaneously disappear after a few weeks. Note that Epstein's pearls look very different than patches of thrush—which are also white and also in the mouth—as seen in chapter 8.

Birth Trauma

Birth trauma generally refers to those events that result in an injury to the infant. The injury can be mild to severe, and the effects can last a few hours, a few days, or a lifetime. The effects of birth trauma have been well studied; consequences may include physical, cognitive, and psychological disorders. Some things—such a bump or bruise—may be immediately apparent, but others—developmental delays, fine motor problems, speech problems, and autism—have all been associated with birth trauma.

Here is a list of the most common types of birth trauma:

- caput succedaneum ("molding") (**Figure 19**)
- cephalohematoma (**Figure 21**)
- bruising and abrasion (**Figure 15, Figure 16, Figure 17**)
- subconjunctival hemorrhage
- facial palsy (facial paralysis)
- brachial plexus injury (usually, Erb's palsy)
- bone fractures, especially fractured clavicle (collarbone)
- oxygen deprivation

Some of these conditions are shown in *The Breastfeeding Atlas*. Because they are all injuries, each could impact the feeding experience.

Try to imagine yourself falling down a flight of stairs, slamming your fingers when closing the car door, or slipping on the ice. What's the first thing you would want to do? I'm guessing you would want to catch your breath, get something to help with your pain, and generally be consoled. You didn't say "eating", did you? A newborn who has experienced birth trauma has much the same reaction. Birth trauma is one form of *noxious stimuli* that can turn infants off from eating.

Caput succedaneum (**Figure 19**) is a swelling of fluid in the scalp. (Note that the fluid accumulates in the scalp, not under the scalp.) It is due to pressure on the fetal head. Such pressure is very often due to prolonged pressure on the fetal head from the dilated cervix or vaginal walls, often in conjunction with a prolonged pushing phase of labor. And, because the amniotic fluid cushions the head, an early rupture of the membranes or having very little fluid in the amniotic sac can create pressure on the infant's head.

When pressing on the swollen scalp, some indentation or dimpling of the flesh can be observed with a caput. The caput almost always crosses the suture line, and, if the newborn is moved from side to side, the fluid moves to the dependent side.

After the swelling subsides a little, the newborn is likely to have a misshapen, "pointy" head. Whereas the swelling is referred to as a caput succedaneum, the resulting pointiness is referred to as *molding*. (This is a fine distinction, but the former refers to the *fluid* in the scalp, whereas the latter refers to the *shape* of the head.) Usually, the caput succedaneum and the molding resolve within several days.

A *Cephalohematoma* (also correctly spelled cephalhematoma) (**Figure 21**) is a bruise—a collection of blood—located beneath the scalp that never crosses the suture line. (A *hematoma* is any collection of blood that pools outside of a vessel.) The location of the bump on the head does not change, even if the newborn's position changes. Like the caput succedaneum, the cephalohematoma is the result of some type of physical trauma, either from the mother's pelvis or from the misuse of assistive devices. However, the newborn is at higher risk for complications, and a slow resolution can be anticipated.

A newborn with a cephalohematoma may have a much more serious problem such as cerebral palsy. But more frequently, a newborn with a cephalohematoma is at high risk for developing jaundice, because newborns are slow to break down excess red blood cells. Early feedings of colostrum are a priority for care. Most cephalohematomas resolve spontaneously, but not quickly. It would not be unusual for a cephalohematoma to persist for three months. Some resolve even later.

People frequently ask me, "How can you tell the difference between a caput succedaneum and a cephalohematoma?" Admittedly, I've seen and taken care of many hundreds of newborns, so it's easy for me! Here, I have described several differences, and with the words as well as the photos (**Figures 19** and **21**) you should be able to see the differences, too.

Positioning is important for all breastfeeding couplets, but it is especially important for the infant with a specific injury. A newborn with trauma to the head would best be held in a position that avoids unnecessary contact or pressure on the head. For example, the newborn with the cephalohematoma might respond better to a more upright breastfeeding position; discomfort may make him entirely unwilling to breastfeed in a traditional cradle hold (see chapter 6) with his head in the crook of the mother's elbow.

Bruising and abrasions are not uncommon. Newborns who are especially large are at high risk for bruising. Those whose deliveries are assisted (such as with *forceps*, a surgical instrument shaped like salad tongs, or with *vacuum extraction* by a cap-like device and negative pressure) are highly likely to have visible bruising and/or abrasions.

A *subconjunctival hemorrhage* is a rupture of small blood vessels located just beneath the eye. Since it's visible on the eye, we may be tempted to assume that a birth injury such as a subconjunctival hemorrhage is unrelated to feeding issues. However, subconjunctival hemorrhages that do not resolve within a day or so may herald underestimated birth complications that are not visible at all. It may be a clue for why a newborn is a reluctant feeder.

A *facial palsy* in the newborn signals an injury to the facial nerve, which may be caused by use of forceps or a face presentation (the face, rather than the back of the head, is delivered first). Drooping of the face or jaw, and uneven lips (and in older infants, an uneven smile) are likely signs of a facial nerve paralysis. Closure of the eye on the affected side might also be noted.

Newborn facial palsy may result in an inability to form a good seal around the breast. If due to birth trauma, facial palsies usually resolve within several weeks. Depending on the severity, breastfeeding may or may not be possible. Protecting the mother's milk supply, and feeding with a special bottle, may be the best strategy. An experienced occupational therapist may be helpful.

A *brachial plexus* injury is one that affects the nerve fibers that run from the spine and through the neck into the arms. The injury can affect any part of the nerve fibers; the extent of damage depends on the location of the injury and how it happened. A breech delivery can result in injury to the brachial plexus. Any infant who has been "stuck" due to size—including large infants and/or those whose shoulders have been stuck in the pelvis (shoulder dystocia) are at high risk for a brachial plexus injury.

The indicators for a brachial plexus injury are highly dependent on which part of the nerve fibers have damage. However, in the most common type—the *Erb's palsy*--the arm hangs by the side and is rotated toward the midline (medially). The forearm is extended and pronated. The arm cannot be raised from the side; the elbow does not flex. The biceps muscle is damaged. Keeping pressure off the affected side may help to improve breastfeeding efforts. So, for example, if his right side is affected, a cradle hold (see chapter 6) in the mother's left arm will likely increase the newborn's pain perception, and decrease his breastfeeding skills

Complete Exercise 2-3, 2-4, and 2-5 to help you better recognize common causes and results of birth trauma.

Feeding implications: It's difficult to give clear strategies for how to help with breastfeeding management with these types of birth traumas, since the extent and type of trauma experienced by one newborn might be quite different from that of another. Here are some basic questions to ask:

- What muscles, nerves, or bones are affected? To what extent are they affected?
- How does this impact holding or feeding?

- How long is the situation likely to continue, and will it resolve spontaneously?
- What behaviors does the newborn display? Grimacing, pulling away, or displaying any other signs of pain should be noted, even if there is no visible birth injury.
- Is the newborn willing to be held or nursed on one side but not the other?
- What can be done to avoid contact or pressure on the affected part or the affected side?
- If milk is left in the breast after the newborn stops suckling, what can be done to protect the mother's milk supply?
- Is expressing milk, and giving it through a bottle or an alternative means a more realistic option?

Although newborns cannot talk, they can communicate! It's important to look at all the clues, and formulate an individualized plan of care that makes sense for the situation, and the family.

Looking Back, Looking Forward

In this chapter, we've talked about sleep/wake states, normal newborn behaviors, normal appearance of the newborn's skin, and birth trauma.

Evidence in the education field shows that writing your own summary helps your retention. The Summarize What You've Learned exercise helps you to do this, so take just a few minutes to complete that exercise now.

By now, if you have viewed the photos carefully, and if you've completed the written exercises, you should feel confident that you can distinguish between normal variants (behavioral states, skin or general appearance, and birth trauma) and identify feeding implications (if any) for the breastfeeding newborn.

Recalling, Reinforcing, and Expanding Your Learning

Have you ever felt frustrated that you "learned" something, but later, can't recall it? That may be because you didn't reinforce the material you learned. And, perhaps what you originally learned isn't enough to get you through the next few decades of practice; sometimes you need to expand your learning. The exercises in this section are designed to help you recall, reinforce, and expand your learning.

What was your main motivation for reading this chapter?

- [x] To study for the IBLCE exam, as a first-time candidate
- [ ] To review for the IBLCE exam, as a re-certificant
- [ ] To improve my clinical skills and clinical management

How soon do you think can use the information presented in this chapter?

- [x] Immediately; within the next few days or so
- [ ] Soon; within the next month or so
- [ ] Later; sometime before I retire

Pro Tip! If you are preparing for the IBLCE exam, it would be wise to pace your studying. Set a target date for when you plan to complete the exercises, and check off them off as you go along.

Done!	Target Date	
☐	________	Learning Exercise 2-1. Terms describing normal and variations of normal well-being in newborns.
☐	________	Learning Exercise 2-2. Comparing four observations that are clues to sleep states.
☐	________	Learning Exercise 2-3. Common examples of birth trauma.
☐	________	Learning Exercise 2-4. Terms to describe technology and issues related to traumatic birth.
☐	________	Learning Exercise 2-5. Differences between cephalohematoma and caput succedaneum.
☐	________	Explore What You've Learned in a Journal
☐	________	Summarize What You've Learned
☐	________	Quick Quiz

Master Your Vocabulary

Unless you the meaning of a word, you cannot fully answer a question about it. Those listed under "key terms" are only a small representation of the words that you might need to know in clinical practice or on the exam. If there are any others that you do not know, you need to look them up now!

Learning Exercise 2-1. Terms describing normal and variations of normal well-being in newborns.

Instructions: Did you download the March of Dimes document (see Additional Resources at the end of this chapter)? You will need it to complete this learning exercise. Write the letter of the correct match next to each item. Answers are in the Appendix.

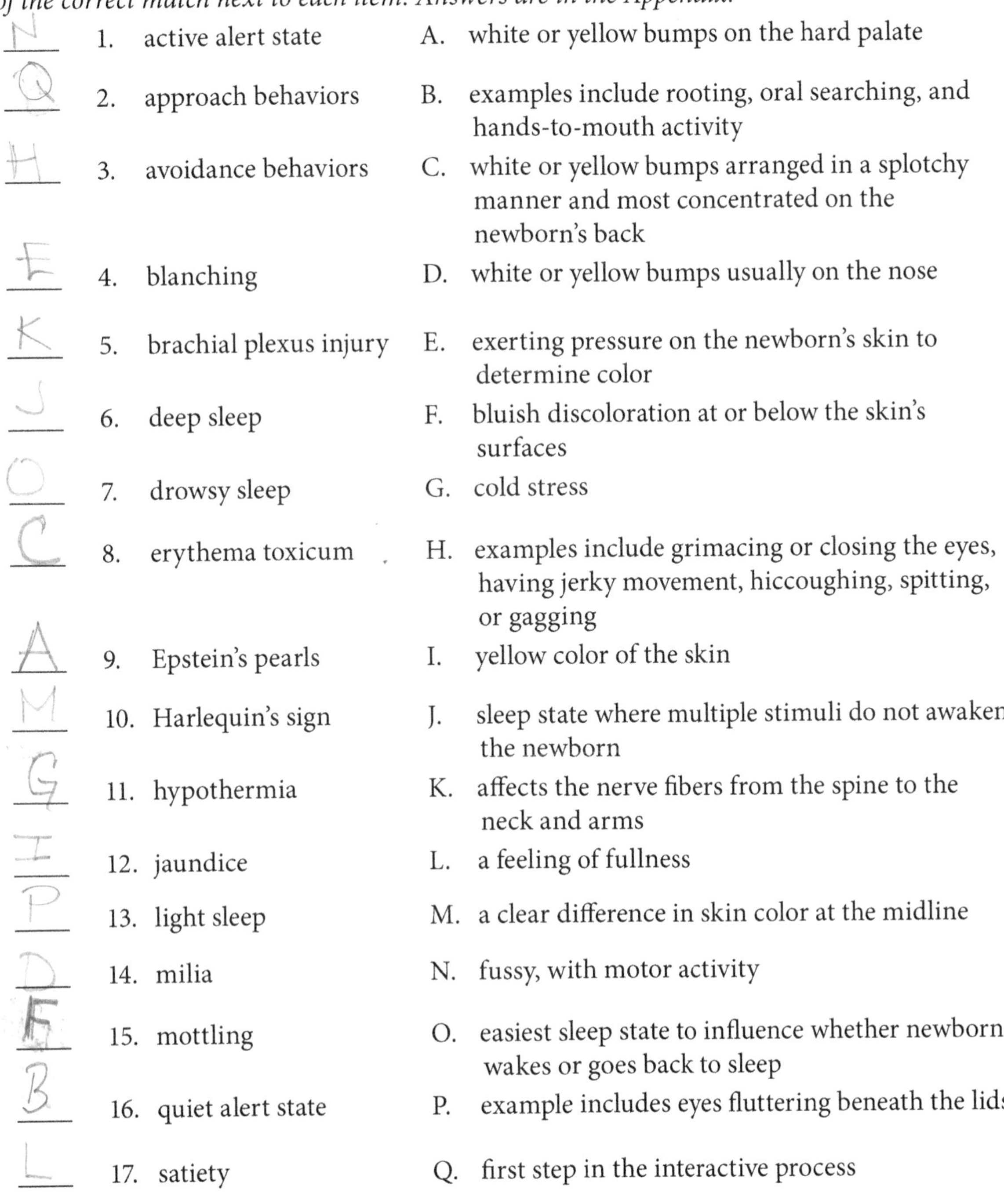

N	1. active alert state	A.	white or yellow bumps on the hard palate
Q	2. approach behaviors	B.	examples include rooting, oral searching, and hands-to-mouth activity
H	3. avoidance behaviors	C.	white or yellow bumps arranged in a splotchy manner and most concentrated on the newborn's back
E	4. blanching	D.	white or yellow bumps usually on the nose
K	5. brachial plexus injury	E.	exerting pressure on the newborn's skin to determine color
J	6. deep sleep	F.	bluish discoloration at or below the skin's surfaces
O	7. drowsy sleep	G.	cold stress
C	8. erythema toxicum	H.	examples include grimacing or closing the eyes, having jerky movement, hiccoughing, spitting, or gagging
A	9. Epstein's pearls	I.	yellow color of the skin
M	10. Harlequin's sign	J.	sleep state where multiple stimuli do not awaken the newborn
G	11. hypothermia	K.	affects the nerve fibers from the spine to the neck and arms
I	12. jaundice	L.	a feeling of fullness
P	13. light sleep	M.	a clear difference in skin color at the midline
D	14. milia	N.	fussy, with motor activity
F	15. mottling	O.	easiest sleep state to influence whether newborn wakes or goes back to sleep
B	16. quiet alert state	P.	example includes eyes fluttering beneath the lids
L	17. satiety	Q.	first step in the interactive process

Conquering Clinical Concepts

Learning Exercise 2-2. Comparing four observations that are clues to sleep states.

Instructions: Using the information in this workbook, and in the March of Dimes download (see Additional Resources at the end of this chapter) and in The Breastfeeding Atlas, complete this exercise using as few words as possible.

	Deep Sleep	Light Sleep	Drowsy	Quiet Alert	Active Alert ("Fussy")	Crying
Bodily Movement	Nearly Still	Some	variable	minimal	variable, smooth movements	↑ w/ motor activity ruddy color
Eye Movement	No	yes, lightly, beneath the lids	occasional	open & bright	open but dull	tightly closed or open
Facial Movements or Expression	No	perhaps briefly	perhaps some	attentive	little/ none	grimaces
Breathing	Smooth, regular	Irregular	Irregular	regular	Irregular	Irregular
Responsiveness and other observations or comments	low	possible	Often easy to awaken infant, or help him to return to sleeping	High, to positive stimuli	present but may be delayed	highly reactive to noxious stimuli

Learning Exercise 2-3. Common examples of birth trauma.

Instructions: Find eight common examples of birth trauma. Letters will go forward and down.

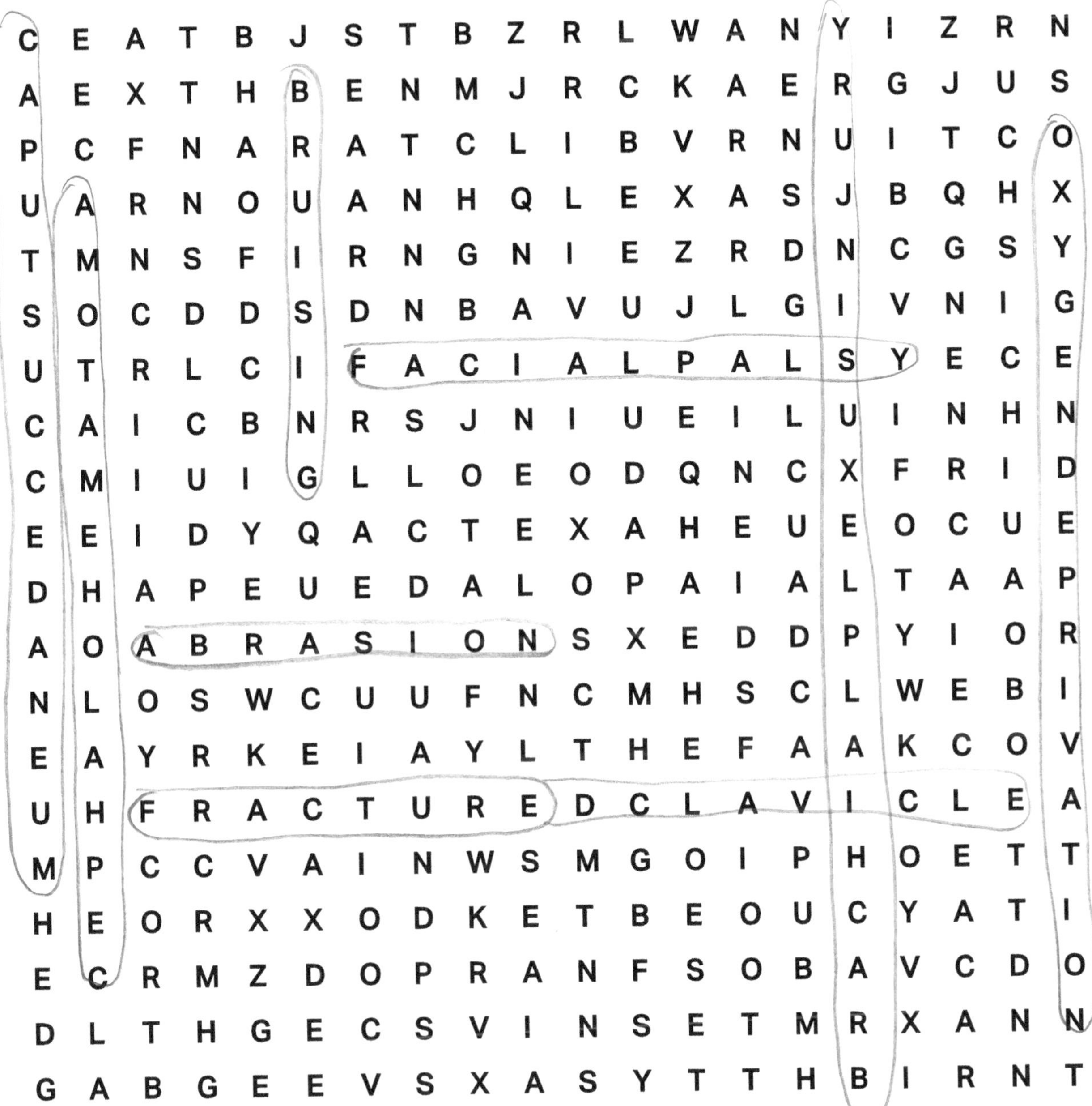

Learning Exercise 2-4. Terms to describe technology and issues related to traumatic birth.

Instructions: Write the letter of the correct match next to each item. Answers are in the Appendix.

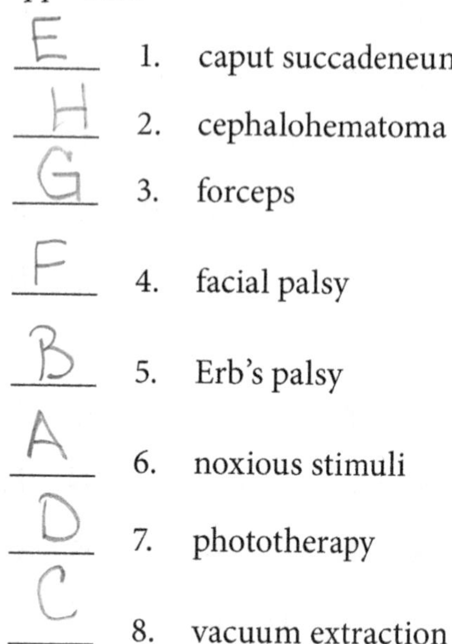

____ 1.	caput succadeneum	A.	Unpleasant experiences
____ 2.	cephalohematoma	B.	Paralysis where arm is rotated medially
____ 3.	forceps	C.	Cap-like device used to assist in delivery
____ 4.	facial palsy	D.	Technology used to help reduce newborn jaundice
____ 5.	Erb's palsy	E.	Collection of fluid that crosses the suture lines
____ 6.	noxious stimuli	F.	drooping of mouth and even the eyelids
____ 7.	phototherapy	G.	Tong-like instrument used to assist in delivery
____ 8.	vacuum extraction	H.	Collection of blood that does not cross the suture line

Learning Exercise 2-5. Differences between cephalohematoma and caput succedaneum.

Instructions: Using content that appeared earlier in this chapter, and the photos in The Breastfeeding Atlas, *write just a few words to describe each of these conditions.*

	Cephalohematoma	Caput succedaneum
Collection of…	blood	fluid
Cross sutures	NO	yes
Location	beneath scalp	within scalp
Result of…	birth trauma inluding assistive devices	pressure on head
Possible complications	jaundice discomfort	"cone head" discomfort
Breastfeeding issue or implications…	positioning to reduce pressure on head "early + often" feed to reduce hyperbili	
Resolves…	within few months	within few days

Explore What You've Learned In a Journal

Multiple studies have shown the benefits of using a learning journal. Among them are greater assimilation and integration of new information, better long-term retention of course concepts, increasing test and exam grades, and a means by which to have continuous feedback about one's own learning.

Name at least three things you learned from this chapter.

- List at least three things you still need to learn, or more fully master, in this chapter.

  birth trauma
  sleep/wake
  jaundica

- Briefly describe how this information fits (or doesn't fit) with what you've seen in clinical practice, what you learned in basic or college courses, or what you've observed in your own experience breastfeeding. (In some cases, you might want to include how the information fits or doesn't fit with what "experts" say, what the media says, or whatever.)

- Describe how you will use any or this information. How might it be related to problems and potential solutions that occur in real life or in clinical situations?

- If you wish, include how you felt about learning this information. Were you overwhelmed? Enlightened? Worried? Something else?

Summarize What You've Learned

The goal of this chapter was for you to be able to distinguish between normal variants (behavioral states, skin or general appearance, and birth trauma) and identify feeding implications (if any) for the breastfeeding newborn.

- Write your own summary of what you just learned in this chapter. What four key observations help you to distinguish one sleep state from another in a photo?

- When seeing a photo, what clues might you see that would indicate feeding readiness?

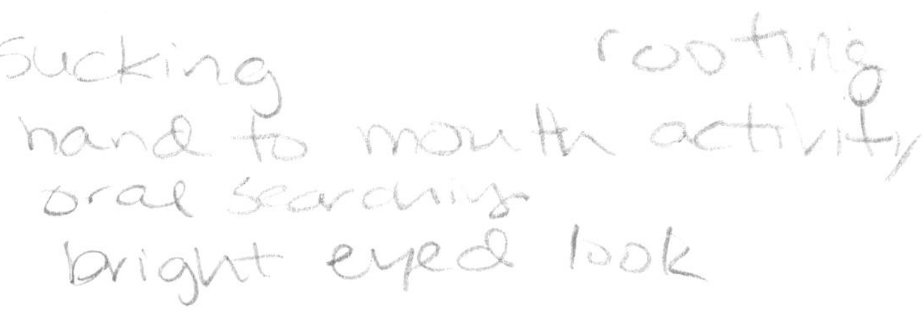

- What might you see that would indicate feeding resistance?

grimace
jerky movements
hiccups
gagging / spitting

- What might you see that would indicate satiety?

looking satisfied / milk drunk

- When you view a photo of normal skin conditions, what clues makes them similar to one another? What makes them different?

- What are some common examples of birth trauma, and their impact on feeding behaviors?

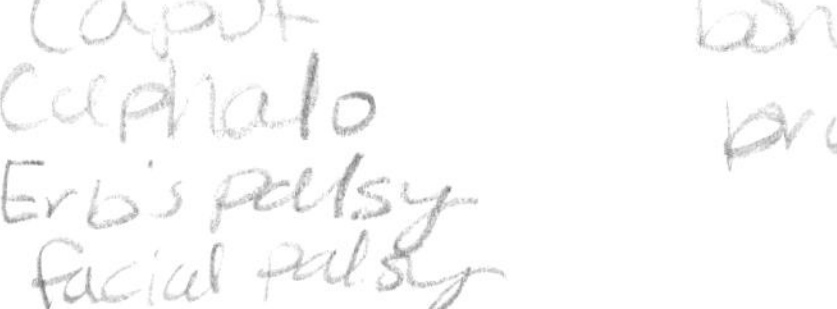

bone fracture
bruising / abraision

Self-Assessment

People often dive into a test before they have thoughtfully reflected on how well they have prepared for it. Instead, it would be helpful if they would take a few moments to give their alter-ego (their "other self") a chance to reflect on how confident they feel about mastering the stated objectives.

Instructions: Take a moment to review the chapter objectives (below). Then rate yourself. How confident are you that you have achieved each objective below?

Objective	Highly Confident	Somewhat Confident	Somewhat Unsure	Completely Unsure
Recognize key features that distinguish one sleep state from another.	○	✓	○	○
Recognize newborn sleep states or behaviors that indicate feeding readiness, resistance, or satiety and their meaning for the caregiver.	○	○	✓	○
Describe newborn jaundice in terms of how to blanch for its presence, the technology to treat it, and its relationship to breastfeeding.	○	✓	○	○
Compare and contrast at least three types of skin conditions that are considered normal in newborns.	○	✓	○	○
Recognize the most common examples of birth trauma (including those related to diagnostic testing and therapeutic intervention) and their effect on feeding behavior.	○	✓	○	○
State the definition of at least 10 terms related to newborn appearance, state, behavior, and general well-being.	○	✓	○	○

On the next page, you will encounter some simple recall questions pertaining to this chapter. These are *not* the application-type questions you will find in the IBLCE exam. However, you cannot *apply* information unless you can fully *recall* that information! You should do these without looking up the answers.

When you finish with the quiz, look up the answers in the Appendix. Then, score your answers, using the Appendix. Finally, you should analyze the results of your quiz. It's not enough to just know what you got right or wrong; you must look at why you got the answers right or wrong.

Quick Quiz Chapter 2

Circle the correct response. For a better understanding of how well you are mastering the material, try answering without looking it up. If you are really stuck, questions come from this workbook and from *The Breastfeeding Atlas* so go back and review the appropriate material. Answers are in the appendix.

1. The most profound state of sleep for the newborn is called deep sleep. The next is light sleep. What is the following state?

   A. active alert

   B. crying

   C. drowsy

   D. quiet alert

2. The word "noxious" means

   A. knocked out

   B. unpleasant

   C. without control

   D. without oxygen

3. Ideally, bilirubin is processed by what organ?

   A. gall bladder

   B. liver

   C. pancreas

   D. spleen

4. Blood that pools outside of a blood vessel is called a:

   A. hemangioma

   B. hematoid

   C. hematoma

   D. hemorrhage

5. The clavicle could be described as which bone?

   A. cheek bone

   B. collar bone

   C. funny bone

   D. jaw bone

   E. tail bone

Analyze Your Own Quiz

- What percentage of the questions did you answer correctly?

80%

- If you got 100% of them right, to what do you attribute your success?

- If you did not get all the questions right, can you identify your learning gap? (Example: Didn't know the information, knew the information but could not remember, knew some information but confused it with similar information, other.)

* sleep/wake cycle info

- Would you have been able to answer the questions as well if you had not read this chapter?

No

- What do you need to do next? (If you got them all right, what you need to do next is celebrate! Even a high-five with your child, a YESSS and a fist-pump in the air, or anything else is good! A small acknowledgement of your success is better than no acknowledgement!)

Additional Resources

1. Academy of American Pediatrics. Management of Hyperbilirubinemia in the Newborn Infant 35 or More Weeks of Gestation. 2004. ***http://pediatrics.aappublications.org/content/114/1/297***

2. Academy of Breastfeeding Medicine. ABM Clinical Protocol #22: Guidelines for Management of Jaundice in the Breastfeeding Infant Equal to or Greater Than 35 Weeks' Gestation. 2010. Available ***http://www.bfmed.org/Media/Files/Protocols/Protocol%2022%20Jaundice.pdf***

3. March of Dimes. Infant Behavior, Reflexes, and Cues. 2003. Available ***https://www.marchofdimes.org/nursing/modnemedia/othermedia/infantBehavior.pdf***

4. March of Dimes. Infant Sleep States. 2003. ***https://www.marchofdimes.org/nursing/modnemedia/othermedia/states.pdf***

5. Reader JM, Teti DM, Cleveland MJ. Cognitions About Infant Sleep: Interparental Differences, Trajectories Across the First Year, and Coparenting Quality. J Fam Psychol. 2017 Jan 5. Uvnas-Moberg K. Physiological and endocrine effects of social contact. Ann N Y Acad Sci. 1997:807:146-863.

Chapter 3
Infant Orofacial Assessment and Feeding Reflexes

Assessment is a major part of any expert's role. Yet, assessment is only helpful when the pertinent data are identified and interpreted. When helping mothers and infants, we can look at information from laboratory and diagnostic tests, interviews, and health histories. But these provide only part of the story. Physical assessment data are critically important when formulating a plan to meet a goal.

When you collect the pertinent data and correctly interpret it, you are much more likely to take the right action or actions to help the breastfeeding family. Sometimes, it may be as simple as reassuring the family that all is well. Other times, it may mean making minor or major adjustments in the feeding plan, or referring the family to a health care provider.

In Chapter 3 of *The Breastfeeding Atlas*, you'll see many photos that will show you the details that differentiate between typical normal conditions, normal variations, and abnormal infant conditions. By studying the photos, considering the context of each situation, and completing the written learning exercises, you will develop the skills to recognize and manage such situations in real life—or on your lactation exam!

I promise, when you finish this chapter, you will be able to determine when it is appropriate to reassure, resolve, or refer the family for congenital oral (and other) anatomical variations in the infant that may (or may not) impact breastfeeding. This topic can feel a little daunting at first, but I'll show you exactly what to look for, and the questions to ask yourself as you look at certain conditions.

Objectives

Given a clinical photo, you will be able to:

- Recognize bony, soft tissue, and neuromuscular alterations of the intraoral and extraoral structures that can affect latch, positioning, and milk transfer.
- Recognize key features of pigmented and vascular birth marks, and describe how they affect your responsibility to help the breastfeeding family.
- Name at least six different types of birthmarks, and recognize how they may affect health or feeding (if at all).
- Describe assessment techniques and findings that indicate optimal or suboptimal functioning of (1) seal of the lips, (2) negative intraoral pressure, and (3) mandibular (jaw) compression of the nipple.

Key Terms

- asymmetry
- buccal mucosa
- craniosynostosis
- frenum (frenulum)
- gag reflex
- hard palate
- hemangioma
- hypertonic, hypertonia
- hypotonic, hypotonia
- lesion
- mandible
- maxilla
- melanin
- melanocytosis
- micrognathia
- natal tooth
- nevus, nevi
- pigmentation
- plagiocephaly
- protrusion
- retrognathia
- retrusion
- soft palate
- symmetry
- tone (tonus)
- torticollis

Data Gathering and Assessment

Data gathering includes reviewing medical records, interviewing the parents, and more. But it also involves physical assessment—and recognizing clues you need to help the breastfeeding family in situations that are normal, variations of normal, or abnormal.

Visual inspection is perhaps the most commonly used means to obtain physical assessment data related to feeding issues. Throughout this chapter, we will focus on visual cues about structure and function and their role in transferring milk from the breast.

Palpation is using one's hands to gain information about a body structure. Palpation can be used to determine whether a structure is intact (for example, a cleft of the palate means the palate is not intact), or to determine a structure's size, shape, firmness, or location. However, knowing when and how to palpate the infant's oral cavity can be tricky. While all newborns should have a thorough oral examination by the physician prior to being discharged from the hospital, additional assessment may be needed later. But because the oral cavity is a highly sensitive part of a newborn's body, he is likely to perceive the oral assessment as intrusive and unpleasant, (**Figure 5** in Chapter 2) and his feeding behavior may be compromised afterwards.

Auditory cues are often overlooked, but can enormously enhance our understanding of the feeding experience. Audible swallowing is almost always reassuring. (Or, more to the point, the absence of audible swallowing is always cause for concern). Other auditory cues are also important. For example, clicking or smacking noises while breastfeeding indicate a problem.

As you begin to assess the oral cavity, there are several observations you should make:

- **What is the color of the structure**? Is it what you would expect, given the infant's ethnic background? Is the color of part of the structure different from the rest of the structure? Is there hyperpigmentation?
- **How is the muscle tone in each structure**? *Muscle tone* is the muscle tension inside of a muscle or a muscle group when it is at rest. Notice tone that is too tense (*hypertonic*) or too limp (*hypotonic*). You might notice that an infant with generalized hypotonia of his body also has specific intraoral structures that are hypotonic. Recall, however, that in the first few hours of life, hypotonicity is characteristic of an infant who has had a traumatic delivery.
- **Is normal tissue present and adequate?** Is there enough tissue, or too much? Is it too thin? Is the tissue functioning as it should?
- **Are lesions present?** Just as we expect normal tissue to be present, we expect abnormal tissue to be absent. A handy but imprecise term, the word *lesion* refers to a discontinuity of tissue or loss of function to a body part. Lesion is a broad term that might be used to mean a sore, a tumor, a cleft, or damaged skin. In the intraoral cavity, the term might include a yeast infection, a blister, Epstein's pearls (**Figure 59**) a cleft, a tongue-tie, or any other number of conditions. Even a *natal tooth* (**Figure 38**)—a tooth that the infant is born with—might be thought of as a lesion because it causes a discontinuity of the gum tissue.
- **How is movement and flexibility?** The human body is meant to be in motion. The tongue and the lips, as well as all orofacial structures should be able to move for successful breastfeeding.
- **What is the size of the structure**? Sometimes, a structure seems to be larger or smaller than normal, or it may look out of proportion in comparison to the size of the infant. The size of the tongue and jaws are particularly noticeable.
- **Are the structures symmetrical?** In human anatomy, the term *symmetry* is**, by definition**, a right-to-left comparison. Symmetry means that two parts, on either side of the midline, are the same. Corresponding structures on one side are the same as on the other side; this is normal. When corresponding structures are not the same, they are *asymmetrical*. The term asymmetrical is frequently misused in the lactation community! Asymmetry—an inequality of right-to-left comparison of structures— is not normal.

The Relationship Between Milk Transfer and Orofacial Structure and Function

Decades ago, my good friend Sarah Danner, RN, MSN, CNM, CPNP, PhD, taught me that optimal milk transfer is dependent upon three factors: a good seal, adequate negative pressure, and good compression. She has also written about it.[1] More specifically:

- The seal must not only be present; it must be adequate. The seal allows negative pressure and holds the nipple and areola in place. (Negative pressure also helps to extract the milk from the breast).[2, 3]

- The negative pressure must be adequate; this is accomplished in part by the motion of the tongue upon the gum and lips, and the areola compressing against the hard palate.
- Good compression and *suckling mechanisms* must be adequate. Milk flows from the nipple, and as a result, the swallowing reflex occurs in the infant. Problems with intraoral muscular movements occur if the tongue does not stabilize the nipple, or if the tongue cannot compress the nipple effectively.

Those three factors are related to the adequacy of the bony and soft tissue structure and neuromuscular functioning. Here, we'll discuss the normal structure and function of the oral structures, and their impact on feeding.

Intraoral and Extraoral Structures

The ability to adequately assess the intraoral and extraoral structures of the infant's mouth is highly dependent upon a fundamental mastery of anatomy and physiology facts. We must also know the difference between normal and abnormal. In this section, we will look at various intraoral and extraoral variations, and their effect on breastfeeding, if at all.

Intraoral Variations

There are several variations of normal that can and do occur intraorally. These may or may not affect successful milk transfer. The most common intraoral variations occur on the lips, the buccal pads (cheeks), tongue, or palate.

Lips

The main muscle in the lips is the orbicularis oris. This muscle enables the lips to create a seal around the nipple/areola, which results in negative pressure (suction). Normally, the lips are flanged around the breast. Good lip "rounding" (**Figure 39**) indicates normal muscle tone and free movement.

Muscle tone—too little or too much—affects the infant's ability to display lip rounding. Compare the normal tone of the lips in **Figure 39** to the excessive lip tone (hypertonia) in **Figure 40**. Note the tightness, or pursed-lip appearance.

Low muscle tone of the lips may occur for several reasons, including general hypotonia, which is characteristically seen in premature infants, those who had a traumatic birth, or those with a neuromuscular deficit. Generalized hypotonia is frequently predictive of low lip tone.

Regardless of the reason, the most glaring consequence of low muscle tone of the lips tends to be impaired ability to achieve a good seal, and thus good negative pressure. Infants with this condition tire easily and may fall asleep before finishing the feeding.

How can we recognize if the orbicularis oris muscle is creating a good seal and adequate negative pressure, or if low muscle tone is a problem? There are many clues, including those which are visual, palpable, and audible.

The Breastfeeding Atlas discusses four main visual clues of low muscle tone of the lips, summarized here:

- An infant with normal muscle tone of the lips should be able to close his lips, while awake or asleep. If he cannot (**Figure 41)** it's likely that the lip muscles are hypotonic.
- Leaking of milk at the corners of the mouth, or on the mother's clothing *during* a feeding, may indicate low lip tone. (Leaking of milk *after* the feeding usually indicates that the infant has fallen asleep with milk in his mouth).
- Drooling in an infant who has not yet begun teething almost always indicates low muscle tone of the lips.
- Muscle tone and lip-sealing should be equal on both sides; asymmetry in these characteristics may indicate a problem with low muscle tone in the lips or, if there is unequal closure, a problem with the jaw (**Figure 34, 35**).

Palpation can also help to determine the degree of tone. When gentle, digital pressure is exerted against the lips, some resistance should be felt. Also, given a rubber nipple (**Figure 46),** the infant should be able to exert pressure on it.

Audible clues of low muscle tone of the infant's lips include clicking or smacking. While these may indicate other problems (including low tone or defects in other oral structures, or less-than-optimal attachment at the breast), low lip tone is a distinct possibility.

Not all lip problems are attributable to muscle tone. There may instead be an oral structure that restricts muscle *movement*, such as a tight labial *frenum* (**Figure 29)** (A frenum, also correctly called a *frenulum*, is a small fold of tissue that restricts or secures a mobile organ**).** Midline structural variations have become common these days. Chapter 17 discusses frenums.

Often, however, the problems noted with the lips are attributable to what *The Breastfeeding Atlas* calls "lip retraction," or what I tend to call "lip bunching." In some cases, the lips are not flanged outward (Figure 28), and in more exaggerated cases, the tissue of the lips may seem "bunched." Either of these situations can result in sucking blisters (**Figure 30).**

Complete Learning Exercise 3-2 to improve your data-gathering skills for intraoral muscle tone.

Buccal fat pads

The sweet round cheeks that make the parents' hearts melt actually serve another purpose. The fat deposits (fat pads) in the cheeks—or *buccal fat pads*—help to provide intraoral negative pressure when the infant uses the buccinator muscle. The thickness of the buccal mucosa can be palpated **(Figure 32)**. If there is less mucosa, there will be less intraoral negative pressure. To compensate, you may see an indrawing or "dimpling" of the cheeks. This creates a smaller "space" which then increases negative pressure. Alternatively, the caregiver can intervene to form this smaller space (**Figure 333, Figure 334**).

Tongue

The tongue's function is to assist with milk transfer, and it must have a full range of motion. This includes being able to:

- elevate (so that it can compress the mother's nipple against the infant's hard palate)
- extend out over the lower alveolar ridge
- form a scoop-shape (i.e., a central groove)
- generate a peristaltic, rhythmic wave that controls the direction of fluids4
- create negative pressure in the mouth

Low tone can also occur in the tip of the tongue (**Figure 44**) and can prevent tongue elevation. (Photo shows infant at 4 days old.). The 17-day old in **Figure 41** has low tone of the tongue, low tone of the lips, and low facial tone. At 5½ weeks old, this infant was able to close her lips (**Figure 42**) following craniosacral therapy.

Palates

The anterior two-thirds of the palate is bony. This is the *hard palate.* In general, it provides stability for the mouth[4] and allows the infant's tongue to compress the mother's nipple, and the milk ducts. If the right and the left palatal shelves fail to meet and fuse around the seventh week of intrauterine life, the infant will have a hole (i.e., a cleft) of the hard palate.

The posterior one-third of the palate is muscular. This is the *soft palate.* As with the hard palate, a cleft can occur. Clefts of either the hard or soft palate substantially affect breastfeeding. Chapter 18 addresses more about clefts of the lip and palate.

Extraoral Variations

Although the intraoral cavity is of utmost importance to successful milk transfer, it is supported by the extraoral structures. It can be difficult to tell initially which problems are related to intraoral structures and which are due to extraoral structures.

In this section, we'll discuss three extraoral structures: The head, neck, and jaw. (A more thorough discussion of head and neck problems are addressed elsewhere.[5])

Head

Newborns have four bones that are connected by sutures, or "soft spots." These bones are the frontal, parietal, temporal, and occipital. The major sutures that connect these bones are the coronal, sagittal, lamboid, and squamous. The sutures of the skull allow the skull to grow as the brain grows.

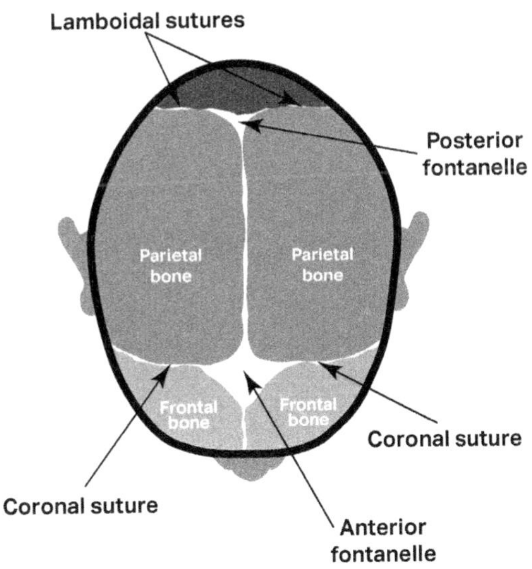

Figure 3-1. Sutures of the newborn skull. Reprinted with permission from Marie Biancuzzo's Lactation Exam Review.

Many head issues (for example, caput succadeneum and cephalohematoma discussed in Chapter 2) typically are related to birthing issues, and have comparatively little impact on the infant's ability to transfer milk. Other issues, such as cranial asymmetry, have much more impact.

Cranial asymmetry (**Figure 20**) is seen in an unusual condition called *craniosynostosis*, in which one (or more) of the sutures in the infant's skull closes early. This occurs in about 1 out of every 2500 births. Asymmetry occurs because the skull attempts to grow parallel to the closed suture, rather than perpendicular to it, resulting in an abnormal head shape.

Note that craniosynostosis results in asymmetry of the skull, not the jaw. Although **Figure 20 is** an accurate representation of one type of craniosynostosis, it is not representative of all types of craniosynostosis. The exact shape of the skull depends on which sutures have prematurely closed.

Craniosynostosis may occur as part of a syndrome, because of a familial trait, or for an unknown cause. This is a serious medical condition that often requires surgery by a specialist. If it is left uncorrected, brain injury may occur. (One of the twins in **Figure 20** underwent surgical correction.) Children with craniosynostosis may have decreased stamina and may require temporary supplementation with expressed milk.

Craniosynostosis should not be confused with *plagiocephaly* (a.k.a. "flat head syndrome"), in which skull sutures are not fused. In plagiocephaly, the head is misshapen, typically at the back, due to repeated pressure to the same area, such as what happens from not having enough "tummy time" and being put "back to sleep." Nearly half of children in the United States have some degree of plagiocephaly; some will need help with breastfeeding.[6] Although they are different conditions, infants who are treated for plagiocephaly also have torticollis.

To gain clarity on the difference between craniosynostosis and plagiocephaly, complete Learning Exercise 3-3.

Neck

A large, strong, paired muscle in the neck contracts and pulls the head towards one side. This is the sternocleidomastoid muscle (SCM). Its name comes from its origin and insertion sites, since it originates at the manubrium of the sternum and the clavicle, and inserts at the mastoid process of the temporal bone, as shown in Figure 5-2 below. It is innervated primarily by Cranial Nerve XI, the spinal accessory nerve.

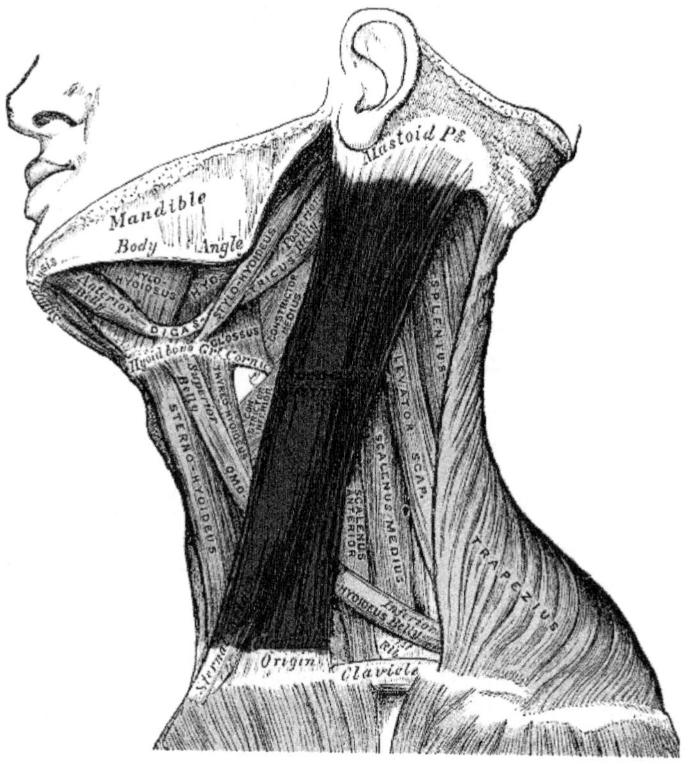

Figure 3-2. The sternocleidomastoid muscle.

Congenital muscular *torticollis* is a stricture of the sternocleidomastoid muscle (SCM). Commonly known as a "wry neck," torticollis is characterized by the stricture of the muscle such that the infant's head is tilted to one side. Often, the stricture of this muscle is attributable to the position the infant assumed in utero. About 75% of the cases of torticollis pull the infant's head to the right, although this is not always the case (**Figure 53**). In my experience, torticollis can range from the obvious to the subtle, and may be overlooked. Sometimes, the best (or only!) tell-tale sign of torticollis is the infant's behavior at his mother's breast. Frequently, infants who have torticollis also have plagiocephaly.

Because of the stricture of the SCM muscle, the infant does not have good range of motion in his neck. As a result, his chin is always pointing more to one side than to the other. He may be perfectly happy to nurse on one side, and the mother may experience no nipple pain in this position. However, when offered the other breast, the infant may seem reluctant, cry, or appear to be in pain. Often, the mother will experience nipple pain when nursing on that side.

There are several different opinions about what position to use in these cases, some of which are mentioned in *The Breastfeeding Atlas* or elsewhere.[7] I espouse two general principles that tend to work: biological nurturing [8] (or so-called "laid back" nursing, a somewhat inaccurate term), or the football position. Both positions allow the infant a little more space to spread out, and he generally does better. Helping the infant to flex his hips (**Figure 54**) can be helpful, too.

Several treatments are available for torticollis. Whether such treatments work, and how quickly they work, often depends on the severity of the condition. Physical therapy, craniosacral therapy, and chiropractic treatments have all been reported to be successful. That said, I know of one child who did not receive help in a timely manner. The mother kept insisting that "something was wrong" but all the healthcare professionals she approached assured her that all was well. When the child was 2 years old, she took him to a craniofacial center several hundred miles away; they said it was too late for less aggressive therapies, and they performed surgery for the very constricted SCM.

Mandible and Maxilla

The *mandible* is the lower jawbone. The bone of the upper jaw is the *maxilla.*

As with all body structures, the jaws should be symmetrical. Asymmetry of the upper and/or lower jaw can be easily observed (**Figure 47**). Note the right-to-left difference whether the mouth is closed (**Figure 34**) or open (**Figure 35).** In **Figure 48**, the mother is providing jaw support.

As page 19 of *The Breastfeeding Atlas* correctly states, *micrognathia* refers to size, whereas *retrognathia* refers to the mandible's position in relation to the maxilla. However, as fetal medicine experts Paladini and colleagues[9] explain, "in most cases, these two abnormalities are concurrent, as a small mandible is by definition abnormally positioned." This condition (**Figure 33**) can occur alone, or with a syndrome such as Pierre Robin Syndrome, and requires some special breastfeeding management. I agree with all the latch-on suggestions on Page 19 of *The Breastfeeding Atlas*, and I would add my own favorite technique to help with this situation: breastfeeding in a biological nurturing position (**Figure 85**). (I have discussed this condition extensively elsewhere.[10])

Muscle Tone and Feeding-Related Movement and Reflexes

Healthy tone in all feeding-related muscles is important for good milk transfer. Here is an overview of the suckling process: The orbicularis oris creates a seal around the nipple/areola. The buccinator muscle helps to create negative pressure. The masseter muscle connects to the mandible and the zygomatic bone (cheekbone), elevating the mandible and raising the lower jaw. With help from the lateral pterygoid and medial pterygoid, the masseter and other muscles help the mandible accomplish three movements:

elevation and depression (up and down), lateral excursion (side-to-side), and *protrusion* and *retrusion* (back and forth). The temporalis muscle has two parts: when the anterior portion contracts, it elevates the mandible (closing the mouth), and when the posterior portion contracts, it results in retrusion of the mandible.

As mentioned in the discussion of lips earlier in this chapter, successful milk transfer relies on the infant's ability to form an adequate seal, exert negative pressure, and compress the nipple/areola. Muscle tone is key.

A generalized low muscle tone throughout the body, or even just in the orofacial region, usually suggests that the infant will have low tone in the lips, tongue, or cheeks. Gentle stimulation exercises can be done to improve muscle tone (**Figure 31).**

Many infants who have generalized muscle hypotonia have sluggish reflexes and very short periods of being alert. Removing the infant's clothing may help to bring them to a more alert state (**Figure 50**). Muscle tone, alertness, and reflexes are all separate functions, but they are often interrelated. Feeding-related reflexes can be hypertonic or hypotonic, with or without generalized muscle tone issues. These might include a depressed rooting reflex **(Figure 49)** or gag reflex **(Figure 51**).

If the infant has hypotonia of any or all the orofacial muscles, she may have a limited ability to transfer all of the available milk to herself. It is very helpful for the mother to compress her breasts manually (**Figure 43**) during the feeding, to augment the infant's efforts.

Birth Marks

The lay term "birth mark" might be better understood by using the scientific term, *nevus.* The term *nevus* (plural, *nevi*) comes from the Latin word, *naevus* or *natus* (born). Originally, such marks were understood to be present only at birth or shortly after. That's almost always the case, but studies have shown that they may sometimes be acquired in later life.

Nevi may interfere with feeding, and even with bonding, especially if they are disfiguring. They may also be mistaken for other conditions, such as signs of child abuse. Any person who is credentialed in healthcare is *obligated* to report suspicion of child abuse. Therefore, a question on child abuse is entirely "fair game" for the IBLCE exam. Be sure you know how to find some clues about characteristics that might help to differentiate a birth mark from child abuse.

There are two types of nevi: pigmented, and vascular.

Pigmented Nevi

Pigmented nevi are those that have a greater than normal amount of *pigmentation* (coloring) in the skin. The pigment that gives skin, hair, and eyes their color is called *melanin.* The amount of melanin in the skin generally determines the color of any pigmented birthmark. People with darker skin are more likely to have pigmented birth marks that appear darker than the skin but are not cancerous.

There are three major types of pigmented nevi: (1) moles (2) Mongolian spots, (3) café au lait spots.

Moles

Moles may be present anywhere on the body, and can sometimes look very similar to an extra nipple. Certainly, a "mole" on the front of the chest—along the milk line—requires further assessment. Moles are usually dark, and they may be raised. **Figure 187** shows an extra (supernumerary) nipple which could easily have been mistaken for a mole during childhood.

Mongolian spots

Mongolian spots may be known as Mongolian blue spots, slate gray nevi, or as congenital dermal *melanocytosis*. Mongolian blue spots seem to be more common in people with dark skin, including people of African, East Indian, or Asian descent.

Mongolian spots are often mistaken for signs of child abuse. In the 5th edition of *The Breastfeeding Atlas*, a large hairy nevus is noted as **Figure 56**, and a Mongolian spot is seen in **Figure 57**.

How can you determine if a mark is a simple birth mark, or an indicator of child abuse? Here are some classic features of Mongolian spots on an infant:

- flat against the skin, with a normal skin texture
- blue or blue-gray in color
- usually 2-8 centimeters (1-3 inches) wide
- irregular shape, with poorly demarcated edges
- usually present at birth, or soon after
- usually located on the buttocks or lower back, and less commonly, on the arms or trunk

Questions to ask yourself as you consider whether a skin condition is a Mongolian spot or a sign of child abuse include:

- When did the lesion appear? If the spot was not present at or shortly after birth and if it developed later, that is worrisome.
- What is the color? The slate-blue color of a Mongolian spot does not change over a few days, although it may fade in adolescence.
- What is the shape or contour? Is it raised or flat? The Mongolian blue spot is flat (no signs of swelling above the surface of the skin), and it is likely to not have clearly demarcated edges.
- What is the location? These are flat and blue-gray and typically appear on the buttocks or lower back, but may also be found on the arms or legs.

Café au lait spots

Café au lait spots are flat, pigmented birth marks. They are so named because of their light-brown color; café au lait is the French term for "coffee with milk." They are also called café au lait macules (a macule being a lesion that is neither elevated or depressed, of any size but usually less than 1 cm), giraffe spots, and coast of Maine spots.

Café au lait spots are pigment-producing melanocytes (melanin-producing cells) in the epidermis (upper layers) of the skin.

These spots can arise from several causes, mostly syndromes. It's unlikely that they have any direct significance or impact on feeding or breastfeeding. (However, the associated syndromes may.) They are usually permanent, and while they may grow or increase in number, they are usually harmless.

Vascular nevi

Vascular nevi are caused by blood vessels that didn't form correctly. Most are harmless, but parents have a substantial grief reaction to them.[11] Only a small percentage of infants have vascular nevi There are three types: stork bites, strawberry marks, and port wine stains.

Stork bites (Nevus Simplex)

"Stork bites" (or angel kisses or salmon patches) are examples of vascular nevi. Stork bites are extremely common; some sources estimate as many as 30-50% of newborns have a stork bite. Larger birth marks of this type are referred to as salmon patches, but they are the same type of lesion and are, as you might expect, smooth and flat with the skin's surface.

Frequently mistaken for erythema or bruising, these are not necessarily present at birth, but they may rapidly and dramatically develop a few weeks later. They are most commonly seen on the forehead, nose, eyelids, or back of the neck, but they can be elsewhere on the body. They are harmless; eventually, almost all lighten and fade completely.

Strawberry mark (Strawberry nevus, hemangioma)

A strawberry mark (**Figure 60**) is another type of vascular birth mark. The medical term is *hemangioma*, which is a collection of blood vessels that are close to the surface. About 5-10% of newborns have a strawberry mark. The condition is more common in girls and in white children. The cause is unknown.

Even though it is termed a "birth mark," a hemangioma may appear several weeks after birth. However, all hemangiomas are visible by the time the infant is 6 months old. Superficial hemangiomas are on the outer layers of the skin, and are typically bright red or purple (**Figure 60**). Deep hemangiomas grow under the skin in the fat, and colors are more muted; they may even be skin color. However, most hemangiomas are mixed—both superficial and deep. A hemangioma on the lips (**Figure 60**) if substantial, could interfere with breastfeeding. Luckily, the one shown here did not. The lesion may start out flat, but grow into a raised red lesion. Sometimes, it may enlarge rather quickly, and then fade. Typically, a hemangioma will fade by the time a child reaches 9 or 10 years of age.

Strawberry marks are most commonly found on the face, scalp, back, or chest, but they can be anywhere. In almost all cases, there is only one lesion on the body. They come in many different sizes and shapes, and most are fairly small. They tend to be harmless. However, the cavernous hemangioma has a soft, spongy feel to it, and it may contain a large amount of blood. If the parents wish, the hemangioma can be treated.

Common treatments include steroid injections, laser removal, or cryotherapy. However, treatment is not without risk, and most physicians advise waiting until the hemangioma fades, as most (but not all of them) do.

Port wine stain (Nevus flammeus)

Like other vascular nevi, port wine stains are caused by a localized area of abnormal blood vessels (capillaries). Of the three types of vascular nevi, these are the least common. About 3 in 1000 infants have a port wine stain.

Port wine stains can be located anywhere, but typically, they are found on the face, neck, scalp, arms or legs. They can be any size, but they do grow with the child. They are smooth and flat, with a shape that makes them appear as though someone splashed wine onto the skin. Usually flat, they can change into a pebbly texture. You may have noticed large port wine stains on singer Tina Turner and musician Billy Corgan (arms) and one on the head of Mikhail Gorbachev.

Unlike the hemangioma, the port wine stain is not bright red. At birth, they are usually pink, and then grow darker. Typically, they are a muted maroon color.

Although port wine stains are sometimes associated with a syndrome or some specific pathology, usually, they are harmless. They can be treated (or masked with makeup) but they never disappear spontaneously.

Here are a few principles to keep in mind about nevi:

- If you or the parent or the provider did not see a mark when the infant was born, its presence a few weeks later is NOT necessarily indicative of abuse.
- Be very familiar with the distinct differences between birth marks, and signs of child abuse.
- Recognize that most birth marks are harmless, many or most fade or completely disappear, and few interfere with feeding.
- Parents feel very isolated when their sons or daughters have a very obvious or disfiguring birth mark. Beware of signs of grief for loss of a perfect child, and/or a possible postpartum depression.

To help you compare these lesions, be sure to complete Learning Exercises 3-4 and 3-5 later in this chapter.

Looking Back, Looking Forward

In this chapter, we've talked about structural alterations that can affect latch, positioning, and milk transfer. We've also learned ways to recognize birth marks, and how they might affect health or breastfeeding (if at all). We've laid a firm foundation for the techniques and findings to deal with suboptimal functioning of the seal of the lips, negative intraoral pressure, and the mandibular compression of the nipple.

By now, if you have viewed the photos carefully, and if you've completed the written exercises, you should feel confident that you can develop the skills to recognize and manage normal conditions, variations of normal and abnormal conditions that affect latch, positioning, and milk transfer.

Recalling, Reinforcing, and Expanding Your Learning

Have you ever felt frustrated that you "learned" something, but later, can't recall it? That may be because you didn't reinforce the material you learned. And, perhaps what you originally learned isn't enough to get you through the next few decades of practice; sometimes you need to expand your learning. The exercises in this section are designed to help you recall, reinforce, and expand your learning.

What was your main motivation for reading this chapter?

- ❍ To study for the IBLCE exam, as a first-time candidate
- ❍ To review for the IBLCE exam, as a re-certificant
- ❍ To improve my clinical skills and clinical management

How soon do you think can use the information presented in this chapter?

- ❍ Immediately; within the next few days or so
- ❍ Soon; within the next month or so
- ❍ Later; sometime before I retire

Pro Tip! If you are preparing for the IBLCE exam, it would be wise to pace your studying. Set a target date for when you plan to complete the exercises, and check off them off as you go along.

Done!	Target Date	Learning Exercise
❑	____________	Learning Exercise 3-1. Vocabulary related to data-gathering, assessment for skin and orofacial structure and function
❑	____________	Learning Exercise 3-2. Recognizing normal and alterations in normal lip tone
❑	____________	Learning Exercise 3-3. Comparison of major differences between craniosynostosis and plagiocephaly
❑	____________	Learning Exercise 3-4. Comparison of Mongolian slate blue spots and indicators of bruising related to physical abuse
❑	____________	Learning Exercise 3-5. Comparison of three types of vascular nevi
❑	____________	Explore What You've Learned in a Journal
❑	____________	Summarize What You've Learned
❑	____________	Quick Quiz

Master Your Vocabulary

You must know the meaning of relevant vocabulary words so that you can understand—and correctly answer—questions about them. This chapter included many, many terms. While you might not need to know them all on your IBLCE exam, you never know which ones you'll need to know!

Learning Exercise 3-1. Vocabulary related to data-gathering, assessment for skin and orofacial structure and function.

Instructions: Write the letter of the correct match next to each item. Answers are in the Appendix.

N	1. asymmetry	A. pigmented birthmark
B	2. buccal pads	B. cheeks
K	3. craniosynostosis	C. lower jaw
I	4. frenum (frenulum)	D. vascular birthmark
D	5. hemangioma	E. e.g., a backward movement of the mandible
R	6. hypertonic	F. muscle tension at rest
G	7. hypotonic	G. overly limp
P	8. lesion	H. position of the mandible in relation to the maxilla
C	9. mandible	I. small fold of tissue that secures an organ
J	10. maxilla	J. the upper jaw
S	11. melanin	K. early closing of newborn skull sutures
L	12. micrognathia	L. a small mandible
Q	13. natal tooth	M. similar on both the right and the left
A	14. nevus	N. dissimilar from right to left
T	15. protrusion	O. stricture of the sternocleidomastoid muscle (SCM)
E	16. retrusion	P. discontinuity of tissue, or loss of function
H	17. retrognathia	Q. a tooth present at birth
M	18. symmetry	R. overly tense
F	19. tone, tonus	S. the pigment that gives skin, hair, and eyes their color
O	20. torticollis	T. e.g., a forward movement of the mandible

Conquer Clinical Concepts

Learning Exercise 3-2. Recognizing normal and alterations in normal lip tone.

Instructions: Summarize your understanding of muscle tone in the lips below. Try to write just a few words that will help you to remember.

Lip Tone

Indicators

- Visual

  Tight pursed lips reveal excessive tone

- Palpable

  Normally some resistance should be felt

- Auditory

  · audible swallowing is reassuring
  · clicking/smacking is NON reassuring

A&P Connections

- Structure: Name of Main Muscle

  oribicularis oris

- Function: Muscle's Main Function

  · enables lips to create a seal around the nipple/areola
  · ideally lips flanged around breast

Clinical

- Reasons

  · general hypotonia
  · traumatic birth
  · neuromuscular deficit

- Consequences

  low tone impairs:
  · negative pressure
  · adequate seal
  Infant often falls asleep

Non-Muscle Problems of Lip

· tight labial frenulum
· lip retraction

Learning Exercise 3-3. Comparison of major differences between craniosynostosis and plagiocephaly

Instructions: On the table below, summarize the difference between craniosynostosis and plagiocephaly. Answers are in the appendix.

	Craniosynostosis	Plagiocephaly
fusion of the skull?	Yes	No
how common	1 in 2500	1/2 kids in US have some form
effects	asymmetry of skull	head misshapen typically @ back
usual intervention	surgery	tummy time
treatment practitioner?	Specialist	regular peds.

Learning Exercise 3-4. Comparison of Mongolian slate blue spots and indicators of bruising related to physical abuse.

Go back and look at the text descriptions of Mongolian spots, and fill in the appropriate column with a few words. Then, using sources from outside, write descriptions about bruising. If you are uncertain about child abuse, consider taking a short course. (A list of available courses, some free, is available at http://www.keepkidssafe.pa.gov/cs/groups/webcontent/documents/document/c_124444.pdf)

	Mongolian spot	Bruising
Color	blue/blue-grey	Blue@begining
Color changes	fade over years	change over days blue, purple green yellow
Location	lower back butt shoulders, upper arms scalp	anywhere
Flat or raised?	Flat	Raised
Size	1-3in	any
Shape	irregular	more regular depending on what was used to strike
Onset/resolution	@birth usually fades over years	present anytime resolves 2wks
Other characteristics?	non-tender	tender

Learning Exercise 3-5. Comparison of three types of vascular nevi.

Instructions: Take a moment to compare the three types of vascular nevi. Use only a few words, but do write your answers! Answers are in the Appendix.

	Stork bite	Hemangioma	Port wine stain
Other names	angel kisses Salmon patch	Strawberry mark	
How common?	extremely common	5-10% newborns	uncommon 3 in 1000 births
Color, shape, size	Smooth, flat w/ Skin surface	Superficial = bright red/purple Deep = more muted	Smooth flat ∆ in pebble structure Pink @ birth get darker, maroon
Most likely location	forehead, nose, eyelids, back of neck	face, scalp back, chest	face, scalp back, chest
Onset, progression, resolution	@ birth or weeks after → almost all fade completely	all visible by 6 mo's.	never disappear spontaneously
Implication for care?	mistaken for erythema or bruising	can be treated but also fade	assoc. w/ pathology usually harmless

Explore What You've Learned In a Journal

Multiple studies have shown the benefits of using a learning journal. Among them are greater assimilation and integration of new information, better long-term retention of course concepts, increasing test and exam grades, and a means by which to have continuous feedback about one's own learning.

- Name at least three things you learned from this chapter.

Diff. between newborn findings

- List at least three things you still need to learn, or more fully master, in this chapter.

- Briefly describe how this information fits (or doesn't fit) with what you've seen in clinical practice, what you learned in basic or college courses, or what you've observed in your own experience breastfeeding. (In some cases, you might want to include how the information fits or doesn't fit with what "experts" say, what the media says, or whatever.)

- Describe how you will use any or all of this information. How might it be related to problems and potential solutions that occur in real life or in clinical situations?

Summarize What You've Learned

The goal of this chapter was to help you determine when it is appropriate to reassure, resolve, or refer the family for congenital oral (and other) anatomical variations in the infant that may (or may not) impact breastfeeding.

Sometimes, the type of information in this chapter can seem much more theoretical than clinical. But you'll need to master both! Take a few moments to summarize: How can you arrange the most salient points into a few bullet points? What type of questions would you expect to see on the exam? How might you use this information for individual clients in your clinical practice?

Main Points

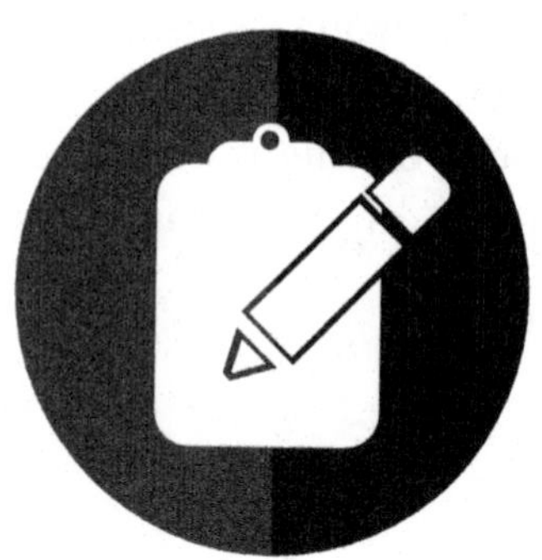

On the test

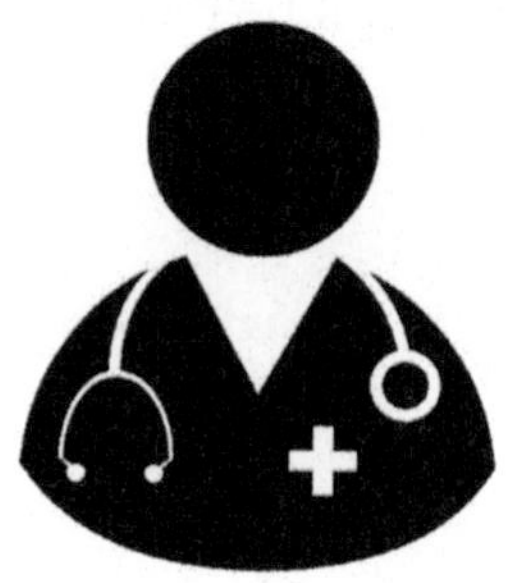

On the job

Self-Assessment and Analysis

People often dive into a test before they have thoughtfully reflected on how well they have prepared for it. Instead, it would be helpful if they would take a few moments to give their alter-ego (their "other self") at chance to reflect on how confident they feel about mastering the stated objectives.

Instructions: Take a moment to review the chapter objectives (below). Then rate yourself. How confident are you that you have achieved each objective below?

Objective	Highly Confident	Somewhat Confident	Somewhat Unsure	Completely Unsure
Recognize bony, soft tissue, and neuromuscular alterations of the intraoral and extraoral structures that can affect latch, positioning, and milk transfer.	❍	❍	❍	❍
Recognize key features of pigmented and vascular birth marks, and describe how they affect your responsibility to help the breastfeeding family	❍	❍	❍	❍
Name at least six different types of birthmarks, and recognize how they may affect health or feeding (if at all).	❍	❍	❍	❍
Describe assessment techniques and findings that indicate optimal or suboptimal functioning of (1) seal of the lips, (2) negative intraoral pressure, and (3) mandibular (jaw) compression of the nipple.	❍	❍	❍	❍

On the next page, you will see some simple recall questions pertaining to this chapter. These are *not* the application-type questions you will find in the IBLCE exam. However, you cannot *apply* information unless you can fully *recall* that information! You should do these without looking up the answers.

When you finish with the quiz, look up the answers in the Appendix. Then, score your answers, using the Appendix. Finally, you should analyze the results of your quiz. It's not enough to just know what you got right or wrong; you must look at why you got the answers right or wrong.

Quick Quiz Chapter 3

Circle the correct response. For a better understanding of how well you are mastering the material, try answering without looking it up. If you are really stuck, questions come from this workbook and from *The Breastfeeding Atlas* so go back and review the appropriate material. Answers are in the appendix.

1. (**Figure 45**). Given what you see here, which suggestion would be MOST helpful to the parents at this time?

    A. skin-to-skin contact

    B. a different type of bottle nipple

    C. a pacifier

    D. a tube-feeding device

2. The main muscle in the lips is the:

    A. buccinator

    B. hypoglossal

    C. masseter

    D. orbicularis oculi

    E. orbicularis oris

3. Which observed characteristics of a newborn would NOT be associated with low tone in the lips?

    A. clicking noises

    B. drooling

    C. generalized hypotonia

    D. jaw asymmetry

    E. unequal closure of the lips

    F. undulating tongue movement

4. To achieve successful milk transfer, the LEAST important factor is adequacy of the:

    A. creation of negative pressure

    B. mandibular compression of the breast

    C. seal of the lips

    D. support from the mother's hand

5. Which birth mark never goes away?

    A. Port wine stain

    B. Stork bite

    C. Strawberry mark

Analyze Your Own Quiz

- What percentage of the questions did you answer correctly?

80%

- If you got 100% of them right, to what do you attribute your success?

- If you did not get all the questions right, can you identify your learning gap? (Example: Didn't know the information, knew the information but could not remember, knew some information but confused it with similar information, other.)

- Would you have been able answer the questions as well if you had not read this chapter?

- What do you need to do next? (If you got them all right, what you need to do next is celebrate! Even a high-five with your child, a YESSS and a fist-pump in the air, or anything else is good! A small acknowledgement of your success is better than no acknowledgement!)

Additional Resources

1. McBride MC, Danner SC. Sucking disorders in neurologically impaired infants: assessment and facilitation of breastfeeding. *Clin-Perinatol.* 1987;14(1):109-130.
2. Geddes DT, et al. Tongue movement and intra-oral vacuum in breastfeeding infants. *Early Hum Dev.* 2008;84(7):471-477.
3. Geddes DT, et al. Tongue movement and intra-oral vacuum of term infants during breastfeeding and feeding from an experimental teat that released milk under vacuum only. *Early Hum Dev.* 2012;88(6):443-449.
4. Wolf LS, Glass R.P. *Feeding and swallowing disorders in infancy: Assessment and management.* 2 ed: Psychological Corporation 1992.
5. Lewis ML. A comprehensive newborn exam: part I. General, head and neck, cardiopulmonary. *Am Fam Physician.* 2014;90(5):289-296.
6. Plagiocephaly and breastfeeding. *RCM Midwives.* 2007;10(1):45.
7. Genna CW. Breastfeeding infants with congenital torticollis. *Journal of human lactation : official journal of International Lactation Consultant Association.* 2015;31(2):216-220.
8. Colson SD, et al. Optimal positions for the release of primitive neonatal breastfeeding. *Early Hum Dev.* 2008;84(7):441-449.
9. Paladini D, et al. Objective diagnosis of micrognathia in the fetus: the jaw index. *Obstet Gynecol.* 1999;93(3):382-386.
10. Biancuzzo M. *Breastfeeding the Newborn: Clinical Strategies for Nurses.* St. Louis: Mosby; 2003.
11. Tanner JL, et al. Growing up with a facial hemangioma: parent and child coping and adaptation. *Pediatrics.* 1998;101(3 Pt 1):446-452.

Chapter 4

Infant Stools and Urine Output

Our primary role is to assist with the infant's intake of his mother's milk, but there's a link between what goes in and what comes out. Therefore, it's important for us to understand output and to be able to explain it to the parents we encounter.

As with topics covered elsewhere in this workbook, we sometimes find ourselves wondering what's normal. It may be that what seems like normal output for one infant may seem like cause for concern with another. Perhaps you've wondered if an infant's loose stool is *too* loose. Maybe a parent has asked you to explain a dusty pink streak in their infant's diaper. What can you say?

I promise, by the time you finish this chapter, you will be able to recognize the key indicators of color, consistency, number, frequency, and volume of urine and stool output and their clinical implications for breastfed infants of various ages.

By viewing the photos in *The Breastfeeding Atlas*, reading the information here, and completing the written activities at the end of this short chapter, you will soon be able to figure out the clinical implications of infants' output—and be able to explain them to parents too!

Objectives

Given a clinical photo, you will be able to:

- Recognize clues to determine if stool or urine output is normal, a variation of normal, or a worrisome condition that requires medical follow-up.
- Compare and contrast meconium, transitional, and milk stools in terms of color, consistency, frequency/timing, number, and volume.
- Name at least five factors that affect whether stool output is normal.
- Distinguish stool/urine output in the diaper from other observations (e.g., oozing from circumcision, pseudo menses, other).
- State the definition of at least seven terms related to newborn output and diaper contents.

Key Terms

- anuria
- oliguria
- brick dust
- meconium stool
- milk stool
- pseudomenses
- transitional stool
- uric acid crystals
- witch's milk

Stool Output

As you might already know, if we are studying the human body's structure and function, there are relatively few exact numbers to describe what is "normal." Rather, there is a range of normal. That range—often called normal parameters—is what we need to keep in mind.

There are several factors to consider when determining what's normal. Before you can draw any useful conclusions about the stools, consider each of these characteristics:

- color
- consistency
- frequency/timing
- number of stools
- volume
- odor

Initially, you may not have access to all of this information. Yet, even when you do, you'll need to figure out what's normal, what's just a variation of normal, and what's cause for concern. There are several factors that affect what makes stool look "normal." The big clues are:

- age of the infant
- what the infant has ingested: human milk, formula milk, medications
- what the mother has ingested: food, medications
- treatments, most notably bili lights
- pathology
- other factors

The age of the infant certainly affects the color, consistency, and volume of stools produced. The number and frequency of stools is especially important. With the exception of the first few days, a breastfed infant should have *at least* three stools per day during the first month of life. A common misconception is that a breastfed infant may go several days without a stool. That is true after the first month, but during the first month, the infant should produce at least three stools per day; otherwise, he is at high risk for failure to thrive.[1]

Let's consider the three types of stools a breastfed infant will produce: meconium, transitional stools, and milk stools.

Meconium Stools

Meconium stools are made up of amniotic fluid and many protective microorganisms. It is the first type of stool newborns pass. (The topic of gut health and "seeding and feeding" is beyond the scope of this workbook; it is covered elsewhere).*

---

* Harman T, Biancuzzo, M. The intergenerational secret service inside you and your baby [Internet radio on iTunes].Born to Be Breastfed. VoiceAmerica Health & Wellness Channel; Nov. 28, 2016.

Color/Consistency: Meconium stools are a dark-green or a tarry-black color (**Figure 61**), and they tend to be sticky and even a little shiny.

Frequency/Timing: A newborn should pass at least one meconium stool within the first 24 hours. If that doesn't happen, the primary care provider should be notified; an obstruction of the gut, although highly unusual, is a possibility that should be explored. Even if the gut is normal, a delay in passing the meconium is well-known to relate to increased serum bilirubin levels, since bilirubin is excreted in the stool. (Note that a vaginally-delivered newborn may pass a meconium stool during the delivery process. Although it should be recorded, sometimes, it goes unnoticed or unrecorded.)

Number: It's difficult to say how many meconium stools a newborn will have. Certainly, a newborn should have at least one meconium within 24 hours of being born. Thereafter, the number varies. Newborns who pass a large volume in one stool usually have fewer stools than those who have a small volume each time.

Volume: The amount shown in **Figure 61** is neither typical or atypical. Sometimes, newborns pass a meconium that is many times that size! Every newborn is different.

Other: Regardless of what the mother has eaten or otherwise been exposed to, the color and consistency of the meconium stool is unaffected. Remember, it consists of amniotic fluid the newborn swallowed while in utero.

Transitional Stools

Sometime after about the first day or so, newborns begin to pass transitional stools. In breastfed newborns, these are made up of some meconium and some of the mother's milk that the newborn has ingested.

Color/Consistency: Transitional stools are olive green, or greenish-brown (**Figure 62**). Try to imagine that the newborn has been swallowing amniotic fluid for many months. Now, he is swallowing milk. As both substances pass through the intestines, the changes in color become apparent.

Those transitional stools that have more meconium and less milk stool will have a more slippery, slimy consistency. Conversely, those that have more of a milk stool will be less slippery. **Figure 63** shows the 24-hour output of a term newborn on Day 3.

Frequency/Timing: Meconium stools give way to transitional stools within a day or two. Some variation is to be expected. It's tough to say; I've sometimes seen a newborn have a massive meconium stool shortly after birth, followed by several good feedings, and a transitional stool within 24 hours of birth. Admittedly, that doesn't usually happen, but it's still within the range of normal.

Number: Studies differ slightly in their conclusions about the "normal" number of stools in the first few days. I give parents a simplistic guideline which is scientifically sound but unencumbered by details: The newborn should pass at *least* one stool on Day 1, at *least* two stools on Day 2, and at *least* three stools by Day 3. Ideally, by Day 4, I want to see a mustard-yellow color; however, that is not always the case. (In my experience, seeing a mustard-yellow stool by Day 4 allows me to predict that the likelihood of jaundice developing is now very, very slim.)

Volume: By Day 4, newborns will produce transitional stools of varying sizes. **Figure 64** shows that one transitional stool is substantially larger than the other; this is normal. Usually, I don't worry too much about size. But if the infant is having very few stools and I am relying on the parents' report, I make sure they understand what "counts." As noted in *The Breastfeeding Atlas*, unless a stool is at least the size of a US quarter (**Figure 65**) it doesn't "count."

Milk Stools and Solid Foods

After the mother's milk moves past the colostral phase, the breastfed newborn produces *milk stools*. Milk stools can have several different appearances, all of which may be normal.

Color/Consistency: When stools are bright yellow and watery (**Figure 66**) parents sometimes describe this as "diarrhea" because it is so liquidy, but in almost all cases, a few bright yellow stools with a watery consistency are not worrisome. (Sustained watery stools, or watery stools that are green, require more follow up.)

Yellow and yogurt-like: This consistency and color in exclusively breastfed newborns is also normal.

Seedy: (**Figure 67**) "Mustard-like seeds" of milk stools are very common, and so are curd-like stools, such as those of a 6-day old (**Figure 68**).

Green: **Figure 69** shows the stool of a 3-week old newborn. Admittedly, a green stool may signal a worrisome situation, but very often, it signals a variation of a normal condition. For example, a newborn who is jaundiced and undergoing photo therapy (Chapter 2, **Figure 27**) may have green stools as the bilirubin is being excreted. Medications, especially antibiotics, are another likely reason for green stools. The consumption of green food or drinks by the mother (or an older infant) may result in green milk stools. Many people associate green stools with an oversupply of mother's milk. That is entirely possible, but I would do much more data-gathering of other signs and symptoms before settling on oversupply as the cause. (Further discussion of oversupply is in chapter 11.) In general, exclusively breastfed infants continue to have stools that are soft and non-malodorous for several months.

Loose, unformed stools are common in the first month or so. Once an older infant starts consuming solids, his stools change again. **Figure 71** shows the output of a 7-month old infant who consumes both his mother's milk and table food. Notice that it is different from the previous photo in terms of color, consistency, and volume. This can be explained by two facts: (1) At six months, the protein of the mother's milk is about 50% casein and about 50% whey, whereas at Day 6, it is about 90% whey and about 10% casein; hence, stools appear more formed. (2) Infants who are consuming soft, semi-soft, or solid food are unlikely to have loose stools.

Frequency/Timing: Figure 70 shows the 24-hour output of an 8-week old exclusively breastfed infant. Note that this type of output would be less typical in an older infant; after about 4-6 weeks, exclusively breastfed infant may go several days—perhaps a week!—between passing stools.

Number: At least one stool on Day 1, at least two stools on Day 2, at least three stools on Day 3, and every day thereafter through the first month. These are the minimum number of stools in that time frame. Usually by Day 4, the newborn will produce 4 or more stools of varying sizes during a 24-hour period; many will pass a stool with each feeding by Day 4 or later.

Volume: Each infant is different. Volume of stool will depend on frequency and number, as well as how much milk—or later, how much solid food—is consumed.

To help you compare and contrast characteristics that typify infant stools, complete Learning Exercise 4-2.

Worrisome Observations About Stools

Blood in the stools (**Figure 73**) may signal a pediatric emergency. Unless you are legally licensed to do so, you cannot diagnose the cause of the bloody stools. However, this should be reported to the primary care provider without delay.

There are several possible explanations for blood in the stool. As Wilson-Clay and Hoover point out in *The Breastfeeding Atlas*, some relatively common reasons include: (1) accidental ingestion of the mother's blood during delivery, or from a sore nipple, (2) small tears in or around the infant's anus or intestine, (3) infection or infectious diarrhea (most notably *Salmonella* or *Clostridium difficile**), (4) allergies or sensitivities to foods that the infant or the mother is ingesting (e.g., dairy products, soy, or other), or (5) other causes. Sometimes, in the first several hours of life, a newborn may have blood in his stool that has a characteristic dark, or "old," appearance. Especially if he was born vaginally, a likely explanation is that he swallowed some of his mother's blood, and is now passing it. Another possibility is that he has ingested blood from the mother's nipple.

Note the color, amount, and location of the blood (i.e., whether it is streaked on the outside of the fecal mass or mixed in with the fecal mass). Streaks on the outside of the fecal mass are more likely to indicate straining at the stool. Streaks of blood mixed with the fecal mass, or accompanied by mucous, are likely to indicate something more serious. Whenever blood is seen in the stool, the diaper should be saved, and the primary care provider notified.

Five worrisome signs that require immediate medical follow-up by the primary healthcare provider:

* *Clostridium difficile* (*C. difficile*) is a spore-forming, anaerobic, Gram-positive bacterium that causes inflammation of the colon. It is a healthcare-associated infection. It is found in the feces, but it can be found in the environment (e.g., touching contaminated surfaces, or affected hands of hospital personnel) or by the oral-fecal route. Infants may be symptomatic, or may have injury to the intestinal mucosa and bloody stools.

- Color: The infant's stool is white, black, or contains streaks of bright red.
- Infant's reaction: The infant screams out in pain or bleeds while defecating.
- Mucous: The presence of mucous, with or without blood, could indicate an infection or a food intolerance.
- Changes: Dramatic changes in stool after introducing a new food or medication may indicate an allergy.
- Consistency: Stool that has a more yogurt-like consistency at around age one year, or more than five runny stools a day after that.

To better gauge the meaning of stool output, determine these five factors:

- the age of the infant
- the timing of the mother's milk "coming in"
- the infant's overall behavior during suckling and at other times
- the mother's intake (food, fluids, or medications)
- the extent to which the infant is breastfed (exclusively, partially, or not at all).

Information that you elicit from the infant's parents in response to questions about the first four factors generally is accurate. However, some parents may hesitate to admit that they have supplemented with formula, for fear of your "disapproval." But if you look carefully at the infant's stool, you will soon be able to determine whether he is exclusively breastfed.

The stool of an infant who has received some formula will have different characteristics than the stool of an exclusively breastfed infant, including:

Color/Consistency: The stool tends to be more brown in color, and it is more rubbery in consistency.

Volume: With the exception of the first or second meconium, most stools passed in the first week or so have relatively little volume. A bigger volume, together with a more brown color, suggests that the infant has received formula supplementation. Infants who are older and exclusively breastfed might pass a large volume of stool if the mother has an oversupply of milk; in that case, the stool will be more green in color and frothy in consistency.

Presence of Blood: Blood in the stool may or may not indicate a formula supplement, but it always requires medical follow up.

Urine Output

Urine output is an important indicator of an infant's wellbeing. In a newborn, no urine output (*anuria*) or very little urine output (*oliguria*) after birth, could be a sign of a genitourinary problem. Also, the amount of urine a newborn passes is an indicator of hydration status.

In the first day or two, details about the newborn's urine output should be observed and recorded. The number of wet diapers produced, and the color of the urine are important facts to note. Generally, the newborn's urine should be clear and a pale yellow, and he should have at least one wet diaper in the first 24 hours.

Keep in mind, though, that you might not have the full picture. A substantial number of newborns pass urine at birth. With a female newborn the instance is likely to go unobserved, and unrecorded. Hence, what we think might be "no urine" actually isn't. Nevertheless, since we can't be sure, if we can't confirm the newborn's urine output, the situation deserves follow-up.

Sometimes, the amount of urine passed by the newborn in the first day or two creates a deceptive picture of the infant's health, such as when it is inflated by the mother receiving a lot of intravenous fluid during labor. The problem isn't one of wet diapers, but of perceived extreme weight loss; newborns carrying a lot of fluid for this reason typically have many wet diapers and lose weight rapidly in the first day or two. The problem is that the infant's weight at birth is presumed to be his "baseline" weight, and the extra fluid he is carrying because of his mother's intravenous fluid intake during labor isn't accounted for.[3]

In this workbook, however, we will assume that "normal" parameters are those which would occur under a more natural set of circumstances. (Remember, the lactation exam is administered worldwide!)

Normal Parameters for Urine

Often, parents hear that breastfed infants should have 6-8 wet diapers a day. However, that is untrue for the first few days. There are certainly factors that could affect the number of wet diapers a newborn has in the first few days. (The amount of fluid his mother received in labor, and the amount of vomitus or blood loss his mother had in labor are, in my experience, the most glaring variables).

As a general rule, however, the newborn should have at least one wet diaper within the first 24 hours of life. Some other easy "rules" to tell parents include: At least two wet diapers by Day 2, at least three wet diapers by Day 3, and at least four wet diapers by Day 4. By Day 5, the newborn should have at least six to eight wet diapers within a 24-hour period, assuming he has been taking in milk (including colostrum) since birth. Urine should be light yellow, or straw-colored.

Brick Dust

Brick dust is a lay term for *uric acid crystals,* which describes output that consists of calcium and uric acid. In the newborn's diaper, this appears as a reddish-orange stain or salmon-color stain. The stain has a dusty, dry appearance (**Figure 72**).

There's scant science to help us understand why some newborns have uric acid crystals and others don't, but most experts agree that it is harmless in the first few days after birth. Although it can appear sooner, brick dust typically appears about two days after birth, with the color of the "dust" getting progressively lighter each day. (In older infants, brick dust is a sign of dehydration). I have never seen brick dust after the completion of Day 4, so if you are seeing it thereafter, or if it is not getting lighter each day, the family should be referred for medical help.

Brick dust, because of its red color, can be confused with other "red" matter that is the diaper. However, these "similar" red splotches are different in terms of their shape, amount, texture, and location. **Figure 74** shows a bloody vaginal discharge, called *pseudomenses.* Note the clues that it is not likely to be from the gut or the stool. Specifically, it has a shiny, slippery, appearance, and it is located in the area of the diaper beneath the vagina. A white vaginal discharge (**Figure 75**) may also be seen in the diaper; it is normal and is caused by the mother's hormones, like the so-called *witch's milk*, which might be seen oozing from a newborn's nipples (**Figure** 57).

Oozing from the circumcision is also red, but it is located in the front of the diaper, the area of the infant boy's penis. The blood stain is a round shape, reflecting the shape of the head of the glans. By comparison, brick dust is usually arranged linearly, from front to back, as shown in **Figure 72**. The blood from a circumcision looks wet and oozing in appearance, whereas brick dust looks "dusty."

Complete Learning Exercises 4-1 and 4-3 to increase and solidify your ability to recognize normal, variations of normal, and abnormal output in breastfed infants.

Looking Back, Looking Forward

In this chapter, we've talked about the normal parameters for stool output and urine output at different infant ages. We've also briefly mentioned other diaper contents.

Evidence in the education field shows that writing your own summary helps your retention. The Summarize What You've Learned exercise helps you to do this, so take just a few minutes to complete that exercise.

By now, if you have viewed the photos carefully, and if you've completed the written exercises, you should feel confident that you can recognize the key indicators of color, consistency, number, frequency, and volume of urine and stool output and their clinical implications for breastfed infants of various ages.

Recalling, Reinforcing, and Expanding Your Learning

Have you ever felt frustrated that you "learned" something, but later, can't recall it? That may be because you didn't reinforce the material you learned. And, perhaps what you originally learned isn't enough to get you through the next few decades of practice; sometimes you need to expand your learning. The exercises in this section are designed to help you recall, reinforce, and expand your learning.

What was your main motivation for reading this chapter?

- ❍ To study for the IBLCE exam, as a first-time candidate
- ❍ To review for the IBLCE exam, as a re-certificant
- ❍ To improve my clinical skills and clinical management

How soon do you think can use the information presented in this chapter?

- ❍ Immediately; within the next few days or so
- ❍ Soon; within the next month or so
- ❍ Later; sometime before I retire

Pro Tip! If you are preparing for the IBLCE exam, it would be wise to pace your studying. Set a target date for when you plan to complete the exercises, and check off them off as you go along.

Done!	Target Date	Learning Exercise
❑	______________	Learning Exercise 4-1. Matching terms related to infant output
❑	______________	Learning Exercise 4-2. Comparison of meconium, transitional, and milk stools
❑	______________	Learning Exercise 4-3 Recognizing and correctly documenting types of infant output.
❑	______________	Explore What You've Learned in a Journal
❑	______________	Summarize What You've Learned
❑	______________	Quick Quiz

Master Your Vocabulary

Learning Exercise 4-1. Matching terms related to infant output.

Unless you know the meaning of a word, you cannot fully answer a question about it. Match the terms in the left column to their definitions in the right column.

-Matching terms related to infant output and maternal hormones.

A	1. anuria	A.	no urine output
F	2. meconium stool	B.	bright yellow
B	3. milk stool	C.	olive green
D	4. oliguria	D.	scant amount of urine
C	5. transitional stool	E.	a dusty pink output
E	6. uric acid crystals	F.	tarry black or dark green
G	7. witch's milk	G.	secreted from a newborn's nipple

Conquer Clinical Concepts

Learning Exercise 4-2. Comparison of meconium, transitional, and milk stools.

Instructions: In this table, write one or two words to describe each type of stool.

	Meconium	Transitional Stool	Milk Stool
Color	tarry black or dark Green	olive green or Greenish brown	bright yellow & watery yellow & yogurt like
Consistency	sticky Shiny	slippery Slimy	loose unformed seedy/space
Frequency/Timing	within first 24hrs	1-2 days	Day 4
Number	at least 1	Day 2 = 2 Day 3 = 3	Day 4 3-4/day first month
Volume	different	at least quarter size	

Learning Exercise 4-3. Recognizing and correctly documenting types of infant output.

Instructions: Write your answers to these questions.

Question	Answer
How will you recognize various clues to determine if stool or urine output is normal, a variation of normal, or a worrisome condition that requires medical follow-up?	Color Infants reaction mucous changes consistency
Name factors that affect whether stool is normal.	age infant timing of mom's milk comming in infants overall behavior mother's intake exclusivety of breastfeed
How can you distinguish stool/urine output in the diaper from other observations (e.g., oozing from circumcision, pseudo-menses, other)?	consistency time appearance amount texture location

Summarize What You've Learned

The goal of this chapter was to recognize the key indicators of color, consistency, number, frequency, and volume of urine and stool output and their clinical implications for breastfed infants of various ages.

Using the main topics in this chapter, write your own summary of what is important for clinical actions. Meaning, it's not just about "recognizing" one type of output from another. It's also about understanding the composition of the output, and knowing what that means for clinical care.

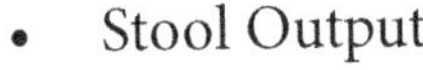

- Stool Output

- Urine Output

- Other Output

Explore What You've Learned In a Journal

Multiple studies have shown the benefits of using a learning journal. Among them are greater assimilation and integration of new information, better long-term retention of course concepts, increasing test and exam grades, and a means by which to have continuous feedback about one's own learning.

- Name at least three things you learned from this chapter.

- List at least three things you still need to learn, or more fully master, in this chapter.

- Briefly describe how this information fits (or doesn't fit) with what you've seen in clinical practice, what you learned in basic or college courses, or what you've observed in your own experience breastfeeding. (In some cases, you might want to include how the information fits or doesn't fit with what "experts" say, what the media says, or whatever.)

- Describe how you will use any or all of this information. How might it be related to problems and potential solutions that occur in real life or in clinical situations?

- If you wish, include how you felt about learning this information. Were you overwhelmed? Enlightened? Worried? Something else?

Self-Assessment

People often dive into a test before they have thoughtfully reflected on how well they have prepared for it. Instead, it would be helpful if they would take a few moments to give their alter-ego (their "other self") a chance to reflect on how confident they feel about mastering the stated objectives.

Instructions: Take a moment to review the chapter objectives (below). Then rate yourself. How confident are you that you have achieved each objective below?

Objective	Highly Confident	Somewhat Confident	Somewhat Unsure	Completely Unsure
Recognize clues to determine if stool or urine output is normal, a variation of normal, or a worrisome condition that requires medical follow-up.	❍	❍	❍	❍
Compare and contrast meconium, transitional, and milk stools in terms of color, consistency, frequency/timing, number, and volume.	❍	❍	❍	❍
Name at least five factors that affect whether stool output is normal.	❍	❍	❍	❍
Distinguish stool/urine output in the diaper from other observations (e.g., oozing from circumcision, pseudomenses, other).	❍	❍	❍	❍
State the definition of at least seven terms related to newborn output and diaper contents.	❍	❍	❍	❍

On the next page, you will some simple recall questions pertaining to this chapter. These are *not* the application-type questions you will find in the IBLCE exam. However, you cannot *apply* information unless you can fully *recall* that information! You should do these without looking up the answers.

When you finish with the quiz, look up the answers in the Appendix. Then, score your answers, using the Appendix. Finally, you should analyze the results of your quiz. It's not enough to just know what you got right or wrong; you must look at why you got the answers right.

Quick Quiz Chapter 4

Circle the correct response. For a better understanding of how well you are mastering the material, try answering without looking it up. If you are really stuck, questions come from this workbook and from The Breastfeeding Atlas so go back and review the appropriate material. Answers are in the appendix.

1. Which shade of green BEST describes a transitional stool?
   A. emerald
   B. forest
   C. lime
   D. olive
   E. pine

2. Which pattern of output would indicate a need for follow-up?
   A. a 2-week-old infant with 2 watery stools and 6 curd-like stools in the past 24 hours
   B. a 3-day-old infant with 10 transitional stools in the past 24 hours
   C. a 3-week-old infant with 2 stools per day for 3 consecutive days
   D. an 8-week-old infant with 11 milk stools in 24 hours

3. Brick dust, if noted, should:
   A. disappear by the second day
   B. gradually decrease each day
   C. increase by Day 3

4. Three of the following observations require medical follow-up for an exclusively breastfed infant in the first month of life. Which one is LEAST likely to need medical follow-up?
   A. blood streaked in the center of a stool
   B. fewer than 3 stools per in a 24-hour period
   C. no urine output within the first 24 hours
   D. several green stools in a 1-day period

Analyze Your Own Quiz

- What percentage of the questions did you answer correctly?

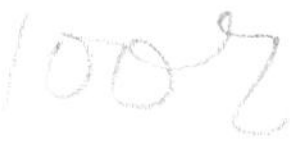

- If you got 100% of them right, to what do you attribute your success?

- If you did not get all the questions right, can you identify your learning gap? (Example: Didn't know the information, knew the information but could not remember, knew some information but confused it with similar information, other.)

- Would you have been able answer the questions as well if you had not read this chapter?

- What do you need to do next? (If you got them all right, what you need to do next is celebrate! Even a high-five with your child, a YESSS and a fist-pump in the air, or anything else is good! A small acknowledgement of your success is better than no acknowledgement!)

Additional Resources

1. Bekkali N, Hamers SL, Schipperus MR, Reitsma JB, Valerio PG, Van Toledo L, et al. Duration of meconium passage in preterm and term infants. Arch Dis Child Fetal Neonatal Ed. 2008 Sep;93(5):F376-9.

2. Chantry CJ, Nommsen-Rivers LA, Peerson JM, Cohen RJ, Dewey KG. Excess weight loss in first-born breastfed newborns relates to maternal intrapartum fluid balance. Pediatrics. 2011;127(1):e171-179.

3. Committee on Infectious Diseases. Clostridium difficile Infection in Infants and Children. Pediatrics. 2013;131(1): 196-200. Available ***http://pediatrics.aappublications.org/content/131/1/196***

4. Courdent M, Beghin L, Akré J, Turck D. Infrequent stools in exclusively breastfed infants. Breastfeed Med. 2014 Nov;9(9):442-5.

5. den Hertog J, van Leengoed E, Kolk F, van den Broek L, Kramer E, Bakker EJ, et al. The defecation pattern of healthy term infants up to the age of 3 months. Arch Dis Child Fetal Neonatal Ed. 2012 Nov;97(6):F465-70.

6. Gupta S, Suresh GS, Paes B, Shivananda S. Assessment of the severity of visible blood in the stool using a cluster of neonatal cases -a quality improvement study. J Neonatal Perinatal Med. 2015;8(4):379-91.

7. Harman T, Biancuzzo, M. The intergenerational secret service inside you and your baby In: Biancuzzo M, ed. Born to Be Breastfed: VoiceAmerica Health & Wellness Channel; 2016.

8. Lawrence RA, Lawrence R. M. Breastfeeding: A guide for the medical profession. 8th ed 2016.

9. Lindower JB. Water balance in the fetus and neonate. Semin Fetal Neonatal Med. 2017 Jan 30. ***https://www.ncbi.nlm.nih.gov/pubmed/28153467***

Chapter 5

Appearance of Human Milk

The infant or child doesn't care what his mother's milk looks like; he only cares about how it tastes and smells and how it fills his belly. Yet, when we express the milk for later feeding, we often focus on what it looks like. We compare today's milk to yesterday's. We make observations about what color it is, how much there is, and more. We ignore the fact that mothers were designed to have the milk suckled, not expressed.

Parents ask lots of questions about human milk. But they're not the only ones who do! You can be sure you'll need to answer questions about it when you take the IBLCE exam!

I promise that when we finish this chapter, you will be able to distinguish between reassuring and worrisome factors when viewing samples of colostrum or human milk at different stages of lactogenesis.

By viewing the photos in *The Breastfeeding Atlas*, and completing the written activities, you'll soon be well on your way to helping parents and professionals know what's okay and what's not.

Objectives

Given a clinical photo, you will be able to:

- State the definition for at least 10 terms related to milk production, including those related to stages of human lactation.
- Name at least two reasons why lactogenesis I may not occur at all.
- List at least eight reasons why a mother might experience a delay in lactogenesis II.
- Describe onset, color, consistency, and volume of human milk as it relates to lactogenesis I, lactogenesis II, and lactogenesis III.
- Relate the differences in milk color, consistency, and volume to clinical implications for counseling and anticipatory guidance.

Key Terms

- autocrine
- colostrum
- dysplasia
- endocrine
- engorgement
- feedback inhibitor of lactation
- foremilk
- galactogogue
- galactopoiesis
- hindmilk
- hypoplasia
- involution
- lactation
- lactogenesis I
- lactogenesis II
- lactogenesis III
- mature milk
- multiparous
- post-glandular
- pre-glandular
- primary hypoplasia
- primiparous
- retained placenta
- rusty pipe syndrome
- secondary dysplasia
- secretory activation
- secretory differentiation
- Sheehan syndrome
- transitional milk

The Process of Lactogenesis I, II, and III

As professionals, it's essential that we understand lactogenesis. The word *lactogenesis* is derived from *lact-* meaning "milk," and *genesis*, from the Greek term meaning "origin, *creation*, or *generation*." *Lactogenesis* is the "process by which the mammary gland develops the capacity to secrete milk."[1] It has three distinct phases: lactogenesis I, lactogenesis II, and lactogenesis III.

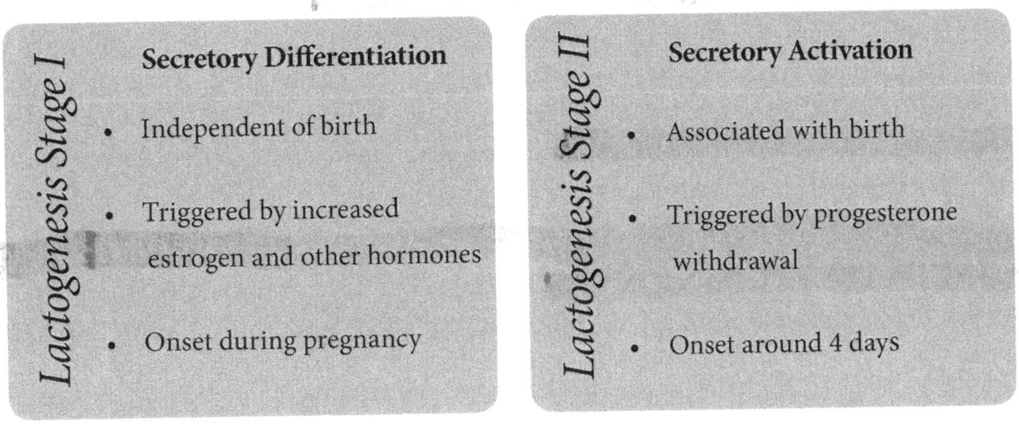

Lactogenesis Stage I	**Secretory Differentiation**
	• Independent of birth • Triggered by increased estrogen and other hormones • Onset during pregnancy

Lactogenesis Stage II	**Secretory Activation**
	• Associated with birth • Triggered by progesterone withdrawal • Onset around 4 days

Figure 5-1. Comparison of lactogenesis I and lactogenesis II. Reprinted with permission from Marie Biancuzzo's Comprehensive Lactation Course.

Lactogenesis I

During pregnancy, profound changes prepare the breasts for lactation. *Lactogenesis I* begins around the middle of pregnancy.[1] Structurally, ductular and lobular proliferation occurs as a result of hormonal influences. Luteal and placental hormones are responsible for the substantial increase in ductular sprouting, branching, and lobular formation.[2] Final stages of mammary growth and differentiation occur, primarily due to progesterone, although prolactin or human placental lactogen may be involved. This cell growth and differentiation is called *secretory differentiation*. Functionally, the gland merely becomes competent for secretion, but it secretes only a colostrum-like substance. Although the gland is structurally competent to secrete milk, it does not because of the hormones associated with pregnancy prevent milk from being synthesized. The high serum levels of maternal progesterone during pregnancy inhibit the secretion of milk until later. (See Figure 5-1 to see a comparison between secretory differentiation and secretory activation.)

After the placenta is delivered, the breasts begin to secrete colostrum. *Colostrum*, the first milk, is a thick substance that most often appears yellow or golden in color (**Figure 77).** However, it might also be clear (**Figure 76**), light brown (**Figure 79**), white, or another color. Colostrum is in the ducts during the latter part of pregnancy and is secreted the first few days postpartum. It is especially important for the newborn, since it is rich in immunoglobulins that support the infant's immature immune system. Also, it has a laxative effect on the gut that aids with the passage of newborn meconium.

Lactogenesis II

Lactogenesis II is "the onset of copious milk secretion" which "occurs during the first 4 days postpartum,"[2] due to the dramatic hormonal changes that occur in the mother's body after the placenta is delivered. This is *secretory activation*.

During the first four days or so after birth, mammary secretions occur by *endocrine* (hormone-based) regulation. Progesterone levels fall sharply. However, they do not reach the levels seen in nonpregnant women for several days. Prolactin levels remain high. The result is often referred to as the *milk "coming in."* The mother usually notices her breasts swelling and feeling tender, as well as a copious volume of milk. This physiologic *engorgement* is both normal and desirable. During lactogenesis stage II, changes in milk volume and composition are significant.

Transitional milk is produced during the very early postpartum period as the colostrum diminishes and the mature milk develops. It's often difficult to say exactly when the mother makes transitional milk, as each mother and each situation is different. One study found that on Day 2, *multiparous* mothers (who have given birth before) produce about 175 ml in a 24-hour period.[3] *Primiparous* mothers—those who have not given birth — may take a little longer.

Dewey et al[4] defined a delayed onset for this stage as that which occurs after 72 hours postpartum. Their study and others agree this is common.[5, 6] Page 33 of *The Breastfeeding Atlas* lists several reasons why lactogenesis II may be delayed. These reasons could be grouped as having to do with parity, labor/birth events, hypertension, supplementation, and obesity/diabetes issues. (Research both supports and refutes a delay in lactogenesis among diabetics; further research is needed.)

However, the more salient questions are: (1) is such a "common" delay normal, and (2) can some of the reasons for delay be modified, and (3) what is the long-term consequence for such delay, if any? We should not be lulled into thinking that because an observation is "common" that is it "normal."

Lactogenesis III

Lactogenesis III, also called *lactation* or *galactopoiesis*, is "the process of milk secretion and is prolonged as long as milk is removed from the gland on a regular basis."[2] The primary hormones that regulate established lactation are prolactin and oxytocin, which are secreted in response to the infant's suckling (or other forms of milk expression, such as pumping or hand expression). Volume of milk appears to be regulated locally by the removal of milk and the *feedback inhibitor of lactation* (FIL).[7] FIL is a chemical that is synthesized by the mammary epithelial cells, and creates a localized mechanism for regulating milk supply.

This local regulation is sometimes referred as *autocrine* regulation of milk.[8] In short, it is said that breastfeeding is based on "supply and demand," with the mother's body increasing the supply of available milk in response to signals of demand (e.g., the infant suckling longer, or more often).

Multiple authors give different perspectives about when the mother produces mature milk. *Mature milk* is produced during lactogenesis III. The energy content may be different from colostrum, as are the proportion of many nutrients. Generally, mature milk includes both foremilk and hindmilk. Multiple studies show that by the end of the first month postpartum, the mother will have about 750-800 ml of milk in a 24-hour period.

Foremilk is the milk that is produced and stored between feedings and released at the beginning of a feeding. It has an appearance similar to skimmed milk, with a characteristic blue tinge.

Hindmilk is milk that is produced during and released at the end of a feeding—it looks more like heavy cream. **Figure 84** shows the "creamy" hindmilk that sits atop the "thinner" foremilk.

Complete Learning Exercises 5-1 and 5-2 to have a clearer understanding of the terms and descriptions associated with lactogenesis I, lactogenesis II, and lactogenesis III.

Involution

Involution occurs when "regular extraction of milk from the gland ceases or, in many but not all species, when prolactin is withdrawn."[1] In other words, it is the natural process that occurs in the mother's breasts when she stops breastfeeding.

Lactation can continue indefinitely, as long as the breast is suckled, or milk is expressed. But in the absence of that stimulation, the mammary glands will involute. When that happens, the concentration of lactose is reduced, the volume of milk secreted by the mammary glands decreases, and electrolytes are elevated.-

Once its intended infant-feeding function is done, the breast begins to involute, much as the uterus involutes after it has performed its intended function of infant-birthing. Whether weaning occurs abruptly or gradually, the mother's milk changes in terms of its volume, and also the quantities of nutritional components and immunologic properties at this time. When the infant suckles less frequently, prolactin levels decrease, and when the breast is not emptied it becomes engorged; blood vessels are compressed, resulting in diminished oxytocin to the myoepithelium. Gradually, the alveoli collapse, although they do not fully involute even after the gland has returned to a resting state.

Volume of Mother's Colostrum and Milk

For decades, research has shown that mothers worry about not having enough milk. That's an understandable worry! Direct breastfeeding is a largely unseen process, with the infant's "food" going largely unseen. Differences in quantities of expressed milk day to day, hour to hour, or mother to mother also may cause concern.

Studies have shown that there are variances not only in milk production but in milk demand. What is "enough" milk for one mother-infant dyad in one situation isn't necessarily enough milk for another mother and infant in a different situation, and vice versa. Therefore, it's important to know the normal parameters for different situations.

Normal Parameters for Volume of Mother's Colostrum and Milk

The "normal" volume of colostrum that a woman produces is best expressed as that amount which adequately meets her infant's needs. Based on the scientific evidence and clinical cases, it may best be expressed as a range.

In a 24-hour period, a woman may produce anywhere from 10-100 ml of colostrum.[2] However, most mothers make about 30 ml of colostrum in a 24-hour period. Physiologist Michael Woolridge[9] showed that a bolus of fluid of about 0.6 ml (**Figure 80**) is likely to trigger the swallow response.

On their first attempt, many mothers are unable to express more than a few drops of colostrum. Very few mothers can express as much as 7 ml. In my experience, a mother who pumps post-delivery may get *nothing* on the first or second attempt; fortunately, volume increases gradually over the first few days. (Hand-expression of the first colostrum, and collection in small, 1 to 2 ml needleless syringes, can boost confidence in a new mother who must express her milk initially.) Some mothers make substantially more colostrum, especially well-illustrated in **Figure 76**.

As milk matures, color changes can be noted (**Figure 81**). Volume changes occur, too. On Day 2, this mother pumped 32 ml of colostrum at 2:00 AM. By the morning of Day 3, note that her milk was a whitish color with a more transparent appearance, characteristic of mature milk.

Mature milk volume is dependent on circumstances. How many weeks of gestation were completed when the mother delivered her newborn? How frequently has her breast been stimulated, and by what method (e.g., newborn suckling, pump, or hand expression)? How well was the breast emptied at those times? What are her circumstances (e.g., birth events, illness, pathology, or other circumstances)? Is she a *primiparous* mother or a *multiparous mother?* How many days, weeks, or months postpartum? Is this volume measured in the morning (when milk volume tends to be greater and fat concentration lower) or in the evening (when milk fat typically is higher and volume lower)? How do the volumes of milk produced by her breasts compare to each other? (Often, one breast does produce a little more than the other, but large differences need further follow up.)

The clinical question is, what parameters are normal, or at least typical? Research results from specific studies are based on multiple populations, conducted with different research methods and even with different equipment. For that reason, I tend to look at all of those numbers, consider my clinical experience, and arrive at a round number that helps me to know when to feel reassured, and when to intervene.

In a 24-hour period, most mothers produce at least 600 ml of milk by seven days after delivery, and 750-800 ml by the end of the month. Depending on several circumstances surrounding their labor and delivery, mothers who have had a cesarean delivery may have a lower volume of milk in the first several days, but they will "catch up" by the seventh day. Mothers whose newborns are unable to suckle—mothers who are pump dependent—should produce at least 450 ml by the end of the week; otherwise, they may be at risk for low production thereafter, and deserve follow-up with effective strategies.[10]

These numbers are not necessarily precise, or ideal! But they give guidance for clinical judgements. Every mother—and every infant—is different.

Possible Explanations for Decreased Milk Volume

Dr. Jane Morton poses a useful framework for explaining problems with lactogenesis.[11] She explains that insufficient milk production can be due to one of three factors:

- *pre-glandular* (e.g., hormonal or profound nutritional or illness situations)
- *glandular* (e.g., primary *hypoplasia*—incomplete or underdevelopment of the gland—or secondary *dysplasia*—abnormal cells that later grow within the tissue or gland)
- *post-glandular* factors (e.g., maternal-infant separation, ineffective emptying, or other management issues)

This framework helps us to understand why sometimes, milk doesn't "come in" at all. This doesn't occur often, but it can and does happen. If the mother has a *retained placenta*—meaning that the placenta (or, more likely, that a fragment of the placenta) was not delivered—lactogenesis will not commence. (Usually, a postpartum hemorrhage heralds a retained placenta. In rare cases, the first indication of a retained placenta is no milk.[12]) Even more rarely, a mother might have *Sheehan syndrome*.[13] This condition is brought on by a massive postpartum hemorrhage so severe that it deprives the pituitary gland of oxygen; hence, there is a dysfunction of the associated hormones and endocrine mechanisms. In the case of Sheehan syndrome, the mother will be unable to produce milk now, or with future childbearing.

Sometimes, milk may have "come in" but was delayed or the volume quickly diminished. By understanding Morton's framework, we can better understand how to help the mother. So, for example, "better breastfeeding management" won't help a woman with primary hypoplasia to make milk or make more milk, but there are a seemingly endless number of strategies to help a woman who has post-glandular issues.

With a thorough understanding of the physiology of lactation, one can understand that there is no substitute for frequent stimulation and adequate draining of the breast. *Galactogogues*—substances thought to improve milk supply but for which evidence is lacking—are often recommended. (Common galactogogues here in the United States include pharmaceutical agents, herbal remedies, or even food—oatmeal has been touted as a galactogogue!)

A recent Cochrane review showed that effective strategies for increasing the quantity of milk include relaxation, music, warmth, massage, initiation of pumping, increased frequency of pumping and a correctly-sized pump flange.[14]

Variations in Color

Milk that is discolored can be worrisome to professionals and parents alike. Some mothers who notice their milk isn't the white color they expect feel so worried that they terminate breastfeeding; some healthcare providers even recommend this. But consider—for every mother who notices her discolored milk, there are probably many other mothers who have discolored milk but never notice it! After all, when the infant is suckling directly at the breast, we don't see the milk before it is consumed. The only time the color is evident is when the mother has expressed her milk.

Milk can come in many different colors. Sometimes, there is no apparent explanation for why the milk is discolored. Sometimes, it is related to medications or pathology. (Read on for discussion of that.)

Colostrum can change color, even within a few hours. Colostrum pumped at two-hour intervals on Day 1 shows the light brown colostrum becoming progressively lighter (**Figure 79**). Similarly, milk pumped within five hours shows that the first one is more yellow; the second is more white/clear (**Figure 81**). Sometimes, there is a distinct difference in color between the milk from the left versus the right breast (**Figure 82**).

Many healthcare professionals worry about discolored milk and want to discard it because they assume the color indicates pathology. In my experience, nonpathological causes—especially food consumption or medications—are a frequent explanation for discolored milk. Green milk (**Figure 83**) is not terribly uncommon. I distinctly remember one mother who proclaimed herself as "the poster child for green vegetables." Her milk was almost always green! For other mothers, green milk is attributable to consuming a green sports drink, even green beer! My take-home message is this: Inquire about food or medications before assuming that discolored milk is due to pathology.

A fairly common cause for discolored milk is so-called *rusty pipe syndrome*. Although clinicians have noticed rusty pipe syndrome in expressed milk for decades, formalized reports have not been published until recently.[15-18] The color of "rusty pipe" milk has a pink/orange or red color, as it indicates the milk from the mother's breasts includes some blood. Although some hospital staff may be tempted to discard rusty pipe colostrum out of fear that it would hurt the newborn, this is unnecessary. (However, if the milk is very dark and thick, it may have so much protein the infant will find it bothersome.)

Apparently, rusty pipe syndrome was named not only because of the characteristic rusty color, but also because of the way the coloring clears. When water has been sitting for a prolonged period in a rusty pipe, it grows increasingly clear the longer that it runs. Similarly, the more the milk of a mother with rusty pipe syndrome is suckled or expressed, the clearer the milk becomes. Rusty pipe syndrome is thought to occur because of vascular engorgement. Some women will never have it.

Figure 78 shows the typical rusty color. However, I have seen rusty-pipe milk that is substantially darker (dark red or brown) and thicker than the sample shown. And, it may be entirely possible that some milk has so little "rust" that it goes unnoticed. There is likely a range of rusty pipe characteristics.

But not all milk coloring has a benign cause. Bright yellow milk (**Figure 261**) or orange milk (**Figure 262**) or even red milk (**Figure 264**) may be seen during a bout of methicillin-resistant staphylococcus aureus (MRSA) infection. (But, lack of discoloration does not mean that MRSA is absent! For more on MRSA, see Chapter 11.) Pink milk may be seen in the presence of *Serratia.*[*]

Yellow milk may result from treatment with nitrofurantoin, an antibiotic commonly prescribed for urinary tract infections. Orange milk may result from treatment with rifampin, an antibiotic used in the treatment of tuberculosis, or it may result from a large consumption of orange-colored vegetables. A full discussion of discolored milk is beyond the scope of this publication.

Looking Back, Looking Forward

In this chapter, we've talked about the process of lactogenesis I, II, and III, as well as the normal parameters for colostrum/milk characteristics.

Evidence in the education field shows that writing your own summary helps your retention. The Summarize What You've Learned exercise helps you to do this, so take just a few minutes to complete that exercise now.

By now, if you have viewed the photos carefully, and if you've completed the written exercises, you should feel confident that you can distinguish between reassuring and worrisome factors when viewing samples of colostrum or human milk at different stages of lactogenesis.

* *Serratia* is gram negative, anaerobic, endosporeforming, rod-shaped bacteria of the Enterobacteriaceae family. The most common genus of this bacteria is *S. marcescens*, a pathogen that often causes a hospital-based infection.

Recalling, Reinforcing, and Expanding Your Learning

Have you ever felt frustrated that you "learned" something, but later, can't recall it? That may be because you didn't reinforce the material you learned. And, perhaps what you originally learned isn't enough to get you through the next few decades of practice; sometimes you need to expand your learning. The exercises in this section are designed to help you recall, reinforce, and expand your learning.

What was your main motivation for reading this chapter?

- ❍ To study for the IBLCE exam, as a first-time candidate
- ❍ To review for the IBLCE exam, as a re-certificant
- ❍ To improve my clinical skills and clinical management

How soon do you think can use the information presented in this chapter?

- ❍ Immediately; within the next few days or so
- ❍ Soon; within the next month or so
- ❍ Later; sometime before I retire

Pro Tip! If you are preparing for the IBLCE exam, it would be wise to pace your studying. Set a target date for when you plan to complete the exercises, and check off them off as you go along.

Done!	Target Date	Learning Exercise
❑	________	Learning Exercise 5-1. Basic terms related to mothers and milk-making.
❑	________	Learning Exercise 5-2. Comparisons of lactogenesis I, II, and III.
❑	________	Explore What You've Learned in a Journal
❑	________	Summarize What You've Learned
❑	________	Quick Quiz

Master Your Vocabulary

Unless you know the meaning of a word, you cannot fully answer a question about it. There were many, many terms in this chapter; you might not need to know them all, but you never know which ones you'll be tested on, or which ones you'll find in the medical record!

Learning Exercise 5-1. Basic terms related to mothers and milk-making.

Write the letter of the correct match next to each item. Answers are in the Appendix.

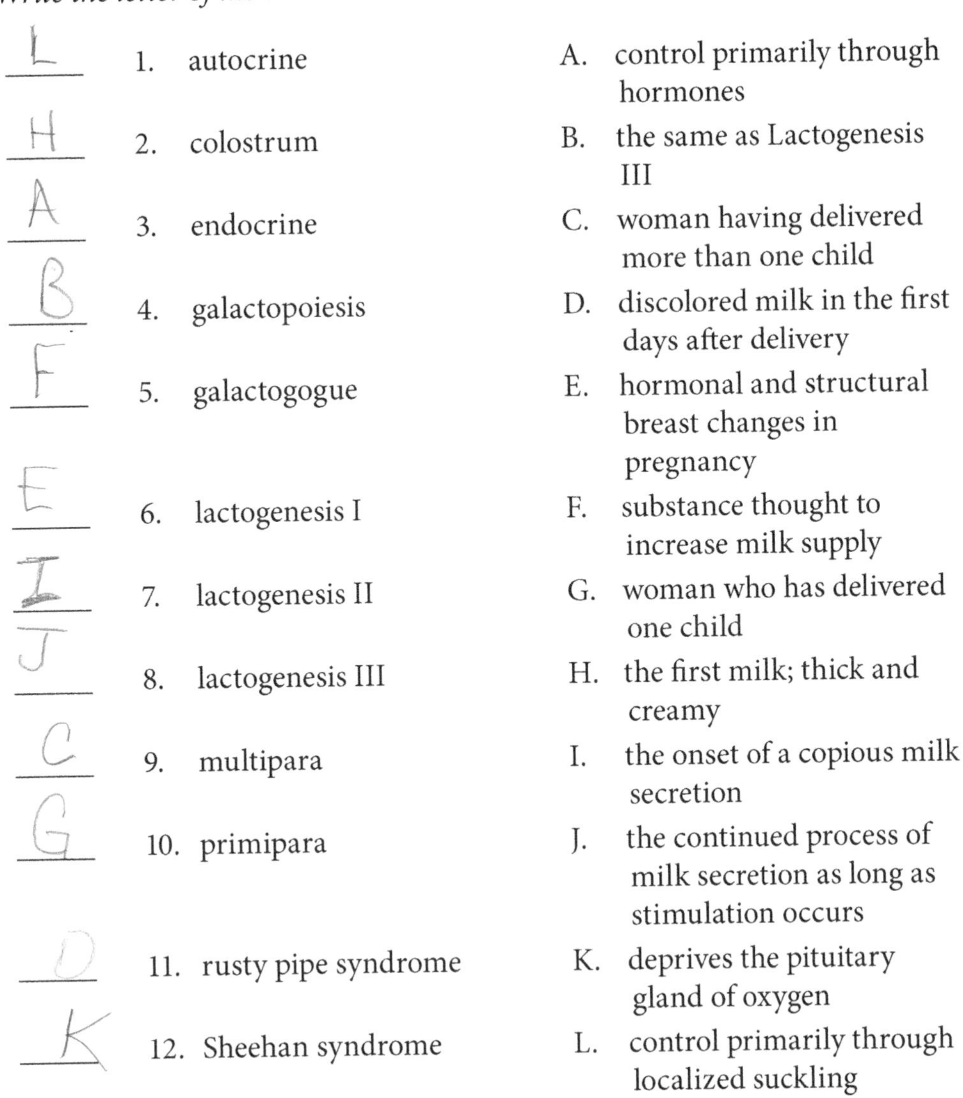

L	1. autocrine	A.	control primarily through hormones
H	2. colostrum	B.	the same as Lactogenesis III
A	3. endocrine	C.	woman having delivered more than one child
B	4. galactopoiesis	D.	discolored milk in the first days after delivery
F	5. galactogogue	E.	hormonal and structural breast changes in pregnancy
E	6. lactogenesis I	F.	substance thought to increase milk supply
I	7. lactogenesis II	G.	woman who has delivered one child
J	8. lactogenesis III	H.	the first milk; thick and creamy
C	9. multipara	I.	the onset of a copious milk secretion
G	10. primipara	J.	the continued process of milk secretion as long as stimulation occurs
D	11. rusty pipe syndrome	K.	deprives the pituitary gland of oxygen
K	12. Sheehan syndrome	L.	control primarily through localized suckling

Conquering Clinical Concepts

Learning Exercise 5-2. Comparisons of Lactogenesis I, II, and III.

Instructions: Complete the table below. Answers are in the appendix.

	Lactogenesis I	Lactogenesis II	Lactogenesis III
Also called...	N/A	onset of copious amounts of milk	lactation or galactopoesis
Onset	mid-pregnancy	3-4 days PP	as long as milk is removed on reg. basis
Typical volume	↓ during pregnancy	Day 2=175mL Day 7=600mL	1 month 750-800 ml/hr
Color	usually yellow	more white	bluish white
Consistency	thick/sticky	fluid	fluid
Primary control is through...	Hormones	Hormones	primarily autocrine
Other comments	Higher in protein, lower in fat	Physiologic engorgement	Some consistency in patterns

Summarize What You've Learned

The purpose of this chapter was to help you distinguish between reassuring and worrisome factors when viewing samples of colostrum or human milk at different stages of lactogenesis.

Sometimes, the type of information in this chapter can seem much more theoretical than clinical. Take a moment to summarize: How can you arrange the most salient points into a few bullet points? How will you use this information for individual clients in your clinical practice? How might this information be important in the bigger world of system-level changes (e.g., procedures, standing orders, etc.) or issues with populations of clients (e.g., writing patient education materials.)

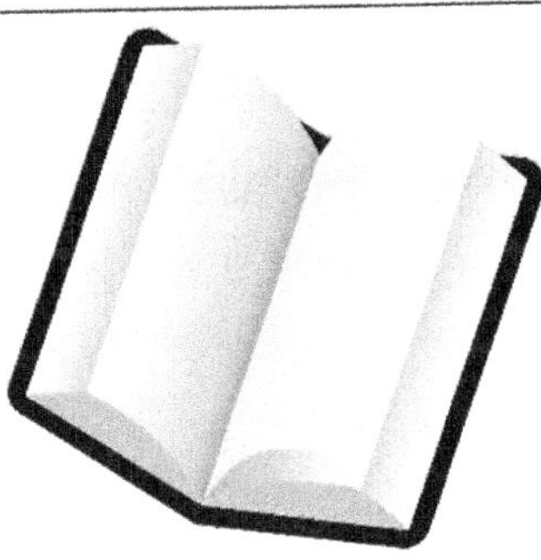

Main Points

On the test

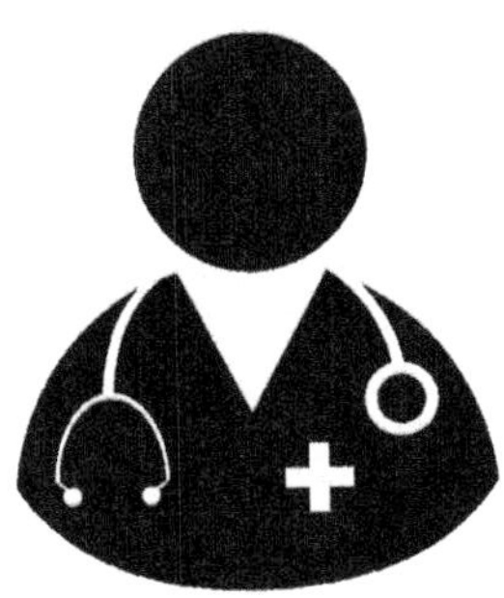

On the job

Explore What You've Learned in a Journal

Multiple studies have shown the benefits of using a learning journal. Among them are greater assimilation and integration of new information, better long-term retention of course concepts, increasing test and exam grades, and a means by which to have continuous feedback about one's own learning.

- Name at least three things you learned from this chapter.

- List at least three things you still need to learn, or more fully master, in this chapter.

- Briefly describe how this information fits (or doesn't fit) with what you've seen in clinical practice, what you learned in basic or college courses, or what you've observed in your own experience breastfeeding. (In some cases, you might want to include how the information fits or doesn't fit with what "experts" say, what the media says, or whatever.)

- Describe how you will use any or all of this information. How might it be related to problems and potential solutions that occur in real life or in clinical situations?

- If you wish, include how you felt about learning this information. Were you overwhelmed? Enlightened? Worried? Something else?

Self-Assessment

People often dive into a test before they have thoughtfully reflected on how well they have prepared for it. Instead, it would be helpful if they would take a few moments to give their alter-ego (their "other self") a chance to reflect on how confident they feel about mastering the stated objectives.

Instructions: Take a moment to review the chapter objectives (below). Then rate yourself. How confident are you that you have achieved each objective below?

Objective	Highly Confident	Somewhat Confident	Somewhat Unsure	Completely Unsure
State the definition for at least 10 terms related to milk production, including those related to stages of human lactation.	❍	❍	❍	❍
Name at least two reasons why lactogenesis I may not occur at all.	❍	❍	❍	❍
List at least eight reasons why a mother might experience a delay in lactogenesis II.	❍	❍	❍	❍
Describe onset, color, consistency, and volume of human milk as it relates to lactogenesis I, lactogenesis II, and lactogenesis III.	❍	❍	❍	❍
Relate the differences in milk color, consistency, and volume to clinical implications for counseling and anticipatory guidance	❍	❍	❍	❍

On the next page, you will some simple recall questions pertaining to this chapter. These are *not* the application-type questions you will find in the IBLCE exam. However, you cannot *apply* information unless you can fully *recall* that information! You should do these without looking up the answers.

When you finish with the quiz, look up the answers in the Appendix. Then, score your answers, using the Appendix. Finally, you should analyze the results of your quiz. It's not enough to just know what you got right or wrong; you must look at why you got the answers right.

Quick Quiz Chapter 5

Instructions: Circle the correct response. For a better understanding of how well you are mastering the material, try answering without looking it up. If you are really stuck, questions come from this workbook and from The Breastfeeding Atlas *so go back and review the appropriate material. Answers are in the appendix.*

1. Of these descriptors for colored milk, which would be the MOST worrisome?
   - A. bright pink
   - B. light brown
   - C. light green
   - D. rusty orange

2. Of these situations, which is most in need of further follow-up?
   - A. Milk from one breast is a slightly different color than milk from the other breast.
   - B. The volume of milk from one breast is twice as much as from the other breast.
   - C. Milk collected in the morning has greater volume than that collected in the evening.
   - D. Milk expressed on Day 3 looks different from milk collected on Day 2.

3. On Day 1, a primiparous mother is preparing to express her milk. She is worried about how much she will obtain. You tell her that in one "sitting" it is likely that she will get:
   - A. 25-30 ml.
   - B. 15-24 ml.
   - C. 8-15 ml.
   - D. 7-14 ml.
   - E. < 7 ml, and maybe only drops.

4. A mother who delivered her infant less than 24 hours ago has expressed the milk shown in **Figure 76**. The amount of milk she has obtained is:
   - A. about as much as might be expected.
   - B. more than might be expected.
   - C. less than might be expected.

5. A mother has delivered a healthy infant at term. He has suckled well since birth. By the end of the first week postpartum, about how much milk does the mother have?

A. 175 ml

B. 350 ml

C. 450 ml

D. 600 ml

E. 800 ml

F. 1000 ml

Analyze Your Own Quiz

- What percentage of the questions did you answer correctly?

- If you got 100% of them right, to what do you attribute your success?

- If you did not get all the questions right, can you identify your learning gap? (Example: Didn't know the information, knew the information but could not remember, knew some information but confused it with similar information, other.)

- Would you have been able to answer the questions as well if you had not read this chapter?

- What do you need to do next? (If you got them all right, what you need to do next is celebrate! Even a high-five with your child, a YESSS and a fist-pump in the air, or anything else is good! A small acknowledgement of your success is better than no acknowledgement!)

Additional Resources

1. Neville MC. Anatomy and physiology of lactation. *Pediatr Clin North Am.* 2001;48(1):13-34.
2. Lawrence R, Lawrence, RM. *Breastfeeding: A guide for the medical profession.* 8 ed 2016.
3. Neville MC, et al. Studies in human lactation: milk volumes in lactating women during the onset of lactation and full lactation. *Am-J-Clin-Nutr.* 1988;48(6):1375-1386.
4. Dewey KG, et al. Risk factors for suboptimal infant breastfeeding behavior, delayed onset of lactation, and excess neonatal weight loss. *Pediatrics.* 2003;112(3 Pt 1):607-619.
5. Chapman DJ, Perez-Escamilla R. Identification of risk factors for delayed onset of lactation. *J Am Diet Assoc.* 1999;99(4):450-454; quiz 455-456.
6. Nommsen-Rivers LA, et al. Delayed onset of lactogenesis among first-time mothers is related to maternal obesity and factors associated with ineffective breastfeeding. *Am J Clin Nutr.* 2010;92(3):574-584.
7. Wilde CJ, et al. Autocrine regulation of milk secretion. *Biochem Soc Symp.* 1998;63:81-90.
8. WHO Working Group on the Growth Reference Protocol and WHO Task Force on Methods for the Natural Regulation of Fertility. Growth patterns of breastfed infants in seven countries. *Acta Paediatr.* 2000;89(2):215-222.
9. Woolridge MW. The 'anatomy' of infant sucking. *Midwifery.* 1986;2(4):164-171.
10. Hill PD, et al. Comparison of milk output between breasts in pump-dependent mothers. *J Hum Lact.* 2007;23(4):333-337.
11. Morton J. Pre-glandular, glandular and post-glandular causes for insufficient milk production. *ABM News and Views.* Vol 92003:13.
12. Neifert MR, et al. Failure of lactogenesis associated with placental retention. *Am-J-Obstet-Gynecol.* 1981;140(4):477-478.
13. Sheehan HL. Postpartum necrosis of the anterior pituitary. *J Path Bacteriol.* 1937;45:189-214.
14. Becker GE, et al. Methods of milk expression for lactating women. *Cochrane Database Syst Rev.* 2016;9:Cd006170.
15. Cizmeci MN, et al. Rusty-pipe syndrome: a rare cause of change in the color of breastmilk. *Breastfeed Med.* 2013;8(3):340-341.
16. Faridi MM, et al. Rusty pipe syndrome: counselling a key intervention. *Breastfeed Rev.* 2013;21(3):27-30.
17. Silva JR, et al. Rusty pipe syndrome, a cause of bloody nipple discharge: case report. *Breastfeed Med.* 2014;9:411-412.

18. Virdi VS, et al. Rusty-pipe syndrome. *Indian Pediatr.* 2001;38(8):931-932.

Chapter 6

Positioning and Latch Techniques

Wouldn't it be ideal if every newborn arrived ready, willing, and able to accomplish the perfect breastfeeding position and latch? Unquestionably, some do, and I have seen them! But in the United States—where most newborns are born in a hospital, often after a medicated birth (for nearly one-third of babies, this means a cesarean delivery), and perhaps some birth trauma—most don't. Consequently, we need to help them to achieve good positioning and latch. Otherwise, the infant goes hungry, the mother experiences problems, and breastfeeding may cease before it has even truly begun.

I promise that by the time you finish this chapter, you will be able to determine how and when to help a breastfeeding couplet to adjust positioning and latch to achieve optimal milk transfer.

Whether you think you've already mastered this skill, or whether you think it's too difficult to learn yet, I urge you to stick with this. By applying a simple, four-step model as you view the clear, crisp pictures in *The Breastfeeding Atlas*, you'll learn how to aid the many mothers and infants who need help with positioning and latch.

Objectives

Given a clinical photo, you will be able to:

- Use the correct terms of movement to describe the infant's position at the breast.
- Describe how neuromuscular reflexes and movement can positively or negatively impact milk transfer.
- Recognize commonly-based breastfeeding positions and the likely reasons to use or avoid them for infants/children of various ages.
- Distinguish between indicators of effective and ineffective latch-on, and make suggestions for improvement.

Key Words

- abduction
- adduction
- biological nurturing
- chin-first latch
- clutch hold
- cradle hold
- cross-cradle hold
- distal
- extension
- flexion
- football hold
- hyperextension
- hyperflexion
- laid-back position
- over-rotation
- pronation
- protraction
- proximal
- retraction
- rotation
- side-lying hold
- straddle hold
- supination
- transitional hold

Reflexes and Movements

Unquestionably, successful milk transfer relies on good positioning and latch; these, in turn, rely on the infant having good feeding reflexes (discussed in Chapter 3) and being capable of a full range of motion. Also important to breastfeeding are primitive neonatal reflexes (PNRs), more than 20 of which have been identified by research midwife and nurse Suzanne Colson, PhD.[1] When the reflexes are intact, and the infant is given the opportunity to use them, he will self-attach to the breast.

An infant's ability to perform basic anatomical movements also impacts good positioning and latch.

Reflexes and movement are based on an understanding of anatomy and physiology, and it's critical for precise communication that we use such terms correctly. Further, in using the right terminology, we can better understand how anatomical parts relate to each other.

The Breastfeeding Atlas uses several terms of movement throughout chapter 6. Perhaps you are already familiar with these terms from previous anatomy coursework. However, terms of movement have somewhat different connotations when used to explain the motion of a knee than when used to describe a nursing infant's movement! I will attempt to describe these terms in a breastfeeding context.

First, let's look at terms to describe movements towards or away from the body's midline. *Adduction* refers to bringing a body part towards the midline, such as when an infant moves his hands or arms towards the midline. That's a sign of engagement, as discussed in chapter 2. *Abduction* involves movement away from the center of the body. Very often, abduction is a stress cue in an infant, as described and shown in chapter 14.

Flexion and extension are movements that occur in the sagittal plane. *Flexion* refers to decreasing the angle between two body parts. In the context of the neck and truck, flexion occurs as the infant moves his chin towards his chest. *Hyperflexion* (sometimes called over-flexion) (**Figure 122**) can occur when the mother uses her hand to push on the back of her infant's head (**Figure 97**), and it interferes with latch, breathing, and swallowing. But sometimes the mother does need to support her infant's head during breastfeeding. In this case, it can be useful to say to the mother: "point your fingers towards the baby's ears" (**Figure 98**), as this reduces the risk of hyperflexion. Note that this hand-on-head pushing can occur regardless of what position the mother is using to feed her infant.

In the context of the neck and trunk, *extension* refers to movement in the posterior direction, when the head tips backwards. Technically, *hyperextension* refers to excessive joint movement that is beyond the normal range of motion. For a breastfeeding infant, hyperextension almost always refers to tipping the head so far back that latch and swallowing are impaired.

In the context of breastfeeding, *supination* would be placing the infant's body supine—on his back. *Pronation* means placing him face-down, on his belly (**Figure 247**).

Rotation usually means movement of limbs around their long axis. However, in Chapter 6 of *The Breastfeeding Atlas*, Wilson-Clay and Hoover use the terms rotation and over-rotation several times to indicate that the infant's head and/or body is not aligned from shoulder to iliac crest (i.e., edge) of the pelvis, as it should be when breastfeeding. This term works well in this context! While breastfeeding, the infant often has his body around the long axis of the mother!

Technically, retraction or protraction refer only to movements of a joint, and the only joints in the body capable of retraction are the shoulder joints (glenohumeral and acromioclavicular joints) and the jaw joint (temporomandibular joint). *Retraction* is a tricky term, though! More casually, the term is used to describe the movement of body parts other than joints—for example, backward movement of the tongue. Retraction can also mean bringing the mandible backwards. Similarly, *protraction* means extending the mandible or tongue forward. In *The Breastfeeding Atlas*, the authors do refer to a "retracted lip," and we can assume they are referring to a lip being "bunched" or drawn backward inward rather than being flanged outwardly, as it should be.

As we move through this section, beware of the movements of the muscles—and how the movements can facilitate or thwart good milk transfer.

Knowing correct terminology is important for your understanding of the body's movements, as well as for your documentation—and your ability to gain credibility with healthcare professionals in other disciplines. To help you truly grasp and use these words, complete Learning Exercises 6-1 and 6-2 now.

Principles for Positioning, Latch, and Milk Transfer

Positioning and latch, while separate topics, are inextricably related. Without good positioning, it is difficult, and may even be impossible for the newborn, to achieve an optimal latch. For nearly three decades, I have consistently used the model developed by Shrago and Bocar in 1990.[2] They recommend evaluating the infant's position and latch though four observations: alignment, areolar grasp, areolar compression, and audible swallowing. Applying their model for ideal breastfeeding, I later articulated the observations that indicate breastfeeding that is *not* ideal, as well as specific strategies for overcoming suboptimal positioning and latch.[3]

Alignment

Good alignment is critical for good positioning. It helps keep the nipple and areolar in the infant's mouth, facilitates the infant's swallowing, and reduces traction or dragging on the mother's nipples.

Citing multiple studies, Redstone & West[4] assert that "alignment of the oral structures for feeding is related to head and neck stability" and that "head position influences the swallow during feeding and reduces the risk of aspiration." They emphasize that "structures that are significantly distal to the oral area influence its functioning." (That is, structures situated away from the mouth influence its functioning.)

Breastfeeding can occur in many different positions, but Shrago and Bocar[2] point out four conditions are key to good alignment.

- *The infant is flexed and relaxed.* Muscular rigidity results in an improper alignment, and poor infant feeding.
- *The infant's head and body are at the level of the breast.* If the infant's head and body are sagging, or the infant is "reaching" for the breast, repositioning is required. (In **Figure 89**, an older infant's body is sagging; in newborns, it is more often the head that is sagging.)
- *The infant's head must squarely face the breast, nose-to-nipple* (**Figure 114**). The infant's nose should be opposite the nipple in the "sniff" position (**Figure 88**), which encourages the infant to lead with the chin. The nipple is tilted upwards *only* until the infant latches. Compare this to **Figure 133,** in which the infant does not start out in the "sniff" position, and his mother experiences nipple trauma. (See Chapter 8 for additional discussion.) Interestingly, when the infant detaches after a successful feeding, this "sniff" position once again occurs (**Figure 130**). If the infant's head is turned laterally, hyperextended, or hyperflexed, he is not squarely facing the breast. Ideally, the infant should be "tummy-to-mummy," and not over-rotated in either direction. If the infant does not squarely face the breast, nipple trauma, as seen in the "creasing" of the nipple (**Figure 113**) is likely to result.
- *The infant's body should be aligned from the shoulder to the iliac crest.* Without such "tip-to-toe" alignment, poor compression of the breast and obstruction of swallowing are likely. Sometimes, the infant's alignment can be fixed if the mother simply hugs the infant's shoulders in closer (**Figure 115**), or draws his buttocks in closer to her.

As you view the photos in this Chapter of *The Breastfeeding Atlas*, you will likely notice that all or nearly all of the alignment problems stem from one or more one of these four conditions.

Areolar Grasp

A good areolar grasp occurs when the infant attaches to the areola, not just the nipple. Simply stated, the infant should *breast*feed, not *nipple*-feed. A good areolar grasp is critical for good milk transfer, and maternal comfort, and it can be identified in several ways:

- *The infant's mouth opens widely.* Wilson-Clay and Hoover specify that a wide mouth should be open at a 150° angle (**Figure 129**). Pursed lips are a strong indicator that the mouth was not open wide enough. Without a wide gape, a likely consequence is nipple trauma (e.g., a "pinched" nipple, as in **Figure 127**). Sometimes, it's difficult to get an infant with a depressed feeding affect to achieve a wide open mouth, and therefore, a shallow latch results (**Figure 124**).
- *Lips are flanged outward* (**Figure 129**). Lips that are pursed or "retracted" (**Figure 125**, **Figure 126**) will result in poor milk transfer and damage the mother's nipple tissue.
- *A complete seal is formed around the areola with strong negative pressure* (**Figure 129**). If the seal is incomplete, the infant can be pulled away from the breast easily, and/or milk will dribble out.
- *Approximately 1.5 inches of areolar tissue is centered in the infant's mouth.* Don't bust out your ruler; this is an estimate, and it is highly dependent on the size of the mother's areola.
- *The tongue is troughed and extends over the lower alveolar ridge.*
- *The chin indents the breast.* In **Figure 112**, you can imagine that when the infant latches, the chin will indent the breast. Compare this to **Figure 123**, in which the infant has already latched but the chin does not indent the breast; in this case, a "chewing" motion is likely to result in poor intake, as well as trauma to the nipple. The importance of the chin to breastfeeding was identified after the Shrago & Bocar's model was published. The newborn should attach by leading with his chin (**Figure 112** and **Figure 116**) and then making contact with the mother's breast; this helps him to gape widely, grasp the nipple, and take in adequate areolar tissue.[5] I call this a *chin-first latch*, both because it conveys the anatomical relationship between the infant's chin and the mother's breast and because the research supports the importance of the chin in proper latch.

Areolar Compression

It's hard to see movement in still photos, but when caring for breastfeeding dyads, we should observe for the infant's mandible to be moving in a rhythmic motion and the tongue to be moving in a wave-like motion. Shrago and Bocar's third criteria—looking for cheeks that are full and rounded—can sometimes be seen in a still photo. (**Figure 119** somewhat demonstrates this.) The converse observation might be more helpful. When cheeks are *not* full and rounded, they look dimpled or indrawn.

Audible Swallowing

Audible swallowing is a sign of effective breastfeeding that you can hear when observing breastfeeding mothers and their infants. However, it is not something you can see. You won't find it in the pages of *The Breastfeeding Atlas*, although you can see it in videos such as those from Stanford University's Department of Medicine. [https://med.stanford.edu/newborns/professional-education/breastfeeding.html]

Specific Positions and Holds

Getting the "right" position for milk transfer is critical for newborns and very young infants. By comparison, older infants seem to be able to breastfeed well in almost any position (**Figure 111**)! As long as milk is being transferred and the mother is comfortable, there is no need to suggest a specific position or critique the finer points. For positioning and latch, your guide should be: "If it ain't broke, don't fix it."

Nevertheless, you'll want to be well-versed in several breastfeeding positions. It's also critical to watch and help mothers, especially primiparae, because lack of good positioning and latch-on has been related to morbidity.[6]

For each of the following positions—or often called holds—we'll look at the circumstances under which it is most likely to be beneficial, reasons for/against using it, and pitfalls to avoid.

Laid Back Position

Although many professionals sometimes have used the words "biological nurturing" and "laid back breastfeeding" interchangeably, Suzanne Colson, PhD clearly distinguishes between them.[7] According to her, *laid back* is a position, whereas *biological nurturing* is a concept with wider implications. In the laid back position, she explains that the mother's head is raised about 20° (**Figure 85**).

Laid back breastfeeding offers the newborn the opportunity to latch on from 360 different angles. It enables him to do head "bobbing," as Colson calls it, which leads to finding the best spot for him. Anyone who has ever seen a newborn struggling to latch may have noticed that putting him in this laid back position can be a game-changer.

For centuries, most breastfeeding images have shown infants in other positions. However, the infants always appear to be well past the first month of life. It may be, as Colson suggests, that newborns are particularly well-suited for this position.

The laid back position is helpful if the mother has an oversupply and/or a forceful milk ejection reflex. (Those situations frequently—but not always—co-exist.) The laid back position is also useful for an infant with micrognathia. (See Chapter 3.) It supports skin-to-skin contact, because the infant's back can be covered with a blanket. And, it is helpful for any mother who simply wants to sprawl out and relax during the feeding.

Cradle Position

The *cradle position* (**Figure 93**) was long a traditional go-to position for all breastfed infants. Mothers who had seen it used by bottle-feeding couplets knew what it looked like, and they assumed it was how an infant fed. However, for a newborn—an infant who is less than 28 days old—it may offer more disadvantages than advantages.

After decades of work caring for breastfeeding mothers and their infants, I am not convinced that the cradle hold is beneficial for newborns. **Figure 86** shows several pitfalls; skin-to-skin contact is possible but awkward, and blankets that are used tend to get in the way. The mother often finds that the infant does not fit well in the crook of her arm, and attempts to make it work result in her "chasing" the infant with her breast. Fortunately, corrective action can help this situation. **Figure 87** shows that the blankets have been removed, and the infant's head is now on the mother's forearm, allowing him to squarely face the breast. The mother's hand is free to support the weight of her breast.

Newborns or small infants often don't fit snugly in the crook of the mother's arm (antecubital fossa). Sometimes, it's helpful for the mother to use a modified cradle position (**Figure 107**) that gives her additional hands-on control of the infant's body. On the other hand, a larger infant may do well with a modified cradle hold in which the mother is supporting the infant's buttocks (**Figure 108**). A variation of the cradle hold is when the infant's head is on the mother's forearm, rather than in the crook of the mother's elbow (**Figure 92**). Because the infant has a greater ability to flex his neck, he can often achieve a much better latch.

Larger infants may have different issues with support. If there is inadequate postural support, larger infants can experience arm stress (**Figure 89**) because the mother's arm is not supporting him, rather than having both arms positioned at the midline (**Figure 91**).

An infant with a birth injury, such as torticollis, may struggle to get comfortable. The mother's arm does not adequately support the infant for good alignment.

Figure 90 shows a deliberate "trapping" of the arm. By looking very carefully at **Figure 90**, you can see that this infant has had abdominal surgery. Using a slightly rotated cradle position to keep pressure off the incision line, the mother had deliberately trapped the lower arm across the infant's body so that the infant does not grab the feeding tube.

Avoid this pitfall: In situations where support is critical, the cradle position can create problems. If a newborn is very small and/or hypotonic, I do not offer the cradle position as an option. These infants simply don't do well in the cradle position, and the mother often becomes very discouraged because the infant finds it difficult or impossible to get a good grasp of the nipple/areolar complex.

Football Position (and variations)

The *football position* is also called the *clutch hold* or position (**Figure 95**). Again, the mother is supporting the infant's head, shoulders, and back, but the infant's feet are aimed towards the bed or chair.

The football hold can be especially helpful after cesarean surgery, because it directs the infant's body away from the area of the incision. The mother has less reason to worry whether her infant might kick her incision. Certainly, it provides better visualization for the latch-on process.

The football hold is often helpful for mothers with large breasts. However, experiences vary for mothers who are morbidly obese; some find it helpful, while others do not. The football hold allows the mother to use a free hand to make a breast "sandwich" (**Figure 117**), which may be a critical step for a mother with large breasts. It also allows her to compress her breast (**Figure 43**) while the infant is suckling, which can be helpful if the infant is weak or hypotonic.

Avoid this pitfall: Sometimes, a vigorously kicking infant may reflexively push his feet against the bed or chair, and push away from the mother. To minimize or prevent this, place a pillow or two behind the mother, vertically rather than horizontally—this creates more space between the infant and the chair. Also, having the infant's buttocks, rather than his feet, against the bed or chair is a variation of the football hold that may help (**Figure 96**).

Cross-Cradle Position

The *cross-cradle position* (often called the *"transitional" hold*, **Figure 104**) is where the mother uses a hand to support the infant's head, neck, and shoulders. In this position, the mother uses the hand on the opposite side of the body from the breast upon which the infant is feeding; for example, the mother uses her right hand to support the infant breastfeeding from the left side, and her left hand to support the infant when he is feeding from the right side.

The cross-cradle position has several advantages over other holds. It works well for infants who are hypotonic or small. It also works well for any mother who feels a little unsure of herself and wants to have a firmer grip on the infant. A big advantage is that the mother can move the infant from one side using the cross-cradle to the other side using the football hold.

Mothers who have exceptionally large breasts often do well with a modification of the cross-cradle hold. The mother may be seated, placing her breast on a table (**Figure 105**) while she supports the infant's head, neck and shoulders. (In the hospital, the over-the-bed table works well for this.) Or, if she has back pain or a sore bottom, she may prefer to remain standing (**Figure 106**) when using this position.

Avoid this pitfall: Because the mother's hand is behind the infant's neck, she may inadvertently push on the infant's head and hyperflex his neck (**Figure 97**), which can cause poor milk transfer, as well as problems with the infant's breathing and swallowing.

Side-lying Position

In the *side-lying position* (**Figure 99**), the mother rests on her side and has a pillow between her knees both for comfort and to prevent her from rolling forward. She offers her infant the breast that is closest to the mattress.

The side-lying position is great for nighttime feeding. It can also be helpful for a mother who has had a cesarean delivery; putting a rolled-up towel beneath a sagging abdomen if necessary (**Figure 101**) can aid in comfort. Similarly, a side-lying position is more comfortable for a mother with a sore episiotomy or painful hemorrhoids.

Infants who are hypertonic, or those who have some type of birth trauma—including torticollis—may do better with a side-lying position. If the infant seems to be squirming, a side-lying position gives some space, allowing him to feel less confined and better relaxed. A side-lying position can also be beneficial if the infant tends to struggle with the fast flow of the mother's milk, when sitting up. In a side-lying position, the flow is slower because the force of gravity is redirected.

Some women with large breasts may find that the side-lying position works better than the football positions. Mothers with especially small breasts may find it doesn't work for them. However, individual experiences may vary, and trial-and-error is advised.

Avoid this pitfall: It's important for the mother and infant to maintain a chest-to-chest or tummy-to-mummy position. In an over-rotated position, the infant's buttocks are rolled towards the mother (**Figure 100**). If the mother falls asleep during breastfeeding, this could increase the infant's risk for suffocation. An infant who is not over-rotated is more likely to become *supine* ("back to sleep"). (Over-rotation and burying of the face can also occur in other positions, as shown in **Figure 94**).

Straddle Hold

The *straddle hold* (**Figure 103**) is my go-to position for infants who are hypotonic, or those who have orofacial structural defects. An occupational therapist who attended my course explained why: *Proximal* (nearby) stability helps to achieve *distal* (more distant) mobility.

Wrap the legs of an older infant around the mother's waist to provide excellent stability for his body. This position is possible but unlikely for newborns, especially preterm or very small infants.

When I teach in a live course, people frequently ask what the difference is between the straddle hold and the football hold. It's a bit difficult to describe. Here are some key differences:

- *The Breastfeeding Atlas* refers to this as the "seated straddle position." That's a good descriptor, because the infant is in somewhat of a sitting position. Whereas the weight of the infant in a football position is largely supported by the mother's arm, the infant in a true straddle hold is more akin to "sitting." (Of course, a young infant does not yet have enough development of his muscles to support himself).
- In the straddle hold, the infant's feet are facing the mother; in the football hold, the infant's feet are behind the mother.
- In the straddle hold, the infant's hips and knees have maximal flexion; in the football hold, less flexion of the hips and knees is likely.
- In the straddle hold, the infant is more perpendicular to the mother's body; in the football hold, he is more at an angle.

The straddle position isn't a good choice if the newborn is especially small, and/or if the mother is obese. Somehow, the "fit" just doesn't seem right.

While there is no one "right" position, getting the right alignment for any position—at least for a newborn—is critical. Complete Learning Exercises 6-3 and 6-4 to better recall and reinforce your knowledge of positioning.

Signs of Hunger and Satiety

Any breastfeeding position is only the "right" one if it works for the mother and infant; that is, if the mother and infant can transfer milk effectively and comfortable. Picking up on Chapter 2, we look for signs of when to breastfeed, and when the infant has fed enough.

Hunger

When infants show hunger signs, they should be offered the breast. However, it's not enough to look only for hunger signs. We also need to observe signs that the infant is transferring milk. An infant who never opens his eyes during the feeding is almost surely transferring little or no milk to himself. This should not be confused with an infant who closes his eyes *after* a good feeding. Closed eyes after feeding (**Figure 119**) are a good indicator that the infant has had a good feeding; note too that this infant is beginning to relax his fist.

Satiety

An infant who has a clenched fist (**Figure 118**) at the beginning of the feeding is hungry. The fist begins to relax after the infant has taken some milk (**Figure 119**). In **Figure 120**, his fist is even more relaxed; he is mostly satisfied, but should be allowed to take his mouth off the breast when he is done feeding.

Figure 121 illustrates an infant who has spontaneously released the breast; his entire body is relaxed, and his open hand is resting on the mother's breast. This infant has enjoyed a good feeding with optimal positioning and latch, as evidenced by his mother's rounded (rather than distorted) nipple. Compare this to **Figure 127**, which is the result of a poor latch.

Infants often spontaneously take themselves off the breast when they are satiated.

Looking Back, Looking Forward

In this chapter, we've talked about how reflexes and movements are related to positioning and latch. And, we've talked about several different positions—when to use or not use them, and some pitfalls to avoid when using them.

Evidence in the education field shows that writing your own summary helps your retention. The Summarize What You've Learned exercise helps you to do this, so take just a few minutes to complete that exercise.

By now, if you have viewed the photos carefully, and if you've completed the written exercises, you should feel confident that you can determine how and when to help a breastfeeding couplet to adjust positioning and latch to achieve optimal milk transfer.

Recalling, Reinforcing, and Expanding Your Learning

Have you ever felt frustrated that you "learned" something, but later, can't recall it? That may be because you didn't reinforce the material you learned. And, perhaps what you originally learned isn't enough to get you through the next few decades of practice; sometimes you need to expand your learning. The exercises in this section are designed to help you recall, reinforce, and expand your learning.

What was your main motivation for reading this chapter?

- ❍ To study for the IBLCE exam, as a first-time candidate
- ❍ To review for the IBLCE exam, as a re-certificant
- ❍ To improve my clinical skills and clinical management

How soon do you think can use the information presented in this chapter?

- ❍ Immediately; within the next few days or so
- ❍ Soon; within the next month or so
- ❍ Later; sometime before I retire

Pro Tip! If you are preparing for the IBLCE exam, it would be wise to pace your studying. Set a target date for when you plan to complete the exercises, and check off them off as you go along.

Done!	Target Date	Learning Exercise
❑	____________	Learning Exercise 6-1. Illustrating directional terms of movement and direction.
❑	____________	Learning Exercise 6-2. Matching anatomical terms of movement and direction.
❑	____________	Learning Exercise 6-3. Reasons to use or avoid positions; possible pitfalls.
❑	____________	Learning Exercise 6-4. Matching specific positions and holds to their descriptions.
❑	____________	Explore What You've Learned in a Journal
❑	____________	Summarize What You've Learned
❑	____________	Quick Quiz

Master Your Vocabulary

Learning Exercise 6-1. Matching anatomical terms of movement to their meaning.

Instructions: Write the letter of the correct match next to each item. Answers are in the Appendix.

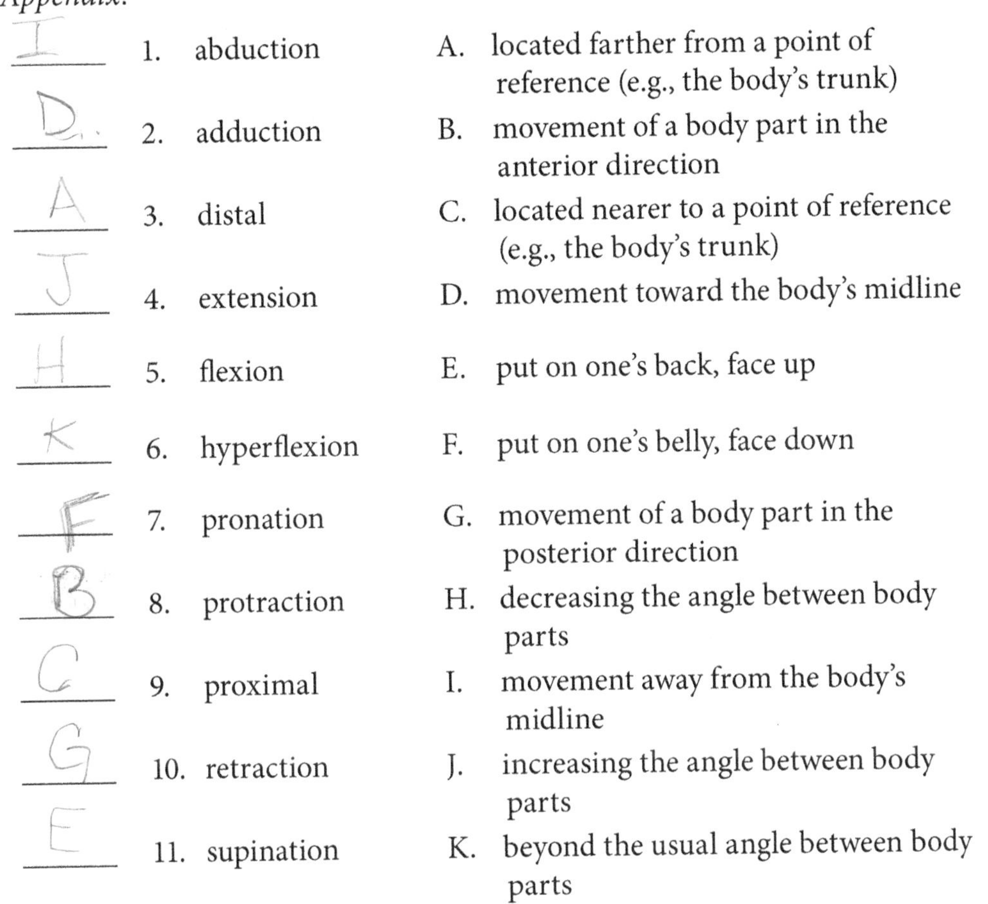

I 1. abduction	A. located farther from a point of reference (e.g., the body's trunk)
D 2. adduction	B. movement of a body part in the anterior direction
A 3. distal	C. located nearer to a point of reference (e.g., the body's trunk)
J 4. extension	D. movement toward the body's midline
H 5. flexion	E. put on one's back, face up
K 6. hyperflexion	F. put on one's belly, face down
F 7. pronation	G. movement of a body part in the posterior direction
B 8. protraction	H. decreasing the angle between body parts
C 9. proximal	I. movement away from the body's midline
G 10. retraction	J. increasing the angle between body parts
E 11. supination	K. beyond the usual angle between body parts

Learning Exercise 6-2. Illustrating anatomical terms of movement.

Instructions: Using stick figures, draw your understanding of many or several of the vocabulary words pertaining to the body's movements. Answers are in the Appendix.

abduction	pronation
adduction	protraction
distal	proximal
extension	retraction
flexion	supination
hyperflexion	hyperextension

Conquer Clinical Concepts

Learning Exercise 6-3. Reasons to use or avoid positions and common pitfalls.

Instructions: Use this workbook and The Breastfeeding Atlas *to summarize the reasons to use or to avoid a particular position, and the common pitfalls. Answers are in the Appendix.*

	Best reasons to use, and/or advantages	Least likely reasons to use	Pitfalls to avoid	Comments and Considerations
Cradle hold	older infant	newborn small infant hypotonic	optimal latch may not occur in infants who needs lots of support	
Cross-cradle (transitional) hold	hypotonic small moms unsure of selves	situation where stress on wrist	mother may push head & hyper flex neck	
Football hold (clutch hold)	C-section large breasts obese		kicking infant may kick off bed/chair	
Side-lying hold	nighttime C-section sore perineum	small breasts	↑ risk suffocation may roll off skin to skin	
Straddle hold	hypotonic orofacial defects	NB small & mom obese	discomfort awkwardness	

Learning Exercise 6-4. Matching specific positions and holds to their descriptions.

Instructions: Write the letter of the correct match next to each item. Answers are in the Appendix.

E	1. chin-first latch	A.	mother is lying down with infant alongside of her
I	2. clutch hold	B.	similar to football, but with infant more "seated"
F	3. cradle hold	C.	infant is held in one arm, while suckling the opposite-side breast
C	4. cross-cradle hold	D.	infant is face down against the mother's body
G	5. football hold	E.	attaches to breast by leading with the chin
D	6. laid-back position	F.	infant is held in one arm, while suckling the same-side breast
A	7. side-lying hold	G.	infant's head is held primarily with the mother's hand
B	8. straddle hold	H.	same as cross-cradle hold
H	9. transitional hold	I.	same as football hold

Exploring What You've Learned in a Journal

Multiple studies have shown the benefits of using a learning journal. Among them are greater assimilation and integration of new information, better long-term retention of course concepts, increasing test and exam grades, and a means by which to have continuous feedback about one's own learning.

- Name at least three things you learned from this chapter.

- List at least three things you still need to learn, or more fully master, in this chapter. Briefly describe how this information fits (or doesn't fit) with what you've seen in clinical practice, what you learned in basic or college courses, or what you've observed in your own experience breastfeeding. (In some cases, you might want to include how the information fits or doesn't fit with what "experts" say, what the media says, or whatever.)

- Describe how you will use any or all of this information. How might it be related to problems and potential solutions that occur in real life or in clinical situations?

- If you wish, include how you felt about learning this information. Were you bored? Overwhelmed? Enlightened? Worried? Something else?

Summarize What You've Learned

The goal of this chapter was for you to be able determine how and when to help a breastfeeding couplet to adjust positioning and latch to achieve optimal milk transfer.

Instructions: Write your own summary of what you just learned in this chapter.

- What terms of movement (related to infant's position at the breast) were new to you?

- How can neuromuscular reflexes and movement positively impact milk transfer?

- How can neuromuscular reflexes and movement negatively affect milk transfer?

- Which breastfeeding positions were new to you? What would be the likely reasons for you to use or avoid them for infants/children of various ages?

- List some indicators of effective latch-on that you would be able to see in a photo.

Self Assessment

People often dive into a test before they have thoughtfully reflected on how well they have prepared for it. Instead, it would be helpful if they would take a few moments to give their alter-ego (their "other self") a chance to reflect on how confident they feel about mastering the stated objectives.

Instructions: Take a moment to review the chapter objectives (below). Then rate yourself. How confident are you that you have achieved each objective below?

Objective	Highly Confident	Somewhat Confident	Somewhat Unsure	Completely Unsure
Use the correct terms of movement to describe the infant's position at the breast.	❍	❍	❍	❍
Describe how neuromuscular reflexes and movement can positively or negatively impact milk transfer.	❍	❍	❍	❍
Recognize commonly-based breastfeeding positions and the likely reasons to use or avoid them for infants/children of various ages.	❍	❍	❍	❍
Distinguish between indicators of effective and ineffective latch-on, and make suggestions for improvement.	❍	❍	❍	❍

On the next page, you will some simple recall questions pertaining to this chapter. These are *not* the application-type questions you will find in the IBLCE exam. However, you cannot *apply* information unless you can fully *recall* that information! You should do these without looking up the answers.

When you finish with the quiz, look up the answers in the Appendix. Then, score your answers, using the Appendix. Finally, you should analyze the results of your quiz. It's not enough to just know what you got right or wrong; you must look at why you got the answers right.

Quick Quiz Chapter 6

Instructions: *Circle the correct response. For a better understanding of how well you are mastering the material, try answering without looking it up. If you are really stuck, questions come from this workbook and from* The Breastfeeding Atlas *so go back and review the appropriate material. Answers are in the appendix.*

1. The cross-cradle hold would should be your FIRST suggestion for an infant in which situation?

   A. fast flow of mother's milk

   B. micrognathia

   C. small or hypotonic infant

2. Hyperflexion of the head is MOST likely to occur when the mother is using which position?

   A. cradle

   B. cross-cradle

   C. side-lying

   D. straddle

3. The side-lying position might be the FIRST choice for a mother who has:

   A. hemorrhoids

   B. short arms

   C. small breasts

   D. small hands

4. An infant was born with torticollis. Which position would you suggest FIRST?

   A. cradle

   B. cross-cradle

   C. football

   D. side-lying

5. If the infant is "over-rotated", a possible risk is:

   A. aspiration

   B. overfeeding

   C. suffocation

   D. underfeeding

Analyze Your Own Quiz

- What percentage of the questions did you answer correctly?

- If you got 100% of them right, to what do you attribute your success?

- If you did not get all the questions right, can you identify as your learning gap? (Example: Didn't know the information, knew the information but could not remember, knew some information but confused it with similar information, other.)

- Would you have been able to answer the questions as well if you had not read this chapter?

- What do you need to do next? (If you got them all right, what you need to do next is celebrate! Even a high-five with your child, a YESSS and a fist-pump in the air, or anything else is good! A small acknowledgement of your success is better than no acknowledgement!))

Additional Resources

1. Colson SD, Meek JH, Hawdon JM. Optimal positions for the release of primitive neonatal breastfeeding. *Early Hum Dev.* 2008;84(7):441-449.

2. Shrago L, Bocar D. The infant's contribution to breastfeeding. *J Obstet Gynecol Neonatal Nurs.* 1990;19(3):209-215.

3. Biancuzzo M. *Breastfeeding the Newborn: Clinical Strategies for Nurses.* St. Louis: Mosby; 2003.

4. West JF, Redstone F. Alignment during feeding and swallowing: does it matter? A review. *Percept Mot Skills.* 2004;98(1):349-358.

5. Widstrom AM, Thingstrom-Paulsson J. The position of the tongue during rooting reflexes elicited in newborn infants before the first suckle. *Acta Paediatr.* 1993;82(3):281-283.

6. Joshi H, Magon P, Raina S. Effect of mother-infant pair's latch-on position on child's health: A lesson for nursing care. *Journal of family medicine and primary care.* 2016;5(2):309-313.

7. Colson S. How Biological Nurturing is Key to Relaxed, Joyful Nursing for Mother and Newborn [Internet radio on iTunes]. *Born to be Breastfed* Phoenix AZ: VoiceAmerica Health & Wellness Channel; January 16, 2017 [cited July 17, 2017]. Podcast: 43 minutes. Available from: ***http://borntobebreastfed.com/?page_id=1192***

Chapter 7

Nipple Inversion, Eversion, & Elasticity

Nipple tissue that is well-everted and easily elongated when suckled is ideal for breastfeeding. However, many women have variations of their nipple tissue. Those with flat, short, or inverted nipples can initiate and continue breastfeeding—and those with long nipples can, too! (We'll discuss that situation in Chapter 10.)

Infants are highly dependent on the stimulation of their palate by the mother's nipple. If they can't sense a nipple on their palate, a host of problems can ensue. Nipples that are very short, flat, or inelastic can make it difficult or impossible for the infant to receive that stimulation. Yet, there are degrees of nipple length, and degrees of tissue elasticity. It takes good clinical management skills to recognize subtle differences.

I promise that when you finish this chapter, you'll be able to confidently recognize the indicators of inelastic or non-everted nipples and their breastfeeding management implications. Be sure to pay close attention to the photos on page 174 of *The Breastfeeding Atlas* and complete the written activities in this workbook, which are designed to help you master this material!

Objectives

Given a clinical photo, you will be able to:

- Discuss how so-called "nipple confusion" may be related to maternal nipple inelasticity.
- Recognize visual indicators and possible consequences of non-everted nipples.
- Differentiate between truly inverted nipples and dimpled inverted nipples.
- Describe at least four clinical management strategies that may be helpful for infants whose mothers have short, flat, truly inverted, dimpled, or inelastic nipples.
- Distinguish between good latching and poor latching by infants using nipple shields.

Key terms

- adhesions
- breast shells
- collagen
- dimpled nipples
- elastin
- everted nipples
- flat nipples
- inverted nipples
- nipple everters
- nipple shields
- protrusion
- sandwich technique
- teacup hold

Elasticity

Body tissue that is more elastic (e.g., more able to stretch and return to its normal state) contains more *elastin*, a protein found in connective tissue. To my knowledge, there are no studies that have looked at the amount of elastin in the nipple tissue. My clinical observations have shown that some mothers have nipple tissue that is more elastic, while others have tissue that is less elastic.

In *The Breastfeeding Atlas,* Wilson-Clay and Hoover present a highly cogent argument that so-called "nipple confusion" may not have to do with the infant being "confused," but rather with the amount of elasticity of the mother's nipples (Page 47). I am inclined to agree. I have seen hundreds of newborns who successfully switch between breast and bottle nipples, but I have also seen hundreds who seemingly cannot. I think it's plausible that more elastic nipple tissue may elongate and stimulate the infant's palate better, causing the sensations between breast and bottle to be more similar.

Often, nipples have more rigidity and structure. Rigidity and structure are usually associated with *collagen*, another protein in connective tissue. It's possible that some women have more collagen in their nipple tissue, but there has been no research in this area.

Nipple elasticity is related to—but different from—nipple *inversion.*

Nipple Inversion and Eversion

As we just saw, elasticity—or lack thereof—is a notable characteristic of human nipples. But nipple eversion or inversion is also a key characteristic of human nipples.

Everted Nipples

An *everted* nipple (**Figure 130**) is one that *protrudes* outward (is above the surface of the areolar skin) whether it is at rest or slightly compressed, even if slightly. The anatomical term, *protrusion* relates to facing outward above the surface of the skin; in this case, that means how the nipple protrudes from the areola.

Inverted Nipples

By comparison, a truly *inverted nipple* is one that is below the surface of the areolar skin, either when it is at rest (**Figure 134**) or when it is stimulated or compressed (**Figure 135**).

You can find, in the medical literature about plastic and reconstructive surgery, definitions for the variations of normal nipple tissue. However, such definitions have little or no clinical relevance for breastfeeding management. Many of the terms used to describe nipples and breasts have changed in use and meaning over the years. In this chapter, I hope to clarify not only what I mean by terms, but how the terms appear to apply to *The Breastfeeding Atlas,* and to clinical care, too.

How Can You Tell?

Many new IBCLCs tell me they feel incapable of distinguishing between inverted and everted nipples. It isn't always easy! The key is looking at how the nipple changes when it is in two situations: (1) whether the nipple is above, below, or at the level of the skin when it is at rest, (2) whether the nipple is above, below, or at the level of the skin when it is compressed or stimulated.

What Happened, and What Will Happen?

An inverted nipple is a condition that occurs during fetal development.[1] The mammary pit of the woman with an inverted nipple did not elevate when she was a fetus; instead, the fibers of the tissue became tied.[1] The tying of these fibers is often referred to as *adhesions*— fibrous bands or structures by which parts abnormally adhere.

Just because a nipple "always" has been inverted doesn't mean it always will be. For some women, breastfeeding can be a means by which the nipple's inversion is reversed; these fibers are released after their infants engage in robust suckling.

For some women, breastfeeding for a few days or a few weeks can help to improve inverted nipples, causing them to be drawn out more easily. Some women find that their nipples don't seem as inverted with a subsequent breastfeeding experience as they did with their first. *The Breastfeeding Atlas* shows a woman who was unable to breastfeed her first two infants, but could breastfeed her third (**Figures 134, 135, 136**). It's possible this could be due to an increase in elastin, at least in some cases. (Even everted nipples have more or less elasticity, as you will see in Chapter 10.)

Severity

Certainly, **Figures 134** and **135** are extreme cases of nipple inversion. Some cases are not nearly as extreme, and can go unnoticed.

Sometimes, we see a nipple that looks everted at rest, and we neglect to check that it stays everted when it is compressed. Inspection or visualization of the nipple can be deceiving; sometimes a nipple that seemingly is everted (**Figure 210**) becomes inverted when it is compressed (**Figure 211**). This is noteworthy, because compression of the nipple/areola complex is key to breastfeeding!

Even when inversion seems less severe, the question remains: Will the nipple stimulate the infant's palate when he starts to suckle? In many cases, it will not.

Consequences of Inverted Nipples

An inverted nipple presents all sorts of problems for the breastfeeding infant. If you watch carefully, you'll see that the infant perceives this problem, and how he reacts.

If the nipple is not everted, the nipple/areola complex is difficult to grasp. Once the infant can draw it into his mouth, it does not stimulate the palate, as is necessary for successful suckling and milk transfer.

In *The Breastfeeding Atlas,* Wilson-Clay and Hoover identify several behaviors that are likely indicators of the infant who is attempting to suckle an inverted nipple. At the risk of seeming redundant, I will summarize those behaviors below, because they are so characteristic, and so important to the overall management of breastfeeding:

- shaking head side to side
- bumping against the breast
- batting with fists
- screaming
- tuning out and falling asleep
- acting bewildered
- acting as if, in the mother's words, "he doesn't like [her]"

Although many nipples are labeled as "inverted," truly inverted nipples are very uncommon. When people refer to "inverted" nipples, it's important to clarify if they are talking about truly inverted nipples, or if they are referring to flat or short, or, possibly, dimpled-inverted nipples, because their clinical management and resolution might be very different.

Dimpled Inverted Nipples

Dimpled nipples (also called *folded nipples*) are a less severe form of inverted nipples. Whereas the truly inverted nipple has tissue that is completely below the surface of the areola, the dimpled nipple has only a "fold" of tissue that is below the surface. Hence, it is sometimes called a "folded" nipple.

To tell the difference between a dimpled nipple and a truly inverted nipple, look at the position of the nipple in relation to the surface of the skin. A truly inverted nipple will be entirely below the surface of the skin (**Figure 134**). A dimpled nipple will be above the surface of the skin (**Figure 138**), but about half of the nipple tissue will be "folded" towards the other half. Here's the tricky part, though. Sometimes, a very short dimpled nipple can be mistaken for a truly inverted nipple. Conversely, a long nipple that is folded may go entirely unnoticed if the fold is small and the nipple narrow.

The mother in **Figure 137** has been pumping her milk. Note that immediately after pumping, the "fold" is not very apparent, but it's clear that the pump has exerted pressure high enough to cause redness and trauma to the nipple. In the next photo (**Figure 138**), taken two minutes later, the characteristic crease or fold can be observed easily, and the redness—which at first glance seems to be reduced—is actually hidden in the fold. Not surprisingly, the mother reports pain. Assume, for a moment, that the mother had been suckling the infant, and the infant exerted as much negative pressure as the pump (which is entirely possible). The appearance may be a bit different, but it's likely you would still see similar nipple trauma.

Sometimes, dimpled nipples can be "pulled out" using the same technique demonstrated by the woman with the truly inverted nipple (**Figure 136**). However, even when dimpled nipples are "pulled out" prior to the feeding, they do not stay everted afterwards.

Flat or Short Nipples

A short or *flat nipple* (**Figure 131**) is at the surface of the skin, or just barely above it. Such nipples can frequently be grasped by full-term, healthy infants who suckle vigorously and seem to draw the nipple out. The nipple stimulates their hard palate, and the feedings go well. (Remember, though, that infants who are hypotonic, premature, or otherwise compromised are unlikely to suckle vigorously, and their feedings on flat or short nipples may not go well.)

Clinical Management of Non-Everted or Non-Elastic Nipples

The first studies of infant suckling at breast were done by Ardran and colleagues in the 1950s.[2] In the 1980s, noted lactation physiologist Michael Woolridge reported that the nipple elongates to 2-3 times its resting length during suckling.[3] More recently, Elad and colleagues[4] made several observations about how the nipple moves in the mouth. Interestingly, they showed that the anterior portion of the infant's tongue moves "as a rigid body with the cycling motion of the mandible" whereas the posterior portion moves in a wave-like motion. And, they showed that the range of motion of the anterior portion of the tongue was approximately 3.7 mm.

Such studies support what we see in clinical care: Breastfeeding can be successful for mothers with many different kinds of nipples—even short or inverted ones, although it might take a bit more work to make it happen, at least initially.

Whether nipples are flat, short, inverted, dimpled-inverted, or everted, the aim of clinical management is the same: to get the nipple everted well enough and have it elastic enough so that it stimulates the infant's hard palate and causes good milk transfer.

Just as experts use different terminology to describe non-everted or non-elastic nipples, they have different and often conflicting opinions on how to manage them. In truth, it's possible that many or all options for management are effective to some degree on some women. Management strategies include the use of special latching techniques, or commercial equipment.

Special Techniques

There are several techniques that can be used to help mothers with inverted nipples. Often nipples that are very short or flat can be compressed, and the mother can use the *sandwich technique* (**Figure 132**) to help the nipple get into her infant's mouth. This is especially important for an infant with a very small mouth. It's called "sandwich" because, just as adults might try to maneuver a thick sandwich into a shape that they can get their mouth around, this same idea is done to help the infant get his mouth around a nipple/areola complex. (Note the large areola in that photo, too.)

Alternatively, a *teacup hold* (**Figure 133**) can be used. In this hold, the mother uses only her thumb and index finger, as if holding the handle of a teacup. The teacup hold is maintained until the infant is latched and suckling in a sustained manner. Like the sandwich hold, the aim of the teacup hold is to make the nipple/areola into a shape that the infant can grasp. A word of caution here: While the mother in **Figure 133** seems to have done well with the teacup hold, it appears to me that her nipple is not severely inverted, nor severely inelastic. Compare her to the mother in **Figure 134** and **135**, for whom I predict the teacup hold would not be sufficient.

Nipple Shields

Nipple shields (**Figure 141**) are soft devices that are worn during the feeding. Luckily, nipple shields have come a long way since the thick material and antique design of yesteryear (**Figure 140**). You're probably thinking that one was made in the Victorian era. No, Wilson-Clay and Hoover point out this shield was purchased in London at a pharmacy (chemist's shop) in 2002!

Nipple shields have been widely debated, in terms of their effectiveness, effect on milk transfer, and possible health risks. Some criticism is warranted. Certainly, the older shields made of thick latex seemed to be associated with decreased milk transfer. However, the thin silicone nipple shields today do not seem to alter infant sucking patterns,[5] and wearing them does not seem to decrease prolactin levels[6], as researchers worried would happen due to decreased direct stimulation of the nipple.

Many manufacturers make nipple shields of various sizes; those in **Figure 141** are 16 mm, 20 mm, and 24 mm in diameter. Confusion abounds about which size to use, and whether the shield should be fitted to the mother's breast anatomy or her infant's mouth.

Powers and Tapia[7] prefer to fit the nipple shield to the mother's nipple; they argue that even a small, preterm infant can open his mouth wide enough to accommodate a 24 mm shield. The authors of *The Breastfeeding Atlas* prefer to fit the nipple shield to the infant's mouth, and they recommend choosing "the shortest available teat with the smallest base diameter" (Page 51). They acknowledge that even if the infant can open wide and initially "accommodate" the large diameter shield, it will be very difficult for him to sustain a seal.

Many mothers and lactation professionals find that some experimentation may be required to find the right fit. In my experience, sometimes the shield you assume to be too small for the mother's nipple might work. By soaking the shield in warm water, you may find that the shield becomes very malleable, enabling it to fit fine on the mother's nipple while being easier for the infant to grasp.

Everyone seems to have a favorite way of applying the shields. I favor turning one-third of the shield inside out before placing it over the nipple (**Figure 142**) and, as mentioned above, soaking the shield —not just rinsing it—in warm water for a few minutes prior.

There are several pros and cons to using a shield; that debate is beyond the scope of this publication. Whether the mother uses a shield or not, positioning and latch are key elements in achieving adequate milk transfer. The aim is to get the infant to latch on with a big open-wide mouth (**Figure 143**). But other signs are important, too, including rhythmic suckling and audible swallowing (see chapter 6). Another indicator that breastfeeding with the shield is going well is the presence of milk in the teat (**Figure 144**).

However, if the infant latches onto the shaft of the shield (**Figure 145**), he cannot adequately transfer milk. This seven-day-old infant lost more than 9 percent of his birthweight, and was still losing weight at the time the photo was taken.

Regardless of how it is applied, or the ratio of benefits to risks, let's say the mother does use the shield. The most clinically-relevant question is: Is the infant getting the milk? You'll need to look for the indicators of adequate milk transfer.

Breast Shells

Not to be confused with breast shields, *breast shells* are rigid devices that are worn between feedings. The shells are often dismissed by lactation consultants because of Alexander's[8] study several decades ago, which showed that they had no benefits. That study, which was replete with flaws, seems to imply that they have no use at all.

In my experience, the efficacy of breast shells depends largely on the brand used, the severity of the nipple inversion, the elasticity of the nipple, when the mother began wearing the shells, and the length of time she wears them each day. (Alexander's conclusions did not consider any of those variables.) Sometimes they help the nipple to evert, sometimes they don't.

Complete learning exercise 7-1 and 7-2 to master basic terms and principles of how to use the shells and shields. Then, complete exercise 7-3 to help you determine if an infant is well latched when using a shield.

Other Commercial Devices

Some mothers might find help for their inverted nipples with one of the available commercial devices. *Nipple everters* are a suction-based device that draws out the nipple prior to attempting latch-on. These are fairly simple to use, and are often effective.

Looking Back, Looking Forward

In this chapter, we've talked about nipple elasticity, nipples that have varying degrees of inversion and eversion, their possible consequences. and some techniques and commercial devices that can be helpful.

Evidence in the education field shows that writing your own summary helps your retention. The Summarize What You've Learned exercise helps you to do this, so take just a few minutes to complete that exercise.

By now, if you have viewed the photos carefully, and if you've completed the written exercises, you should feel confident that you can now recognize the indicators of inelastic or non-everted nipples and their breastfeeding management implications.

Recalling, Reinforcing, and Expanding Your Learning

Have you ever felt frustrated that you "learned" something, but later, can't recall it? That may be because you didn't reinforce the material you learned. And, perhaps what you originally learned isn't enough to get you through the next few decades of practice; sometimes you need to expand your learning. The exercises in this section are designed to help you recall, reinforce, and expand your learning.

What was your main motivation for reading this chapter?

- ❍ To study for the IBLCE exam, as a first-time candidate
- ❍ To review for the IBLCE exam, as a re-certificant
- ❍ To improve my clinical skills and clinical management

How soon do you think can use the information presented in this chapter?

- ❍ Immediately; within the next few days or so
- ❍ Soon; within the next month or so
- ❍ Later; sometime before I retire

Pro Tip! If you are preparing for the IBLCE exam, it would be wise to pace your studying. Set a target date for when you plan to complete the exercises, and check off them off as you go along.

Done!	Target Date	Learning Exercise
❑	________________	Learning Exercise 7-1. Vocabulary words for terms related to inversion, eversion, and elasticity
❑	________________	Learning Exercise 7-2. Using shells and shields
❑	________________	Learning Exercise 7-3. Determining if the infant using a shield is well latched
❑	________________	Explore What You've Learned in a Journal
❑	________________	Summarize What You've Learned
❑	________________	Quick Quiz

Master Your Vocabulary

Unless you know what a word means, you cannot fully answer a question about it. There were many, many terms in this chapter; you might not need to know them all, but you never know which ones you'll need to know!

Learning Exercise 7-1. Vocabulary words for terms related to inversion, eversion, and elasticity.

Instructions: Write the letter of the correct match next to each item. Answers are in the appendix.

B	1. adhesions	A. soft device worn during the feeding
J	2. breast shells	B. fibrous bands
L	3. collagen	C. completely below the skin's surface
H	4. dimpled nipple	D. neither above nor below the skin's surface
K	5. elastin	E. device that uses suction to draw out the nipple
I	6. everted nipple	F. tissue or structure that faces outward
D	7. flat nipple	G. maneuvers the nipple/areola into a shape that can be more easily grasped
C	8. inverted nipple	H. some of the nipple skin is folded
E	9. nipple everter	I. protrudes above the skin's surface
A	10. nipple shield	J. rigid devices worn between feedings
F	11. protrusion	K. protein that gives tissue stretchiness
G	12. sandwich technique	L. protein that gives tissue rigidity and structure

Conquering Clinical Concepts

Learning Exercise 7-2. Using shells and shields.

Instructions: Here are three questions. Unscramble the sentences below to get the answers!

1. When would a nipple shell be worn?
   Shell should be worn during preg or after delivery. It can only be worn between feedings
2. What happens if the mother has a non-everted nipple?
   If mom's nipple has little or no elasticity it is unlikely to provide adequate stimulation to infant's palate.
3. If you use a large-size nipple for an infant with a small mouth, what result can you predict?
   Although infants can initially accomodate a large diameter shield it is difficult for them to sustain an adequate seal around it.

1. worn / could / feedings. / shell / only / can / delivery. / after / during / either / or / However, / worn / A / be / be / between / / it / nipple / pregnancy

2. mother's / palate. / unlikely / to / elasticity, / to / little / a / is / infant's / provide / stimulation / has / it / the / adequate / nipple / If / or / no

3. shield, / initially / around / Although / large-diameter / to / seal / can / it / adequate / for / an / them / / infants / is / difficult / sustain / a / "accommodate" / it.

Learning Exercise 7-3. Determining if the infant using a shield is well latched.

Instructions: Use the following questions to help you complete the table below:

- Infant's gape: At what angle of "open" do you expect to see? This is a review and reinforcement of what as mentioned in chapter 6.
- Where will the lips be, in relation to the shield if the infant has a good latch? Where will the lips be if the infant has a poor latch on the shield? (Check out page 52 of *The Breastfeeding Atlas* to help with your answer.)
- Will you see (or hear) rhythmic sucking?
- Will you see milk inside of the shield's "nipple" (i.e., teat)?
- What do you expect to see with weight gain?
- What other indicator or indicators might you look for that are not mentioned here, or in the corresponding chapter of *The Breastfeeding Atlas*?

In the table, write the words or phrases that describe what you would be most likely to observe about when the infant is well-latched, or when he is poorly latched?

	Infant is latched well	Infant is poorly latched
Mouth, gape	big gape wide open mouth	Small gape
Where will the lips be?	on the body of the shield	on shaft of shield
Rhythmic sucking?	Rhythmic sucking audible swallowing	non-rhythmic little or no swallowing
Milk inside the shield's teat?	Yes	NO
Weight Gain	Yes	NO

Summarize What You've Learned

The goal of this chapter is to help you confidently recognize the indicators of inelastic or non-everted nipples and their breastfeeding management implications.

Relatively few studies have been conducted on inelastic and non-everted nipples. However, the aim of this chapter was to help you recognize the indicators of nonelastic or noneverted nipples in patients and (for instances such as the IBLCE exam) photos, as well as options for clinical management. There are many unanswered questions.

Sometimes, it's good to summarize our KWL: **K**new or know, **W**ant to know, or need to **L**earn?

Instructions: Below, address your KWL. What do you now know? What more would you like to know? What did you learn that was new to you?

Knew	Want to Know	Learn

- How can you use this chapter's information to help breastfeeding families in your practice?

- Where can you learn more?

Explore What You've Learned in a Journal

Multiple studies have shown the benefits of using a learning journal. Among them are greater assimilation and integration of new information, better long-term retention of course concepts, increasing test and exam grades, and a means by which to have continuous feedback about one's own learning.

- Name at least three things you learned from this chapter.

- List at least three things you still need to learn, or more fully master, in this chapter.

- Briefly describe how this information fits (or doesn't fit) with what you've seen in clinical practice, what you learned in basic or college courses, or what you've observed in your own experience breastfeeding. (In some cases, you might want to include how the information fits or doesn't fit with what "experts" say, what the media says, or whatever.)

- Describe how you will use any or all of this information. How might it be related to problems and potential solutions that occur in real life or in clinical situations?

- If you wish, include how you felt about learning this information. Were you bored? Overwhelmed? Enlightened? Worried? Something else?

Self-Assessment

People often dive into a test before they have thoughtfully reflected on how well they have prepared for it. Instead, it would be helpful if they would take a few moments to give their alter-ego (their "other self") a chance to reflect on how confident they feel about mastering the stated objectives.

Take a moment to review the chapter objectives (below). Then, using a scale from 1 to 4, rate yourself. Write the number that best describes your confidence level.

Objective	Highly Confident	Somewhat Confident	Somewhat Unsure	Completely Unsure
Discuss how so-called "nipple confusion" may be related to maternal nipple inelasticity.	❍	❍	❍	❍
Recognize visual indicators and possible consequences of non-everted nipples.	❍	❍	❍	❍
Differentiate between truly inverted nipples and dimpled inverted nipples.	❍	❍	❍	❍
Differentiate between truly inverted nipples and dimpled inverted nipples.	❍	❍	❍	❍
Describe at least four clinical management strategies that may be helpful for infants whose mothers have short, flat, truly inverted, dimpled, or inelastic nipples.	❍	❍	❍	❍
Distinguish between good latching and poor latching by infants using nipple shields.	❍	❍	❍	❍

On the next page, you will see some simple recall questions pertaining to this chapter. These are *not* the application-type questions you will find in the IBLCE exam. However, you cannot *apply* information unless you can fully *recall* that information! You should do these without looking up the answers.

When you finish with the quiz, look up the answers in the Appendix. Then, score your answers, using the Appendix. Finally, you should analyze the results of your quiz. It's not enough to just know what you got right or wrong; you must look at why you got the answers right or wrong.

Quick Quiz Chapter 7

Instructions: Circle the correct response. For a better understanding of how well you are mastering the material, try answering without looking it up. If you are really stuck, questions come from this workbook and from The Breastfeeding Atlas *so go back and review the appropriate material. Answers are in the appendix.*

1. Although it is only speculation, one could make a strong argument that nipple confusion might be related to:
   - A. frequency of using a bottle nipple
   - B. infant temperament
   - C. maternal nipple elasticity
   - D. the brand of the bottle's nipple

2. A nipple that does not easily elongate is likely to have:
   - A. a wide diameter
   - B. higher amounts of tissue collagen
   - C. higher amounts of tissue elastin

3. An inverted nipple first occurs:
   - A. during fetal life
   - B. as soon as the placenta is delivered
   - C. at the onset of puberty
   - D. during the first trimester of pregnancy

4. A breast shell would be worn only:
   - A. between feedings
   - B. during feedings
   - C. during pregnancy
   - D. if the nipple skin is damaged

5. The MOST likely consequence of a nipple with little or no elasticity is:
   - A. a slow or absent milk ejection reflex
   - B. poor stimulation to the infant's palate
   - C. spitting and gagging during the feeding

Analyze Your Own Quiz

- What percentage of the questions did you answer correctly?

- If you got 100% of them right, to what do you attribute your success?

- If you did not get all the questions right, can you identify your learning gap? (Example: Didn't know the information, knew the information but could not remember, knew some information but confused it with similar information, other.)

- Would you have been able to answer the questions as well if you had not read this chapter?

- What do you need to do next? (If you got them all right, what you need to do next is celebrate! Even a high-five with your child, a YESSS and a fist-pump in the air, or anything else is good! A small acknowledgement of your success is better than no acknowledgement!)

Additional Resources

1. Lawrence R, Lawrence, RM. *Breastfeeding: A guide for the medical profession.* 8 ed 2016.
2. Ardran GM, et al. A cineradiographic study of breast feeding. *British Journal of Radiology.* 1958;31(363):156-162.
3. Woolridge MW. The 'anatomy' of infant sucking. *Midwifery.* 1986;2(4):164-171.
4. Elad D, et al. Biomechanics of milk extraction during breast-feeding. *Proc Natl Acad Sci U S A.* 2014;111(14):5230-5235.
5. Woolridge MW, et al. Effect of a traditional and of a new nipple shield on sucking patterns and milk flow. *Early Hum Dev.* 1980;4(4):357-364.
6. Chertok IR, et al. A pilot study of maternal and term infant outcomes associated with ultrathin nipple shield use. *J Obstet Gynecol Neonatal Nurs.* 2006;35(2):265-272.
7. Powers DC, Tapia, V.B. Clinical decision making: When to consider using ta nipple shield. *Clinical Lactation* 2012;3(1):26-28.
8. Alexander JM, et al. Randomised controlled trial of breast shells and Hoffman's exercises for inverted and non-protractile nipples. *BMJ.* 1992;304(6833):1030-1032.

Chapter 8
Nipple Lesions

"Sore nipples" are a common complaint among breastfeeding mothers, but it can be a tricky one to solve. Unless you can determine the root cause of the soreness, finding a successful solution will be highly unlikely.

In this chapter, you'll see that "sore" nipples fall into four main categories. When you understand the characteristics that typify each of the categories—and learn to ask the right questions—you'll be able to give invaluable help to breastfeeding mothers. (For a more in-depth analysis of this topic, see my self-learning module, *Sore Nipples: Prevention and Problem-Solving.*)[1]

It may seem daunting. But trust me on this! By truly immersing yourself in the 36 extraordinary close-up color photos in Chapter 8 of *The Breastfeeding Atlas* (plus images of lesions in other chapters!) and by completing the exercises I've provided here, you'll soon begin to see characteristics of sore nipples that you probably haven't noticed previously.

By the end of this chapter, I promise that you'll be able to determine a corrective strategy for nipple lesions based on precise clues that best indicate one of four main causes: physiologic tenderness, latch-related or pump-related trauma, immune reaction, or infection and what to do about it.

Objectives

Given a clinical photo, you will be able to:

- Classify multiple images of "sore nipples" as being caused or complicated by one of four main reasons.
- Gather and interpret distinguishing data about nipple lesions and their relationship to layers of the epidermis, dermis, and hypodermis.
- Describe 11 different primary lesions in terms of size, flat or raised, solid or fluid-filled, involved skin layers, diameter, and shape, and several examples of each that might be seen on the breast.
- Match commonly-seen nipple/breast lesions to a commonly-used strategy to prevent, minimize, or treat such lesions.
- Recognize lesions that can be resolved with simple treatments, and those that require referral for medical help.
- State the definitions of at least 50 terms related to nipple lesions.

Key Words

- abrasion
- acral
- antihistamine
- atopic
- autotransmission
- benign
- biphasic
- blanched
- bleb
- blister
- blocked (plugged) nipple pore
- candidiasis
- compression stripe
- corticosteroids
- crusts
- cyanotic
- cyst
- dermatitis
- dermis
- eczema
- edema
- epidermis
- erosion
- erythema
- excoriation
- exudate
- fissures
- hand, foot, and mouth disease
- herpes simplex virus (HSV)
- histamine
- hives
- impetigo
- infection
- inflammation
- keloid
- lesion
- maceration
- Montgomery glands
- necrotic
- Paget disease
- pH
- plaque
- primary skin lesions
- psoriasis
- purulent
- Raynaud disease (Raynaud phenomenon)
- sanguineous
- scale
- secondary skin lesions
- serous
- subcutaneous tissue
- steroid
- thrush
- triphasic
- ulceration
- urticarial, urticaria
- vasoconstriction
- vasodilation
- vasospasm
- vesicle
- yeast

Skin and Its Layers

There are three layers of skin: The *epidermis*, the *dermis*, and the *hypodermis* (also called *subcutaneous* skin). See **Figure 8-1** below.

Epidermis

The prefix "epi" means "on" or "upon" and "dermis" means skin. From the Latin word "strata" meaning horizontal layer, the epidermis consists of five separate layers.

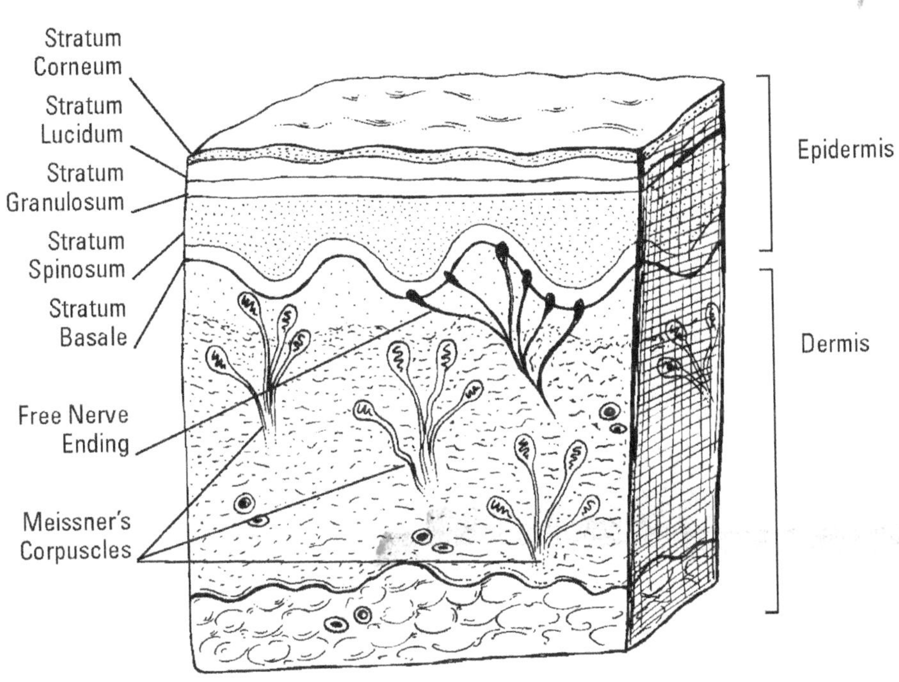

Figure 8-1. Layers of the skin. From Biancuzzo, M. (2016). Sore Nipples: Prevention and Problem-Solving. Gold Standard Publishing. Used with permission.

Because it is not necessary for you to memorize the layers of the skin in order to support the breastfeeding mother, these were not identified as key terms for the chapter. (But if you wish to, here's a good mnemonic: "**C**ome, **l**et's **g**et **s**un**b**urned.") However, if you understand the basic function of the layers, it helps to understand both the subjective (e.g., pain) and the objective (i.e., healing) factors that relate to "sore nipples."

- **Corneum** consists of cells that are dead or desquamating. (Think of the word "coroner," who determines the cause of death. Originally, the word referred to an officer who protected the royal family (a.k.a. the "crown"). Indeed, the chief function of the stratum corneum is to protect the organism. (This layer is also called the "horny layer".)
- **Lucindum**: Flat cells that are present only in the palms and the soles of the feet. (In essence, then, nipples have only four layers in the epidermis, rather than five.)
- **Granulosum**: Diamond-shaped cells that produce a waxy material to help "waterproof" the skin.

- **Spinosum**: Polygonal cells that help bond other cells together.
- **Basale**: Columnar epithelial cells that produce new cells. The new cells move up to the stratum corneum to replace its sloughed-off cells.

Here's the basic principle: When a wound extends into the deeper skin layers, it is more painful, and slower to heal.

Dermis

Below the epidermis is the *dermis*. It consists of tough tissue that is made up mostly of collagen. (Recall the discussion about elastin and collagen in chapter 7.) The dermis contains:

- nerve endings, which are sensitive to pain, pressure, touch and temperature
- sweat glands, which produce sweat in response to heat and stress
- sebaceous glands, which secrete sebum—an oil that keeps the skin moist and soft and acts as a barrier against foreign substances—into hair follicles
- hair follicles
- blood vessels, which dilate in response to heat (vasodilation) and narrow in response to cold (vasoconstriction)

Hypodermis (Subcutaneous)

The *hypodermis* is below the other skin layers. (The prefix "hypo" means "under" or "beneath"). The hypodermis consists mostly of fat. It is also correctly referred to as the *subcutaneous tissue*. The hypodermis helps insulate the body from heat and cold, provides protective padding, and serves as an energy storage area.

Skin Lesions

Before moving on, we should review the meaning of the term *lesion*. As explained in chapter 3, a *lesion* refers to a discontinuity of tissue or loss of function to a body part. In this chapter, we will be discussing only those lesions that occur on the skin.

There are three basic types of skin lesions: primary, secondary, and special lesions. By knowing these classifications, you will be more able to recognize which type of lesion your client has, and the implications for clinical care.

The same types of skin lesions can result from different disease processes. For example, one type of skin lesion—a macule—could be a freckle or a café au lait spot. (See chapter 3 for more detail.) Good interview questions can often help you to elicit a history that fits with the lesion's appearance. History, along with details of the lesion's appearance, will help you to determine what to do next—if anything.

Describing Skin Lesions

Only those who are licensed by the state to diagnose conditions may do so legally. Usually, this means that a physician or his legally-recognized, contracted designee (e.g., a physician's assistant) must make any diagnosis. However, others involved in healthcare should be able to give a good description of a skin lesion.

A skin lesion should be described in as much detail as possible. In general, this includes:

- What is its relationship to the skin's surface? Is the lesion flat, raised, or depressed?
- What is the size of the lesion? Is it smaller or larger than 1 cm?
- Is it solid or fluid-filled? If it is fluid-filled, is the fluid clear (*serous*), bloody (*sanguineous*) or is it pus (*purulent*)?
- What is the shape and configuration of the lesion? Is there one solitary lesion or a group of lesions? There are ten different shapes and configurations of lesions; the details of these are beyond the scope of this publication. (For more details, see the "Shapes & Configuration" page on the LearnDerm site.*) In breastfeeding mothers, it's common to see shapes such as round or oval, linear and configured as grouped (clustered), polycyclic, or scattered.
- What is the color or pigmentation? Redness (*erythema*) is common, but sometimes, the tissue is *blanched* (white) or *cyanotic* (blue). Some lesions show hyperpigmentation, such as a nevus (**Figure 190**) whereas others show hypopigmentation.
- How would you describe the borders? Are the borders well-defined or vague? Are the borders regular or irregular?
- What is the texture of the lesion? Rough? Smooth? Dimpled?
- Where are the lesions located and distributed? For example, eczema is more likely to be located on the dry parts of the body, whereas yeast is more likely to be on moist parts of the body.

Primary skin lesions

Primary lesions are directly associated with a disease process. These lesions include changes in color or texture. They may be present at birth, or they may be acquired over time.

Table 8-1 summarizes and compares different types of primary skin lesions. They are named using established dermatological terminology. One lesion could be indicative of multiple different disease processes.

---

* VisualDx. "Shapes & Configurations." LearnDerm site. Available at ***https://www.visualdx.com/learnderm/shape-configuration***. Accessed July 29, 2017.

	Description: elevated, flat, or depressed?	Size/ diameter	Comments
bulla	fluid-filled (clear) with clearly-defined borders	> 1 cm	Compare with vesicle *Example: large blister*
burrow	tunnel formed in the skin that appears as a linear mark		result of an infestation of the skin with parasites such as mites from scabies
macule	flat, discolored; may be any shape	< 1 cm	Compare with patch *Examples: freckles, some rashes (e.g., smallpox)*
nodule	raised, solid	> 1 cm	Compare with tumor Located in the epidermis, dermis, or subcutaneous tissue *Examples: small tumor, Epstein's pearls*
papule	solid, raised, distinct borders	< 1 cm	Compare with plaque *Examples: Warts, acne, pimples*
patch	flat, discolored	> 1 cm	Compare with macule *Examples: Salmon patch (birthmark), measles, flat moles*
plaque	solid, raised, flat-topped shape	> 1 cm	Often has a fuzzy or velvety texture or appearance *Examples: yeast infection, psoriasis*
pustule	elevated fluid-filled lesion with clearly-defined borders that contains pus	< 1 cm	most commonly infected, but may be sterile *Examples: folliculitis (commonly infected) or pustular psoriasis (may be sterile.)*
telangiectasia	blood vessels near the surface		*Example: spider veins*
tumor	solid, located in the dermis, epidermis, or subcutaneous tissue	> 2 cm	Larger than a nodule. Often mistaken for a cyst or abscess. *Examples: adenomas or fibromas (Note: tumors are NOT necessarily cancerous.)*
vesicle	raised, fluid-filled (clear) with clearly-defined borders	< 1 cm	Compare with bulla *Example: Herpes, which often appears as a group of vesicles on an erythematous base*
wheal	raised, with color changes, with edema in the upper layers of the epidermis; often red and itchy		*Examples: hives, insect bites, allergic reaction*

Table 8-1. Summary and comparison of primary lesions, with examples.

Secondary lesions

Secondary lesions may result from some primary lesions, or from some other factor, such as scratching, trauma, or infection. Opinions vary about how many types of lesions are "secondary" in nature, but these eight are commonly identified: atrophy, crust, erosion, excoriation, fissure, lichenification, scale, and ulceration.

Atrophy is seen when the skin becomes thin or has a smooth or finely wrinkled surface. (It is unlikely to occur on the breasts of a woman in her childbearing years.)

Crusts (a.k.a. *scabs*) are formed by blood, pus, and serum (or a mingling these) on the surface of an ulcer of other type of wound. (*Serous* means watery, and *sanguineous* means bloody.) One example is **Figure 179**.

Erosion refers to a red excoriation that goes through part or all of the epidermis. It may have a serous fluid, and it almost always develops after a blister or pustule ruptures. You might find it difficult to identify **Figure 153** as erosion, since it is already partially healed, and therefore the features of a true lesion, as it originally presented, are difficult to see.

Excoriation is a where a few (but not all) layers of epidermis are abraded or rubbed off.

Fissure is a narrow, linear split that dips down through the deep epidermal layer and possibly the dermis. A fissure on the nipple almost always occurs after a compression stripe. (**Figure 151**).

Keloid scar tissue, such as is shown in a scar from incising an abscess (**Figure 257**) shows the characteristic reddened, scar tissue that extends over the borders of the original incision. (See page 96 for details of the case.) Keloid tissue is not always classified as a secondary lesion.

Lichenification is skin that has become hardened or thickened as a result of a chronic skin disease (e.g., chronic eczema).

Scale refers to the outermost layer of skin (*stratum corneum*) being heaped up with dry, "flaky" skin that often looks like a fish scale.

Ulceration is the formation of a depression in the tissue that goes down from the dermis into the hypodermis (subcutaneous) tissue. It is not as narrow as a fissure, but it is deeper than an erosion. (Ulcerations can also be classified as a type of wound.)

Special Lesions

Special lesions are those that don't readily fall into the primary or secondary category. This might not be an exhaustive list—again, authorities can vary in how they define various types of lesions—but I've frequently seen these 15 types classified as "special": abscess, burrow, caruncle, comedo (blackheads), ecchymosis, excoriation, folliculitis, furuncle, maceration, milia (whiteheads), petechiae, sebaceous cysts, telangiectasia (which are sometimes classified as primary lesions), ulcers, and wen.

If you find yourself feeling like you still haven't recovered from the lists of primary and secondary lesions, don't panic! Focus on the "special" lesions that, in my clinical experience, are more likely to be associated with lactating women.

An *abscess* is a localized collection of pus in the fatty or connective tissue, often accompanied by *edema* (swelling) and inflammation and frequently caused by bacteria. Refer to chapter 11 in this workbook for more details, and observe several examples of an abscess of the breast, shown on page 185 of *The Breastfeeding Atlas.*

Ecchymosis is, in plain language, a bruise. It is a flat, round, purplish patch on the skin that is larger than 3 mm in diameter. (Note: *Petechiae* are similar, but smaller than 3 mm in diameter.) Bruising sometimes happens when an infant "drags" on the breast tissue. This can be solved by having the mother provide firm and consistent support to the infant's head during feeding. However, a bruise may result from another cause, such as physical abuse, or after a surgery (**Figure 279**).

Folliculitis is an infection or inflammation of the hair follicle. Mammals have hair (some more than others, as shown in **Figure 208**) so although it's unusual for a breastfeeding mother to have a folliculitis, it can and does happen.

Maceration can be described best as "water-logged" skin. If you've ever spent too much time in the bath tub and then had white, wrinkled skin, it's because your skin has been in contact with excessive amounts of fluid for a long period of time. You might see this on the nipples or breasts of a woman who leaks milk constantly and doesn't change her nursing pads often. You might also see it if a woman does not dry well after bathing. Although it is okay to rinse the nipples with water or saline after feeding or pumping, they should be patted dry to avoid maceration.[2]

Milia aren't likely to be on the breast or the nipples. Sometimes called "white heads," milia are tiny inclusion cysts. They are common in the newborn (such as on the infant's nose in **Figure 5**) and are really just trapped vernix. Milia tend to disappear within 2-3 months.

Petechiae are tiny hemorrhages under the skin. They are usually 0.5 to 1 mm in diameter. These purplish-red spots on the skin (or elsewhere, such as the nailbeds or mucous membranes) are not raised. Often, they are harmless. Sometimes, however, they can be attributed to such causes as low platelet count, vitamin deficiency diseases, or adverse drug reactions. Petechiae aren't usually found on the mother's chest, but I mention these because petechiae on the newborn's back or trunk can signal any of several serious pathological conditions and should warrant follow-up.

Sebaceous cysts are, first of all, *cysts*. By definition, a *cyst* is an abnormal membrane sac that contains a semi-solid, liquid, or gaseous material. A sebaceous cyst (**Figure 171**) is one that contains the oily or waxy matter from nearby sebaceous glands. Not all experts agree that sebaceous cysts are true lesions, but they are a skin condition you may see.

Ulcers occur when the epidermis and the upper papillary dermis are damaged. Ulcers tend to be wider and deeper than fissures, which tend to be more linear and shallow. An ulcer always results in a scar. It can be caused by any type of skin trauma (e.g., heat, cold, electrical, chemical, pressure—including bacteria, viral or fungal or parasitic) and many more causes. Refer to the skin diagram, and look at **Figure 271**, which is an excellent example of how the epidermis and thin, upper layer of dermis have been damaged.

Other odd lesions aren't usually mentioned in those lists of "special" lesions, but you should call your attention to other discontinuations in the tissue, such as *skin tags* (**Figure 180**), *blebs* (**Figure 169, 170**) and *compression stripes* (**Figure 149**). We'll discuss those later.

Causes of Nipple Lesions

Remember that primary lesions—on the nipples are elsewhere—absolutely are associated with a disease process. You probably remember that one primary lesion can indicate more than one disease process. This is quite different than nipple lesions that are caused by trauma—which, in my experience, are the most likely explanation for "sore nipples." Yet some "sore nipples" aren't attributable to either pathology or trauma. We'll discuss all of this in greater detail.

Transient, Physiologic Changes

Sometimes, nipple soreness is the result of transient, physiologic changes associated with the childbearing cycle. Hormones can heighten nipple sensitivity, such as when it results in nipple tenderness shortly after a woman becomes pregnant. Also, if a multiparous woman becomes pregnant while she is still lactating, she will notice that nipple tenderness especially while nursing. Similarly, nipple tenderness may occur once the mother's menstrual cycle has been re-established and she is ovulating. All these examples can be explained by the normal, physiologic changes that accompany hormonal fluctuations.

During the first few postpartum days, or towards the end of a feeding, a mother may especially note nipple tenderness. This is the time when she has relatively little milk in her ducts, and she is likely to notice some transient discomfort. This happens. It is not unusual. Although negative pressure is not the primary means by which milk is transferred, the infant will exert more negative pressure and swallow less frequently when the ducts are not full; thus, the negative pressure will be relieved less frequently. Interestingly, changes in sucking patterns were first explained by Gunther[3] in 1945; more recently, the difference in sucking patterns was confirmed in an ultrasound[4] study by Geddes. Therefore, until the ducts are filled more completely and swallowing occurs more frequently, some mild discomfort may be present. Especially in the first few days, this situation is not worrisome if the newborn is latching on correctly.

Classic studies and clinical experience confirm that such soreness usually peaks around Day 3 postpartum, when engorgement occurs.[5,6] Why is this so? It's likely that, prior to physiologic engorgement and the milk "coming in," the infant exerts greater negative pressure with fewer times of releasing that pressure. Further, engorgement causes the breast tissue to distend (**Figure 148**) and, along with other variations of the nipple, appears to contribute to nipple soreness.[7] Finally, the nipples are shortened when the breast is engorged, which can make latching on a little more difficult for the infant. Generally, nipple pain peaks when physiologic engorgement appears, and then usually diminishes significantly.

Complete Exercises 8-1 and 8-2 to be able to correctly describe lesions.

Nipple Trauma

To my knowledge, there are no statistics to shed light on the number of mothers who develop nipple lesions due to nipple trauma. However, my clinical experience suggests that during the first month or so, the vast majority of "sore nipples" result from trauma due to latch issues, or possibly, the pump.

When I use the term "sore nipples," I generally mean soreness due to trauma. However, not everyone uses the term that way, so when someone—a mother or a professional—reports "sore nipples," it's critical to look at the nipple carefully and methodically. Nipple soreness that results from other causes looks *very* different from soreness that has been caused by trauma.

"Trauma" implies an injury from a force outside of the mother. For example, if the infant attaches or detaches from the breast in a suboptimal way, a wound may result. Similarly, if the pump or pump apparatus is used in a suboptimal way, a wound can result. Such wounds are due to external mechanical causes rather than internal physiologic or pathologic causes.

Many wounds are acute, and can be healed with good clinical management. Others are chronic, and require a meticulous 3-step healing process.[8] Many wounds have some sort of *exudate*—a mass or serosanguinous material, including cellular debris—that has seeped out of the wound during the healing process. Often, chronic wounds cannot heal because *necrotic* (dead) tissue causes the accumulation of bacterial (cellular) debris during the inflammatory process and fuels bacterial growth.[8] Hence, it's important to first prevent nipple trauma, and second, find ways to resolve nipple wounds if they are present. *The Breastfeeding Atlas* (pages 59-60) gives some guidance.

Most "sore nipples" that are attributable to a traumatic cause can be described as one of these three classic types of wounds:

Abrasions result from a rubbing, scraping or wearing down of the epidermis. For example, if you have ever fallen on some rough grass or a rough pavement, you've probably experienced a "brush burn"— an abrasion. Similarly, if the mother's nipple has been repeatedly rubbed against the infant's hard palate, the mother would have an abrasion.

Lacerations are wounds that create a tear in the skin. On a mother's nipple, this linear tear is preceded by a linear compression stripe, (**Figure 113**) which is typically lighter in color than the rest of the nipple. This happens when the skin is folded onto itself because the nipple has been pinched during a poor latch (**Figure 149**). When the skin tissue breaks apart, a more clearly-defined, linear, open tear results, and as it begins to heal, a scab (**Figure 150**) will soon become apparent. However, if it does not heal completely, pathogens can invade the broken skin, and the laceration can become infected (**Figure 155**).

Ulcers are concave depressions in the epidermis and some of the dermis with an irregular size and shape. Ulcers are different from *fissures* (thin, linear tears in the epidermis). Sometimes, an ulcer occurs on the mother's nipple (**Figure 154),** and these need additional treatment.

Erosions (**Figure 153**) are wider than fissures, and they are located only in the epidermis.

Blisters (**Figure 174**) result from high negative pressure, such as from the infant suckling or the pump. Recall, too, that blisters then break open.

Contusions are ecchymotic spots—bruises—without skin breakage. However, in addition to discoloration, they have *edema* (swelling).

These are perhaps not the only types of wounds that occur, but they are by far the most frequent types of wounds seen in breastfeeding mothers, and all are mentioned in *The Breastfeeding Atlas*. The question is, what causes such wounds?

Most lacerations of the mother's nipple or breast occur when the infant does not have a deep latch. Sometimes, correction is a matter of education and patience. However, an infant may not be able to achieve a deep latch because of an anatomical disorder, such as tongue-tie (**Figure 365**).

Biting is another reason a laceration can occur. In a newborn, this may occur because the mother attempts to pull the infant off her breast without first breaking the suction (**Figure 181**). Understandably, the gums will still be clamping down on the nipple, and a laceration will result. In an older infant—especially those with teeth—biting occurs when active suckling has ceased. For example, biting can occur during a feeding when the infant is distracted, and moves his head without detaching from the nipple. It can also occur as a feeding is ending, or has ended.

Engorgement, is not a true "cause" for nipple damage, but because the nipples are typically shorter, the infant may have more difficulty achieving a deep latch, making nipple trauma is more likely (**Figure 147**). Also, engorgement makes the nipple skin taut, and hence, more vulnerable to injury.

Excessive negative pressure (i.e., "suction") is also a cause of injury to the tissue. Excessive negative pressure is exerted when the infant is unable to exert adequate mechanical pressure to remove milk. There are several reasons why high negative pressure might be exerted by the pump; common examples include turning the suction to a setting that is too high, or using a flange that is too small. With excessive negative pressure, a blister can form on the nipple (**Figure 174**).

Treatments for Nipple Trauma

Over the years, several treatments for traumatized nipple skin have been proposed. Some are supported by weak evidence, while others have no evidence whatsoever. A short list of options includes creams and ointments, moist wound patches, protective methods (e.g., breast shells), moist tea bags, and many more. One meta-analysis showed that no topical agent was superior to another, and that correct latch-on was key to the prevention of nipple trauma.[9] Similarly, another meta-analysis showed that such treatments had no benefit over doing nothing, or applying the mother's milk to her nipple.[10]

More recently, a silver-impregnated cap (**Figure 156**) was tested with 40 lactating subjects who had nipple fissures.[11] Although there was no statistical difference in healing between the control group and the experimental group at Day 2, differences were noted at Day 5 and Day 7 of the experiment. The study included only a small group, but the results suggest an option very different from previously-used treatments.

Infection

Infection is the process whereby microorganisms invade and multiply in a place where they are not normally present, or become overgrown in their normal location. For example, *Staphylococcus aureus* is normal flora on the skin, but it is not normally present in the milk ducts or ductules. Candida is normally present in the vagina, but an overgrowth of candida—in the vagina, or elsewhere in the body—is not normal. Infection occurs when the body's innate or specific immune systems have not succeeded in protecting the body.

Infections on the nipple are usually bacterial, viral, or fungal. It should be noted that one type of infection can co-exist with another type of infection (e.g., a bacterial and a fungal infection) (**Figure 163**), highlighting the need for a thorough evaluation of the lesion.

Candidiasis

Candida is a fungus that is normally present in the mouth, gut, and vagina. However, an overgrowth of candida is called *candidiasis* (or sometimes, candidosis). The lay term *yeast* is used to describe an overgrowth of candida on the breasts or vagina, whereas *thrush* is used to describe an overgrowth of candida in the mouth.

Observe location and distribution of the lesion if you suspect candidiasis. A lesion that is on the areola but not on the nipple is highly unlikely to be a yeast infection. That is, candidiasis will be present on the nipple and spread to the areola, but not the other way around. Candidiasis is almost always in a moist area.

In the infant's mouth, a white *plaque* may be visible, usually on the tongue (**Figure 157**), at the buccal pads (**Figure 158**), or below the upper or lower lips (**Figure 159**). "White spots" located elsewhere in the intraoral cavity are highly unlikely to be candida. The white plaque may also be in the diaper area.

The white plaque of yeast may be visible on the mother's nipples; if this is the case, it is usually in a "swirling" shape, following the crevices of her nipple. It might also appear at the nipple/areolar junction. White plaque is more visible on a dark-skinned woman, and more difficult to detect in a light-skinned woman. All too often, clinicians who do not spot the plaque assume that the mother does not have a yeast infection, leading to misdiagnosis, undertreatment, or both.

Very often, the white plaque may not be visible on the mother's nipple. The nipple may appear bright red, purple-red, or bright pink (**Figure 162**). Almost always, the lesion is shiny, and the mother will complain of itching or burning.

Complete Exercise 8-3 related to candidiasis and "white spots".

There are many treatments for candidiasis, both systemic and topical. A remedy that has lost popularity in the United States, but is well-recognized in other parts of the world, is gentian violet. Gentian violet is a dye. It was not originally developed to treat thrush, but it is used topically for that purpose, and it is highly effective against bacteria, fungi and parasites.[12] It can be applied to the infant's mouth (**Figure 160**) or to the mother's nipples **Figure 161**. Those who use or recommend gentian violet for mothers or infants affected with candidiasis should see *The Breastfeeding Atlas* for some important cautions and practical guidelines about using gentian violet.

Viral Infections

A virus is a minute infectious agent that exists within the host's living cell. Unlike a bacterium, a virus is never "friendly"; it is always pathogenic. And, a virus does not reproduce itself; rather, it relies on dismantling the immune system of the host. Like bacteria, however, viruses can be spread through several different modes—for example, through contact with carrier insects, by touch, or by droplet (coughing). Here, we'll confine the discussion about viruses to those examples that affect breastfeeding and are shown in *The Breastfeeding Atlas.*

Herpes

Herpes simplex virus (HSV) may be either HSV Type 1 (HSV-1) or HSV Type 2 (HSV-2). HSV-1 is most likely to be transmitted by oral-to-oral contact (which may include "cold sores"), but it can also cause genital herpes. HSV-2 is a sexually transmitted infection that causes genital herpes.

Herpes is highly contagious. Caution must be taken to ensure that the newborn is not in contact with the herpetic lesions. It may be possible to avoid or cover the lesions while breastfeeding. If not, breastfeeding should be interrupted until the open lesions are healed. However, herpes—like other viruses—is not necessarily transmitted from one individual to another. It is entirely possible for a person with a cold sore on her lip to touch her breast, causing a lesion there. This is called *autotransmission.*

A herpetic lesion on the breast (**Figure 178**) is caused by the same organism as the common cold sore, and has similar signs and symptoms. As is typical of any *vesicle*, a herpetic vesicle is a small (< 1 cm), circumscribed (having definite boundaries) elevation of the skin that contains liquid that forms on the skin's surface, enlarges, breaks open, and then becomes ulcerated. With herpes, it is likely that there will be a cluster of vesicles, rather than just one (**Figure 178**). Typically, the affected area is itchy and painful. The HSV virus isn't "cured". Without medical treatment, the virus stays within the nerves. Therefore, the signs and symptoms may be inactive for a while, but they will recur.

Impetigo

Impetigo is a bacterial infection. The causative pathogen is usually strains of staphylococcus and streptococcus. Impetigo occurs when bacteria enter skin that is already broken in situations such as an eczema flare-up or insect bites. Technically, there are two types of impetigo but we'll consider only the more common nonbullous type here. (The bullous type is less common.)

Impetigo is highly contagious. Impetigo is easily spread by direct contact with those who are infected, or, less frequently, may also be spread by indirect contact with inanimate objects (such as sheets.)

Lesions are around the nose and mouth (or possibly the extremities), and begin as papules, and then become vesicles. Later, the lesions burst, and a crust forms. In nonbullous impetigo, the crusts are honey-colored. (In nonbullous type the crust color is more brown.)

The lesions may be itchy but not painful. Sometimes impetigo can be recurrent.

Treatment depends on whether the impetigo is bullous or nonbullous, the extent of the lesions, or the likelihood of mass spreading (e.g., a sports team.) Most times, topical mupirocin (Bactroban™) or retapamulin (Altabax) is adequate treatment for single lesions of nonbullous impetigo or small areas of involvement. Otherwise, systemic antibiotics are likely to be prescribed.

Since *The Breastfeeding Atlas* does not show photos of impetigo, why have we spent so much time learning about its characteristics? That's because herpes lesions and impetigo lesions are similar in appearance. Care should be taken that the two conditions are not confused.

In at least one case, a tragic outcome occurred because herpes was mistaken for impetigo.[13] The newborn had a lesion on her chin upon discharge from the hospital, but it was presumed to be impetigo. Multiple members of the healthcare team expressed the opinion that it was impetigo, but no one sought to test for the existing pathogen. (This should have been done, and would have required action by the only member of the team licensed to diagnose conditions—the physician.) Nine days later, the infant died from what proved to be herpes.

Complete Learning Exercise 8-4 to see the similarities and differences in these two lesions.

Hand, Foot, and Mouth Disease

Hand, foot, and mouth disease (HFMD) is caused by a coxsackievirus, A type of enterovirus, Coxsackievirus may be either type A, or type B. Type A includes HFMD. It is highly contagious. It usually occurs in children under 5 years old, but it can also occur in older children and adults.

HFMD should not be confused with "hoof and mouth disease," which is caused by a different virus, and, although highly contagious in cloven-hoofed animals, rarely occurs in humans.

Typically, *acral* distribution of the lesions—that is, their presence on the distal extremities (hands, feet, and head) and protrusions such as the nose, ears, penis, or nipples—occurs with HFMD. Those affected by the virus tend to have an erythematous, maculopapular rash. That is, the rash has both macules (flat lesions that are discolored, usually red) as well as papules (raised bumps). If you look carefully, you will see both aspects of the maculopapular rash in **Figure 179**. The rash, and other symptoms such as fever, typically last 7-10 days.

Notice how the herpes lesions differ from the HFMD lesions. A herpes lesion is a vesicle with visible fluid, often configured in a cluster. The HFMD lesions are macular and papular, and are not arranged in a tight cluster.

Bacterial Infections

Infections are often accompanied by *inflammation*, the presence of reddened, swollen, hot, and often painful tissue. Inflammation and infection are different.

Inflammation is a protective mechanism; it's part of our body's innate immune system that creates heat to burn out foreign invaders. Infection, on the other hand, *is* the foreign invader. Look carefully at the infected Montgomery gland (**Figure 176**) in one mother, and the inflamed Montgomery glands in (**Figure 177**) in another mother.

While it's difficult to be certain with only a photo, **Figure 176** looks very much like a pustule. It looks like a fluid-filled elevated lesion with clearly-defined borders less than 1 cm in diameter—the classic definition of a pustule. Beneath the surface, the pus within the pustule is visible. Furthermore, although warm soaks can be a good first step for this situation, the lesion did not improve with the warm soaks. After treatment with antibiotics, the mother squeezed out fluids: white, thickened milk, followed by pus, then blood, then a serous fluid. Everything in this story—including the photo—completely fits with the description of an infection.

Figure 177, however, is different. There is no true "lesion" here. The Montgomery glands do enlarge during pregnancy. The enlargement shown here is greater than usual, and may appear even more dramatic because of the "rubbery" texture that Wilson-Clay and Hoover observed. Certainly, there is redness that is indicative of inflammation. However, there is no sign of infection. It's important to keep in mind the difference between a Montgomery gland that is enlarged and swollen, versus one that has a lesion.

Bacterial infections are frequently due to *Staphyloccocus aureus*. Although *S. aureus* is normal flora on all human skin, infection occurs when the organism moves from the skin to other structures. Sometimes, there is no full-blown infection, but there is substantial inflammation.

Immunological Conditions

Some, but not all, people may experience a condition in which the immune system overreacts. This may occur all the time, or some of the time. For example, stress is a well-known trigger for over-reactions of the immune system.

Skin lesions that occur on any adult can show up on the breasts of lactating women. Here, we'll discuss lesions that occur with eczema, psoriasis, allergic reactions, and nipple vasospasm.

Atopic Dermatitis (Eczema)

The term *atopic* comes from the Greek atopia; *a* meaning "without" and *topia* meaning "place." Hence, atopic refers to the reaction being out of place. More specifically, atopic means the condition has a predisposition toward developing a certain allergic reaction. Some believe that atopy has a hereditary component, but all agree that atopy refers to an IgE-mediated reaction. As such, the allergic reaction occurs at the second—not the first—exposure.

Multiple sources, including the American Academy of Allergy, Asthma, and Immunology, define *atopic dermatitis* as a chronic or recurrent inflammatory skin disease. More specifically, these sources say that atopic dermatitis is one type of eczema. (It should be understood that eczema is not one condition, but rather, about five different conditions, therefore no one specific lesion is associated with eczema.) The most common type of eczema is atopic dermatitis.

Atopic dermatitis can be classified as either acute or chronic, and the distinction may affect its appearance. With acute eczema, lesions are red and perhaps blistered or swollen. With chronic eczema, the lesion is usually darker than the surrounding skin and thickened. This thickening is referred to as *lichenification*.

Her physician correctly diagnosed the woman in **Figure 166** with eczema on her nipples and areolae. However, a word of caution: There are many stories (see page 105 of *The Breastfeeding Atlas*) of women who have had breast lesions diagnosed as eczema, when in fact, they had Paget disease. The lesions look very similar. However, whereas the eczema is a nuisance, *Paget disease* is a cancerous lesion. The prognosis is good if the lesion is accurately diagnosed and treated early, so lesions on the nipple/areola that have an eczema-like appearance should be carefully evaluated by a physician, and, perhaps, confirmed with a second opinion from a physician specializing in dermatology.

Allergic Contact Dermatitis (a.k.a. Contact Irritant Dermatitis)

Often called "contact dermatitis," this condition is better understood as allergic contact irritant dermatitis. Dermatitis (*derm* means skin, and *itis* means inflammation) occurs when an irritant comes in contact with the skin, and the person experiences an allergic reaction.

Unlike a true allergy, however, this is not a direct, overactive, immune response with the release of antibodies. Rather, the irritated skin tends to occur only where contact with the irritant occurred; the irritant and the resulting reaction causes localized inflammation and damage to the skin's surface faster than the body can repair cells or grow new ones. The response can be immediate when the trigger is in contact with a particularly harsh irritant; it may also occur in response to repeated exposure to a less harsh chemical (such as a laundry soap). Skin that has been repeatedly rubbed can also exhibit a contact dermatitis.

Some individuals are more or less reactive to a substance than others. Potential irritants can be found in soaps, shampoos, lotions, perfumes, cosmetics, hair dyes or straighteners; all are common culprits. Contact with plants is another source for irritation. Many people are allergic to latex rubber, a plant product found in some types of gloves worn by healthcare workers. Citrus fruit (especially the peel) can be an irritant, as can many medications, especially those that are applied to the skin.

A contact dermatitis can result in hives (a type of wheal). The mother in **Figure 165** has *hives* caused by a reaction to topical applications of nystatin, an antifungal drug.

Often, women who are suffering from "sore nipples" are urged to apply some type of nipple cream. Over the years, few have been proven to be helpful, including the popular "all-purpose nipple ointment."[10] However, we know with certainty that reactions to nipple cream (**Figure 164**) can and do occur. Presumably, something in the product may be an irritant, and the substance adds to rather than alleviates the mother's pain.

Poison ivy dermatitis is one particular kind of contact dermatitis caused by contact with urushiol, an oil found in the poison ivy, poison oak, and poison sumac plants. Many people are highly allergic to the plants' oils and should avoid contact with them. Severity of reaction can vary, and for some people, washing off within 30 minutes of contact with the oil will help to prevent or minimize the "rash" that develops.

The poison ivy "rash" may be first seem papular; later, it appears as vesicles or weeping vesicles or even bullae. Other experts call the reaction hives; a type of wheal. (Although the term *urticaria* and hives are often used interchangeably, they are not equivalent. There are several types of urticaria, classified according to whether they are acute or chronic.)

The lesions (**Figure 168**) are uncomfortable, but the fluid from the vesicles is not contagious, so breastfeeding may continue.

Psoriasis

Psoriasis is a chronic autoimmune condition that results in skin cells multiplying about ten times faster than normal. Eventually, the cells reach the skin's surface and die. This forms red plaques, covered with white scales, on the skin. The lesions start as small papules, but eventually, these coalesce and form scaling plaques.

Most frequently, psoriasis is found on especially dry body parts—the scalp, elbows and knees, for example—but psoriasis can and does occur on the nipple and/or areola (**Figure 167**). The photo shown here, while accurate and perhaps even typical of one of many types of psoriasis, is by no means the only presentation of psoriasis. For example, inverse psoriasis is found in the folds beneath the breasts (or other skin folds in the body). Although it is often mistaken for a yeast infection, it is not.

Usually, cortisone creams are applied directly to the skin to relieve psoriasis. Topical cortisone creams are made of synthetic corticosteroid hormones. Like the natural corticosteroid hormones produced by the adrenal glands, these creams effectively reduce inflammation. Phototherapy with ultraviolet B is considered a safe treatment also.[14, 15]

Vasospasm of the Nipple

Sometimes, a mother may experience *vasospasms* in her nipples. *Vaso* means "blood vessel(s)" and *spasm* means "an abnormal, involuntary and possibly continuous muscular contraction." Although Dr. Raynaud[16] described vasospasm of the fingers and toes, he did not address vasospasm of the nipples. Still, it is often casually referred to as *Raynaud phenomenon.* Ideally, we should all take a cue from *The Breastfeeding Atlas* and other sources that more correctly refer to this as *nipple vasospasm.*[17-20]

The exact cause of nipple vasospasm is unknown. It may or may not occur in women who have experienced Raynaud phenomenon in the fingers or toes. It occurs in primiparae as well as multiparae. Multiparae who have experienced it while nursing their firstborn may or may not experience it with subsequent infants. Some women have it in both breasts; some in only one breast. It has been associated with use of labetol[21] but I am familiar with cases in which the woman received substantial doses of labetalol but never experienced nipple vasospasm while nursing. I also recall a case of a woman who experienced painful nipple vasospasms early in her third trimester of pregnancy although she had never nursed before. In short, I have been unable to identify a pattern of how or to whom vasospasm occurs.

Unlike other "white spots" on the nipple, the white color of a vasospasm tends to occupy a substantial portion of the nipple (**Figure 172**). The lesion may not be white; it may be cyanotic. That's because vasospasm of the nipple has a *biphasic* (2-phase) or *triphasic* (3-phase) presentation (color changes of white and/or blue and red). Sometimes, there is a sort of "crinkling" of the skin that occurs at the nipple-areolar junction (but that is not seen in **Figure 172**).

Eliciting a good history can be helpful in identifying the cause of the "white spot." A typical trigger for a nipple vasospasm is a sudden change of temperature. A woman may experience vasospasm when she comes out of the shower (where the temperature is about

105° F) or has her nipple move from her infant's mouth (about 98° F) to the ambient room air (where the temperature is around 71° F). I remember one woman who said that even opening the refrigerator door triggered her nipple vasospasm—and she was fully clothed.

Many remedies, including warm therapy and medications, have been used. However, authors of *The Breastfeeding Atlas* credit lactation consultant Diana West with the idea of manually squeezing the nipple (**Figure 173**) so that some blood enters into the nipple vasculature, thereby relieving the pain.

Other lactation-related lesions

Like a report of "sore nipples," a report of "white spots" deserves careful investigation and highly organized inspection. Where are the white spots? When did they start? Are they truly white, or might they be more off-white or yellow? What size and shape are the white spots? Where are they in relation to the skin's surface? (Usually at or above, but could perhaps be below the skin's surface.) Does the mother report the lesion to be painful (**Figure 169**) or not painful (**Figure 170**). Does she say that anything—including breastfeeding—exacerbates or alleviates the pain? Does the pain persist after the feeding has ended?

A *bleb* (**Figure 169**) is a blocked (plugged) nipple pore. (It is not to be confused with a *blocked (plugged) duct*, which will be discussed in Chapter 11.) The exact cause is unknown. A bleb is easy to identify because it is a single, solitary white dot on the tip of the nipple and it is less than 1 mm in diameter.[22] (For perspective, consider that most medium-point ball-point pens are about 1 mm in diameter.) The bleb is usually hard and exquisitely painful, especially when the infant suckles. Very rarely, a bleb occurs in the first month or so postpartum, but most appear much later. They often persist for weeks. Some resolve spontaneously; others require intervention by a physician.

A sebaceous cyst might be described as a white spot (although it is likely to be more of a yellow-white). The term *sebaceous cyst*, although widely used in the medical field, is sometimes a bit of a misnomer. The "sebaceous cyst" (**Figure 171**) may or may not qualify as a true sebaceous cyst. A true sebaceous cyst is filled with sebum, but that presumes that the cyst originates from a sebaceous gland. Such glands are located throughout the body, including the areola. *Montgomery glands* are hybrid glands that release both milk and sebum. (Note that the cyst shown is very near to but perhaps not within the Montgomery gland.) When milk gets stuck, rather than being released, an enclosed cyst is formed (**Figure 171).** Like any other gland, Montgomery glands may become inflamed (**Figure 177**) or infected (**Figure 176**).

The "white spot" shown in **Figure 170** defies explanation. The mother denied pain or symptoms of a blocked duct, so we must rely on what we can see. I agree with authors Wilson-Clay and Hoover that the lesion's lack of symmetry rules out a bleb. Further, their rule-out can be confirmed by the size of the white spot. Admittedly, it's difficult to judge from photo, but this "white spot" appears to be much larger than a bleb, which by definition is <1 mm in diameter. There's more to learn and ponder here, though!

Within the areola are the apocrine sweat glands and Montgomery glands. Typically, there are some 1-20 such glands within the areola, and this woman appears to have extremely few areolar glands. In a fascinating study, Doucet and colleagues[23] showed that primiparae who have fewer areolar glands are more likely to have a delayed onset in lactation, and their infants are likely to have slower weight gain. We are not told what this woman's parity is, but it's tempting to think that the presence of this "white spot" is somehow related to her delayed onset of lactation and the scarce number of glands within her areola.

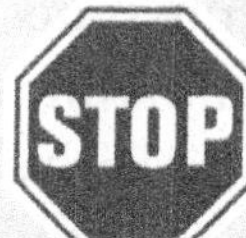

Complete Exercise 8-5 to help you understand conditions that are associated with skin lesions.

Looking Back, Looking Forward

In this chapter, we've looked at four main reasons why lactating mothers have sore nipples, ways to differentiate between the types of lesions, and how to augment that information with relevant interview questions. We've matched characteristics of different types of infectious lesions to their likely causes, and then to examples in the photos. We've seen how, by matching lesions to the right strategies, we can help to resolve such problems or refer them to someone who can. And, oh, did we ever take on a *huge* vocabulary list for all of this!

Evidence in the education field shows that writing your own summary helps your retention. The Summarize What You've Learned exercise helps you to do this, so take just a few minutes to complete that exercise now.

By now, if you have carefully viewed the images on pages 175-180 of *The Breastfeeding Atlas*, and if you've completed the written exercises here, you should feel confident that you can determine a corrective strategy for nipple lesions based on precise clues that best indicate one of three main causes: physiologic tenderness; latch-related or pump-related trauma; immune reaction; or infection) and what to do about it.

Recalling, Reinforcing, and Expanding Your Learning

Have you ever felt frustrated that you "learned" something, but later, can't recall it? That may be because you didn't reinforce the material you learned. And, perhaps what you originally learned isn't enough to get you through the next few decades of practice; sometimes you need to expand your learning. The exercises in this section are designed to help you recall, reinforce, and expand your learning.

What was your main motivation for reading this chapter?

- ❍ To study for the IBLCE exam, as a first-time candidate
- ❍ To review for the IBLCE exam, as a re-certificant
- ❍ To improve my clinical skills and clinical management

How soon do you think can use the information presented in this chapter?

- ❍ Immediately; within the next few days or so
- ❍ Soon; within the next month or so
- ❍ Later; sometime before I retire

Pro Tip! If you are preparing for the IBLCE exam, it would be wise to pace your studying. Set a target date for when you plan to complete the exercises, and check off them off as you go along.

Done!	Target Date	Learning Exercise
❑	________	Learning Exercise 8-1. Matching common skin lesions to their description.
❑	________	Learning Exercise 8-2. Recognizing prefixes, roots, and words.
❑	________	Learning Exercise 8-3. Identifying those "white spots" on nipples.
❑	________	Learning Exercise 8-4. Comparison of herpes and impetigo lesions.
❑	________	Learning Exercise 8-5. Conditions associated with skin lesions.
❑	________	Explore What You've Learned in a Journal
❑	________	Summarize What You've Learned
❑	________	Quick Quiz

Master Your Vocabulary

Learning Exercise 8-1. Matching common skin lesion to their descriptions.

Instructions: Write the letter of the correct match next to each item. Answers are in the Appendix.

Q 1. abrasion
T 2. bleb
F 3. blister
B 4. compression stripe
O 5. crusts
S 6. cyst
R 7. erosion
P 8. erythema
J 9. excoriation
M 10. fissures
L 11. hives
C 12. keloid
N 13. lesion
I 14. maceration
D 15. plaque
G 16. scale
K 17. ulcer
E 18. urticaria
H 19. vesicle
A 20. wheal

A. raised area, with color changes and edema in the upper layers of the epidermis
B. long, linear discoloration of the tip of the nipple
C. late-appearing proliferation of skin that extends beyond the edges of the wound
D. solid, raised lesion with a flat-topped shape that is greater than 1 cm in diameter
E. one type is the hive
F. filled with clear fluid, and characterized by with clearly-defined borders often due to excessive negative pressure
G. heaped-up layers of the outer layer of skin
H. less than 1 cm elevation of the skin that contains liquid that forms on the skin's surface and then enlarges, breaks open, and then becomes ulcerated
I. "water-logged" skin
J. serous fluid through all or part of the dermis; almost always develops after a blister or pustule ruptures
K. depression in the tissue that goes down from the dermis into the hypodermis
L. a type of wheal; red and itchy after an allergic reaction
M. thin, linear tear usually in the epidermis
N. a discontinuity of tissue or loss of function to a body part
O. formed by blood, pus, and/or serum on the skin's surface
P. redness
Q. rubbing, scraping or wearing down of the epidermis
R. wider than a fissure and located only in the epidermis
S. an abnormal membrane sac that contains a semi-solid, liquid, or gaseous material
T. solitary white dot on the tip of the nipple that is less than 1 mm in diameter

Learning Exercise 8-2. Recognizing prefixes, roots, and words.

Instructions: Memorize the prefixes and suffixes below. They are often used in medical terminology. Then, uses that prefix or suffix in the left-most column write a word that appears in this chapter (or other chapters) that best illustrates the use of that or suffix.

Prefix/Suffix	Meaning	Word in this chapter (or other) chapter
-ema, emia	blood	erythema
-itis	inflammation	mastitis dermatitis
-osis	condition or disease	prognosis, diagnosis, ecchymosis
-phasic	having phases	biphasic
a-	not; without	atypical, asymptomatic
ab-	away from	abnormal
aller-	denoting something as different	allergy
anti-	against	antifungal, antibiotic
bi-	twice; double	biphasic
cya-	blue color	cyanosis
cutane-	skin (Latin)	subcutaneous
derm-	skin (Greek)	epidermis, subdermis
ec(t)-	out, away	telectasia
epi-	on; upon	epidermis
erythr(o)-	redness or being flushed	erythemia
hist-	tissue	histamine
hyper	above	hyperpigmentation
hypo	beneath	hypodermis
necr(o)-	death	necrotic
ser-, sero-	watery; fluid	serous
tri	three	triphasic
-ule	small, diminutive	nodule
urt-	herbaceous plant with jagged leaves and stinging hairs	urticaria
vas(o)-	duct; blood vessel	vasoconstriction
-ema, emia	blood	erythemia

Conquer Clinical Concepts

Learning Exercise 8-3. Identifying those "white spots" on nipples.

Instructions: Look carefully at the white spot shown in **Figure 170**. *Give three reasons why this does NOT look like yeast.*

- Round in shape.
  White plaque from yeast is more likely to follow skin crevices.

- Not raised off skin.

- ~~Te~~ Texture is not velvity

Learning Exercise 8-4. Comparison of herpes and impetigo lesions.

Instructions: Use a word or a short phrase to describe the lesions found in these diseases.

	Herpes	Impetigo
Lesion type (appearance)	clustered vesicles	clustered vesticles followed by honey colored crusts
Lesion distribution	lip, nose face	lip, nose face, breasts
Lesion size	<1cm	<1cm
Associated sensation	tingling itching painful	itchy painless
Causative pathogen	Viral Herpes Simplex	Bacterial: Strep or Staph
Effectively resolved with…	antiretroviral tx	abx
Recurrent?	Signs/symptoms recur	unlikely
Contagious?	Highly	Highly
Transmission	Direct contact sexual oral Droplet autotransmission	Direct contact (touching) Indirect contact inanimate objects surfaces

Learning Exercise 8-5. Conditions associated with skin lesions.

Instructions: Match the condition to its description.

G 1. blocked (plugged) nipple pore

F 2. candidiasis

A 3. contact dermatitis eczema

C 4. hand, foot, and mouth disease

D 5. herpes simplex virus (HSV)

E 6. impetigo

H 7. Raynaud disease (Raynaud phenomenon)

B 8. Paget disease

A. occurs when the skin is exposed to an irritant, resulting in inflammation and damage

B. cancerous lesion of the nipple skin

C. viral infection with acral distribution of the erythematous, maculopapular rash

D. viral infection with vesicles with visible fluid, often configured in a cluster

E. highly contagious bacterial infection that is around nose and mouth, in which lesions rupture, ooze for a few days, then form a yellow-brown crust

F. fungal infection that is commonly found on the mouth, nipples, or vagina

G. identifiable by a solitary white dot of less than 1 mm in diameter on the tip of the nipple

H. autoimmune disease that has a biphasic or triphasic discoloration of the nipples due to vasoconstriction

Explore What You've Learned in a Journal

Multiple studies have shown the benefits of using a learning journal. Among them are greater assimilation and integration of new information, better long-term retention of course concepts, increasing test and exam grades, and a means by which to have continuous feedback about one's own learning.

- Name at least three things you learned from this chapter.

- List at least three things you still need to learn, or more fully master, in this chapter.

- Briefly describe how this information fits (or doesn't fit) with what you've seen in clinical practice, what you learned in basic or college courses, or what you've observed in your own experience breastfeeding. (In some cases, you might want to include how the information fits or doesn't fit with what "experts" say, what the media says, or whatever.)

- Describe how you will use any or all of this information. How might it be related to problems and potential solutions that occur in real life or in clinical situations?

- If you wish, include how you felt about learning this information. Were you overwhelmed? Enlightened? Frustrated? Worried? Something else?

Summarize What You've Learned

The goal of this chapter was to help you determine a corrective strategy for nipple lesions based on precise clues that best indicate one of four main causes: physiologic tenderness, latch-related or pump-related trauma, immune reaction, or infection) and what to do about it.

Instructions: Write your own summary of what you just learned in this chapter.

What are four main reasons for "sore nipples"?	
Given those four main reasons, jot a few "clues" of the most common types of lesions associated with each.	
When systematically looking at a lesion, what sorts of descriptors would you be sure to observe?	
Quick, quick! Just write the commonly-encountered lesions that may be present in a lactating mother.	
For which lesions would it be MOST important to refer to a physician?	
What 10 terms did you encounter that were new to you (or maybe, terms that you had never really understood but have more fully mastered?)	1. 2. 3. 4. 5. 6. 7. 8. 9. 10.

Self-Assessment

People often dive into a test before they have thoughtfully reflected on how well they have prepared for it. Instead, it would be helpful if they would take a few moments to give their alter-ego (their "other self") at chance to reflect on how confident they feel about mastering the stated objectives.

Instructions: Take a moment to review the chapter objectives (below). Then rate yourself. How confident are you that you have achieved each objective below?

Objective	Highly Confident	Somewhat Confident	Somewhat Unsure	Completely Unsure
Classify multiple images of "sore nipples" as being caused or complicated by one of four main reasons.	❍	❍	❍	❍
Gather and interpret distinguishing data about nipple lesions and their relationship to layers of the epidermis, dermis, and hypodermis.	❍	❍	❍	❍
Describe 11 different primary lesions in terms of size, flat or raised, solid or fluid-filled, involved skin layers, diameter, and shape, and several examples of each that might be seen on the breast.	❍	❍	❍	❍
Match commonly-seen nipple/breast lesions to a commonly-used strategy to prevent, minimize, or treat such lesions.	❍	❍	❍	❍
Recognize lesions that can be resolved with simple treatments, and those that require referral for medical help.	❍	❍	❍	❍
State the definitions of at least 50 terms related to nipple lesions.	❍	❍	❍	❍

On the next page, you will some simple recall questions pertaining to this chapter. These are *not* the application-type questions you will find in the IBLCE exam. However, you cannot *apply* information unless you can fully *recall* that information! You should do these without looking up the answers.

When you finish with the quiz, look up the answers in the Appendix. Then, score your answers, using the Appendix. Finally, you should analyze the results of your quiz. It's not enough to just know what you got right or wrong; you must look at why you got the answers right or wrong.

Quick Quiz Chapter 8

Circle the correct response. For a better understanding of how well you are mastering the material, try answering without looking it up. If you are really stuck, questions come from this workbook and from *The Breastfeeding Atlas,* so go back and review the appropriate material. Answers are in the Appendix.

1. Of these lesions, which is almost always associated with an infection?
   - A. macule
   - B. nodule
   - C. papule
   - D. pustule

2. A white, painful spot occurs on the tip of the mother's nipple during and after she finishes breastfeeding. She denies itching or burning. Her pregnancy and birth history are unremarkable. Management of this problem is MOST likely to focus on resolving what condition?
   - A. bleb
   - B. candidiasis
   - C. nipple vasospasm
   - D. sebaceous cyst

3. Which of these descriptors applies to a herpes lesion, but not to a lesion associated with hand, foot, and mouth disease?
   - A. acral distribution
   - B. elevated from skin surface
   - C. highly contagious
   - D. tightly-clustered lesions

4. Oral thrush can occur anywhere in the mouth, but of the locations listed below, the LEAST likely location is
   - A. in the throat
   - B. inside of the cheeks
   - C. inside of the lips
   - D. on the tongue

5. **Figure 149** is most likely due to:
   - A. blocked nipple pore
   - B. candidiasis
   - C. poor latch
   - D. poorly-fitting flange

Analyze Your Own Quiz

- What percentage of the questions did you answer correctly?

- If you got 100% of them right, to what do you attribute your success?

- If you did not get all the questions right, can you identify your learning gap? (Example: Didn't know the information, knew the information but could not remember, knew some information but confused it with similar information, other.)

- Would you have been able to answer the questions as well if you had not read this chapter?

- What do you need to do next? (If you got them all right, what you need to do next is celebrate! Even a high-five with your child, a YESSS and a fist-pump in the air, or anything else is good! A small acknowledgement of your success is better than no acknowledgement!)

Additional Resources

1. Biancuzzo M. Sore Nipples: Prevention & Problem-Solving 2016.
2. Fernandez R, Griffiths R. Water for wound cleansing. *Cochrane Database Syst Rev.* 2012(2):Cd003861.
3. Gunther M. Sore nipples, causes and prevention. *Lancet.* 1945;249:590-593.
4. Sakalidis VS, et al. A comparison of early sucking dynamics during breastfeeding after cesarean section and vaginal birth. *Breastfeed Med.* 2013;8(1):79-85.
5. L'Esperance C. Pain or pleasure: the dilemma of early breastfeeding. *Birth Fam J.* 1980;7(1):21-25.
6. Hewat RJ, Ellis DJ. A comparison of the effectiveness of two methods of nipple care. *Birth.* 1987;14(1):41-45.
7. Coca KP, et al. Factors associated with nipple trauma in the maternity unit. *J Pediatr (Rio J).* 2009;85(4):341-345.
8. Gokoo C. A Primer on Wound Bed Preparation. *The Journal of the American College of Certified Wound Specialists.* 2009;1(1):35-39.
9. Morland-Schultz K, Hill PD. Prevention of and therapies for nipple pain: a systematic review. *J Obstet Gynecol Neonatal Nurs.* 2005;34(4):428-437.
10. Dennis CL, et al. Interventions for treating painful nipples among breastfeeding women. *Cochrane Database Syst Rev.* 2014(12):Cd007366.
11. Marrazzu A, et al. Evaluation of the effectiveness of a silver-impregnated medical cap for topical treatment of nipple fissure of breastfeeding mothers. *Breastfeed Med.* 2015;10(5):232-238.
12. Maley AM, Arbiser JL. Gentian violet: a 19th century drug re-emerges in the 21st century. *Experimental dermatology.* 2013;22(12):775-780.
13. Field SS. Fatal Neonatal Herpes Simplex Infection Likely from Unrecognized Breast Lesions. *J Hum Lact.* 2016;32(1):86-88.
14. Bae YS, et al. Review of treatment options for psoriasis in pregnant or lactating women: from the Medical Board of the National Psoriasis Foundation. *J Am Acad Dermatol.* 2012;67(3):459-477.
15. Barrett ME, et al. Raynaud phenomenon of the nipple in breastfeeding mothers: an underdiagnosed cause of nipple pain. *JAMA dermatology (Chicago, Ill.).* 2013;149(3):300-306.
16. Queille Roussel C, et al. A prospective computerized study of 500 cases of atopic dermatitis in childhood. I. Initial analysis of 250 parameters. *Acta-Derm-Venereol-Suppl-Stockh.* 1985;114:87-92.
17. Coates MM. Nipple pain related to vasospasm in the nipple? *J Hum Lact.* 1992;8(3):153.

18. Lawlor-Smith L, Lawlor-Smith C. Vasospasm of the nipple--a manifestation of Raynaud's phenomenon: case reports [see comments]. *Bmj.* 1997;314(7081):644-645.

19. Page SM, McKenna DS. Vasospasm of the nipple presenting as painful lactation. *Obstet Gynecol.* 2006;108(3 Pt 2):806-808.

20. Buck ML, et al. Nipple pain, damage, and vasospasm in the first 8 weeks postpartum. *Breastfeed Med.* 2014;9(2):56-62.

21. McGuinness N, Cording V. Raynaud's phenomenon of the nipple associated with labetalol use. *J Hum Lact.* 2013;29(1):17-19.

22. Lawrence R, Lawrence, RM. *Breastfeeding: A guide for the medical profession.* 8 ed 2016.

23. Doucet S, et al. An overlooked aspect of the human breast: Areolar glands in relation with breastfeeding pattern, neonatal weight gain, and the dynamics of lactation. *Early Human Development.*88(2):119-128.

Chapter 9
9-Congenital and Acquired Variations of the Breasts and Nipples

There is a clear mandate to assess the mother's breasts during pregnancy.[1] Many of us won't see the woman until she is breastfeeding, but we still need to assess her breasts. In either situation, we need to know what's a variation of normal, and what that might mean for breastfeeding and lactation.

Human breasts come in a variety of shapes, sizes and other characteristics. Most are sure to be considered "normal," but there are many conditions that may affect a woman's ability to breastfeed, or her experience of breastfeeding. Consequently, we need to know how to assess the mother's breasts and counsel her about her anatomical variances as part of our support of the breastfeeding dyad. But there many variances, aren't there?

Even if you've had many years of experience, you might not be able to recognize or document certain conditions. Is it macromastia or hypermastia? Micromastia or hypoplasia? And if you struggle to remember the difference between amazia, athelia, and amastia, maybe it's time for you to master all of this, and much more!

I promise that by the time you finish this chapter, you will be able to recognize characteristics of multiple congenital and acquired nipple/breast variations and their implications for clinical breastfeeding management.

By viewing the photos on pages 179-181 of *The Breastfeeding Atlas*, and by completing the learning exercises here, you'll be able to master all of that! So hang on tight, and come take this ride with me!

Objectives

Given a clinical photo, you will be able to:

- State the definition for at least 25 terms related to structural variations of the breasts.
- Recognize visual clues of multiple congenital or acquired breast tissue variations and how (or if) they will affect breastfeeding and lactation.
- Distinguish between anatomical breast variations that have similar appearances but are in fact different in terms of their underlying causes and implications for breastfeeding and lactation.
- Suggest techniques to ensure optimal milk transfer with selected anatomic variations.

Key Words

- accessory nipples
- amastia
- amazia
- athelia
- axilla
- congenital
- corpus mammae
- double nipples
- ecchymosis
- ectopic nipples
- flaccid, flaccidity
- genetic
- granulation tissue
- hyperadenia
- hypermastia
- hyperplasia, hyperplastic
- hyperthelia
- hypomastia
- hypoplasia, hypoplastic
- infrasubmammary, submammary
- keyhole incision
- lesion
- macromastia
- mammoplasty
- micromastia
- Montgomery glands
- periareolar
- polythelia
- striae gravidarum
- supernumerary
- symmastia
- tail of Spence
- tubular breasts

Assessment of the Corpus Mammae

Anything that can happen to a nonpregnant, nonbreastfeeding woman (such as an injury) can also happen during pregnancy and lactation. But those topics are outside the scope of this chapter. The discussion in this chapter focuses on conditions of the human breast as they relate to pregnancy and/or breastfeeding and lactation.

Like all other glands in the body, the mammary gland begins to develop during fetal life. Therefore, variations of normal or more serious issues are present at birth. Conditions that are present since birth are called *congenital.**

Congenital conditions that directly affect breastfeeding include inverted nipples and extra nipples, as discussed in Chapter 7. There are several other conditions, however, and their descriptive terms are frequently misused. The most accurate source for correct terminology is found in Lawrence & Lawrence.[2 p. 40]

Amastia is a unilateral or bilateral condition in which the mammary gland and possibly the nipple are absent.[3]

---

* Many people confused the word *congenital* with the word *genetic*. *Congenital* means that a condition is present at birth or appears shortly afterwards, and that it may or may not lessen or change over time. *Genetic* means that a condition is passed through the genes; most are life-long and can be managed but not cured (e.g., sickle cell disease, Tay-Sachs disease, ventricular septal defect).

Amazia is a condition in which the breast is absent but the nipple is present, which can result from radiation therapy and is therefore not congenital.

Athelia is lack of a nipple on a breast.

Hyperadenia is mammary tissue without a nipple which is also referred to as *hypermastia*.

Symmastia is webbing between the breasts, at the midline. Breastfeeding is entirely possible.

During preadolescence, the breasts begin to enlarge in the human female. As the breast tissue continues to change over the next several years, congenital conditions that may have been overlooked at birth may become more obvious. Congenital conditions of the breasts are not caused by the event of pregnancy or lactation, but they can affect lactation.

Early in the first trimester of pregnancy, hormones cause the ductular and lobular structures of the mammary gland to proliferate. As lactogenesis progresses internally, external changes become more visible. Because the upper outer quadrant of the woman's breast has the greatest amount of glandular tissue, enlargement in this area is especially noticeable. After delivery, changes occur in the size and contour of the breast.

Many people confuse the *corpus mammae* (that is, the body of the breast) with nearby structures. More commonly known as the armpit, the *axilla* is space below the shoulder through which vessels and nerves enter and leave the upper arm. The *tail of Spence* (Spence's tail, axillary tail) is not actually in the body of the breast, but rather, it is an extension of mammary tissue into the axilla.

As described in Chapter 5, physiologic engorgement occurs around the third day after delivery. It is a normal and reassuring sign (as opposed to absence of physiologic engorgement during lactogenesis, which is a non-reassuring sign). Engorgement tends to extend beyond the corpus mammae and into the axilla (**Figure 182**). This is common. It can occur anywhere that mammary tissue is located.

Hyperadenia i.e., *hypermastia*—a congenital condition of extra mammary tissue, a remnant of tissue anywhere along the galactic band—can occur in the axilla (**Figure 183**) and may or may not be accompanied by an extra nipple. If there is excessive mammary tissue in the axilla, it is likely to become engorged, especially if there is no outlet for the milk, and mastitis can occur. Sometimes, there is no nipple (**Figure 183**, **Figure 184, and 185**). These remnants are not connected to the primary breasts.

To distinguish between a breast with a normal amount of mammary tissue extending into the axilla and hypermastia, look at several clues, including location, color, leaking, and timing. Note that in **Figure 182**, the tissue looks to be most distended on the mother's chest and less distended in the axilla. This is normal engorgement.

If milk is leaking, mammary tissue is present. (However, note that the reverse is *not* true. Absence of leaking milk does *not mean that mammary tissue is absent.*) The timeline is also a clue. Although it is certainly possible for engorgement to occur at 1 month postpartum (**Figure 183**), such a situation is atypical and unlikely to occur. On the other hand, engorgement at Day 3 is highly likely. Of course, a combination of extra tissue and engorgement (**Figure 184**, **Figure 185**) is also possible.

Size

Hormonal changes should cause the breasts to enlarge during pregnancy. Specifically, luteal and placental hormones during pregnancy stimulate proliferation of the lactiferous ducts and the alveoli. These changes cause the breasts to increase in size, sometimes significantly beyond the mother's pre-pregnancy size.

Changes in the breast size should occur during pregnancy. However, a lack of dramatic changes in the mother's breast size is not immediate cause for alarm. Mothers with physiologically normal but small breasts can produce milk just as well as those with larger breasts.

Micromastia

Micromastia is the medical term for small breasts. Few of us would tell our clients they have "micromastia," for good reason! Heightening a mother's worry about her breast size and ability to breastfeed is pointless. Our role is to recognize the difference between micromastia and *hypoplasia*. Small, or "micromastic" breasts have adequate glandular tissue, but relatively little fat and connective tissue. In contrast, hypoplastic breasts are lacking in glandular tissue. These are key differences.

Underdeveloped Breasts

"Small" breasts might be mistaken for those that are actually underdeveloped. **Figure 191**, **Figure 192**, **Figure 193**, and **Figure 194** all show hypoplasia of the gland. *Hypoplasia* (from the Greek, *hypo-* "under" + *plasis* "formation") is underdevelopment or incomplete development of any tissue or organ. Originally termed "insufficient glandular tissue" development by Dr. Marianne Neifert[4], hypoplasia that affects the mammary gland is called *hypomastia* (referring to the specific gland.) Hypoplastic breasts are often associated with the inability to conceive (**Figure 191**).

How can you determine if it's hypoplasia, or just "small" breasts? **Figure 191** shows a mother with a wide space between her right and left breasts. Admittedly, the size of her breasts is a bit difficult to determine from the photo, but she has a very wide space between her breasts, which can signal insufficient development. (She is also using a supplemental device, which is an imprecise but possible clue that she does not have enough milk.) In **Figure 192**, there is asymmetry between the breasts, with a marked difference in size between the right and the left breasts. In **Figure 193**, there appears to be little tissue beneath the areola. All of these can be indicators of breast hypoplasia.

Will the mother with breast hypoplasia have enough milk to feed her infant? There's no certain response to this question. The woman in **Figure 191** had a history of infertility and did not go through pregnancy prior to breastfeeding her adopted infant; she was unable to produce enough to exclusively breastfeed the child. The woman in **Figure 193** produced only about eight ounces of milk daily.

Macromastia

Macromastia (**Figure 201, Figure 218**) is the medical term for large breasts. Of course, the term "large" cannot be quantified, since no "normal" breast size has been scientifically established. It's important to realize that breast size tends to be an indicator of the amount of fatty and connective tissue, not the glandular tissue.

Whereas the prefix *macro* means "large" or possibly "long", the prefix *hyper* means "excessive". So large breasts are not referred to as "hyper" anything. You may have heard of *hyperplasia* in pathology reports about breasts. That means there is growth of cells within the ducts and/or lobules of the breast that is not cancerous. Simply stated, hyperplasia is about the unseen glandular tissue, not fatty and connective tissue that make the breasts appear large. Try not to confuse hyperplasia, which unseen, with *hyperadenia*, which is visible.

Be careful not to confuse "engorged" breasts—which are larger temporarily due to physiologic changes of breastfeeding—with large, or macromastic, breasts. Engorgement makes the breasts larger than their baseline size; with macromastia, the largeness *is* the baseline. Compare the features of macromastia in **Figure 218** in this chapter with the features of an engorged breast in **Figure 240** and **Figure 241** shown in Chapter 11.

Clinical Implications for Breastfeeding with Macromastia

Mothers with macromastia should be reassured that—absent any serious glandular problem—they can successfully breastfeed.

Large breasts do not necessarily produce more milk. The external size of the breast is determined more by the fat and connective tissue surrounding the gland than by the gland itself. Some opt for breast reduction surgery (*mammoplasty*, sometimes called a mammaplasty or mastoplasty), which can affect a woman's ability to breastfeed.

Mothers with large breasts may find common problems to be exaggerated during lactation. They may have more back aches, neck aches, and tingling in the fingers when their breasts are full of milk, and heavier. Shopping for a correctly-sized bra—difficult for any woman with macromastia—can be even more difficult for women when their breasts are enlarged due to lactation. Often, they settle for a size that is too small, which puts them at risk for plugged ducts and/or mastitis. At some point, most women want or need to breastfeed in public, and those with larger breasts may find it more difficult to do so comfortably.

While suckling their infant, the mother with macromastia may include such difficulties as seeing her infant during the feeding, or trouble with shaping the breast and areola so that her infant can achieve an adequate grasp. Women with especially large breasts often (but not always!) have very short nipples. Also, because there is more tissue, large breasts are heavy, and so the mother needs to make sure the breasts do not rest on the newborn's chest, especially if he is a premature infant or one who is having difficulty breathing.

Complete Learning Exercises 9-1 and 9-2 to help you master the correct terminology.

Helpful Strategies

Please refer to Chapter 6 to review discussion of breastfeeding positions, particularly those that work well for women with large breasts. Trying out different positions is a common step in breastfeeding, regardless of the mother's breast size. Mothers of newborns should be reminded that positions that seem difficult during the first weeks may become easier as their milk supply stabilizes (and engorgement eases), and as their child grows in size and strength. They may find themselves trying different positions throughout their breastfeeding journey.

Mothers with macromastia should be reminded to continue providing firm and consistent support for their infant's head, neck and shoulders for many weeks, because their breast is so large and heavy. My good friend Debi Bocar, RN PhD IBCLC, teaches that such support is necessary until the infant's head is as big as the mother's breast. I agree with that advice, even though some mothers may find that it can be a few months to meet this milestone!

Some mothers, especially those with large breasts and short arms, tire of supporting their breast so often. They may wish to use an infant carrier such as a sling to provide supplemental support during breastfeeding.

I frequently recommend that mothers with macromastia use a washcloth, or even a rolled up receiving blanket or towel, between their breast and torso while breastfeeding to provide support—in addition to their hands. Without adequate support, gravity may pull the nipple out of the newborn's mouth; he may clamp down on the nipple to keep from losing the nipple to gravity's pull. This technique can also help support the breast's weight when the mother is expressing her milk, either by hand or by pump.

Shape

Typically, the shape of the woman's breast remains largely unchanged during her pregnancy. Most often, they could be described as conical, convex, or pendulous. In any of these cases, the shape is unlikely to interfere with the woman's ability to breastfeed. A woman with *hypoplastic breasts*, however, may experience lactation difficulty. **Figure 196** shows a breast shape that could be best described as *tubular* or cylindrical. Many women with tubular breasts are unable to fully lactate.[5]

Upon palpation, normal breast tissue tends to feel somewhat firm during pregnancy or lactation, as you might expect a gland to feel. Breasts that feel soft or malleable might be underdeveloped. Although the term *flaccid* typically refers to weak or hypotonic muscles, it can be used to describe a breast that feels flabby and can be easily compressed (**Figure 197**).

Symmetry

As discussed in Chapter 3, the word symmetry means that corresponding structures are the same on one side as they are on the other side. When corresponding right-left structures are not the same, they are asymmetrical. Normally, breasts should appear more or less symmetrical in size and shape, although research has shown that the underlying structures may not be truly symmetrical.[6].

It is common for the mother's breasts to appear symmetrical before and during pregnancy but become slightly asymmetrical during lactation; sometimes, the mother will complain that she feels "lopsided." This typically indicates that the infant suckles more frequently or more efficiently on one side than on the other. As long as the infant is getting enough milk and growing well, this development is typically harmless. Mothers can be assured that it tends to create temporary wardrobe issues, but many women find their breasts even out over time.

However, marked breast asymmetry is a different matter. It may be the result of atypical breast development in fetal life. If there is not enough breast tissue in one breast, asymmetry results. After puberty, the asymmetry will become apparent.

Whether a woman with asymmetric breasts can produce enough milk for her infant is unpredictable. The mother with asymmetrical breasts in **Figure 194** did not have enough milk, and her infant was diagnosed with failure to thrive. However, the woman with asymmetrical breasts in **Figure 195** had a normal milk supply. Some women who can only breastfeed from one breast (due to prior breast surgery, injury, or another reason) can still exclusively breastfeed their infant; others find they must supplement.

Is there a difference in the amount of milk each breast produces? Yes. Some mothers with asymmetrical breasts, although "nursing" on both sides, provide only a small amount of milk from one breast, and rely on the more well-developed breast for production. Such mothers often find, when pumping, that more milk can be expressed from the larger breast.[7] (Studies have shown differences in milk volume expressed between breasts, even from mothers with visibly "matching" breasts.[7, 8])

It's hard to tell whether differences in production are due to physiological differences, or variance in breastfeeding behavior. Some women who have asymmetrical breasts may feel less confident in their ability to breastfeed successfully, some might overprioritize breastfeeding on the "smaller" side and inadvertently cause a decline in production on the other side. Some might wean early due to health care professionals or others telling them they "can't" breastfeed, and some might never initiate breastfeeding.

When it comes to mothers with asymmetrical breasts, it's important not to rush to draw conclusions about whether they can breastfeed.

General Assessment of the Skin

Assessment of the skin includes making observations about the appearance, color, and pigmentation; texture and tautness; and presence of any lesions on the breast. Healthy breast skin should appear smooth, soft, and intact. Mammary ducts are an internal structure, but **Figure 186** shows that a duct can be very close to the surface of the skin. This duct had a milk pore that enabled milk to drip through the skin.

During pregnancy, *striae gravidarum* (stretch marks) appear in various areas of the woman's body, and these may be especially noticeable at the outer aspects of the breasts. These marks are the result of stretching of the tissue during pregnancy; they are not caused by breastfeeding. While the mother may consider them to be unsightly, they have no effect on breastfeeding.

Texture and Tautness

The skin of the mother's breast should appear to be about the same color as the rest of her torso, and the color of the two breasts should be the same. During the postpartum period, any red streaking could possibly be a sign of infection and therefore requires follow-up. *Ecchymosis* on the nipple/areola, discoloration due to bleeding beneath the skin, is often due to latch-on problems (such as the infant "dragging" down on the nipple/areola).

Vascularity

Vascular changes during pregnancy are significant. During a singleton pregnancy, total body blood volume increases by about 45%, and the richer supply available to the breasts dilates the vessels beneath the skin. Venous congestion may be more obvious in the primigravida. As pregnancy progresses, the skin appears thin and veins are visible just beneath the skin. Venous congestion may be especially evident during engorgement.

Lesions

Lesions on the breast are usually a cause for concern. As you recall from previous chapters, *lesion* is a broad term that might be used to mean a sore, a tumor, a cleft, or damaged skin. In general, lesions on the breast are the result of a congenital issue, pathology, or trauma from a poor attachment or detachment. Especially during the early days of lactation, lesions on the nipples—blisters, fissures, ulcers, and other lesions—are almost always the result of incorrect latch-on. Chapter 8 discusses breast lesions in more detail.

Assessment of the Areola and Areolar Skin

As with assessment of the breast's skin, assessment of the areola includes observations about appearance, color, and pigmentation, and size, shape, and symmetry. Clues for assessment are identified here.

Appearance, Color and Pigmentation

Typically, the areola is centered on the breast. Hair on the areola (**Figure 205**) is normal and harmless. The mother should be cautioned not to pull the hairs out, as the trauma from doing so could lead to infection.

The color of the areola varies according to the color of the woman's skin. Normally, the areola is somewhat lighter in color than the nipple, and it becomes more pigmented during pregnancy and lactation. During the postpartum period, the color of the areola should be only slightly lighter than the color of the nipple; a more noticeable difference may signal a fungal infection.

Once again, pigmentation is an issue. As discussed in Chapter 3, pigmented nevi are birthmarks. It is unusual to find nevi on the nipple or areola, but certainly, it is possible (**Figure 190**).

Size, Shape and Symmetry

The areola on the right breast should be symmetrical to the areola on the left, in terms of size and shape. During pregnancy, the areola typically increases in diameter from about 34 to 50 mm. The *Montgomery glands* (tiny glands within the areola) also become more prominent during pregnancy.

Assessment of the Nipple and Nipple Skin

As with assessment of the breast's skin, assessment of the nipple includes observations about appearance, color, and pigmentation; size and shape of the nipple; symmetry; discharge or secretions; and elasticity. Clues for assessment are identified here; issues of clinical management for nipple size (width and length) are described in Chapter 10, and clinical management for lesions on the nipple are discussed primarily in Chapter 8.

Appearance, Color and Pigmentation

Changes in hormones during pregnancy and lactation cause nipples to become more erectile, and to change in color. While, as a quick thumbing-through of *The Breastfeeding Atlas* shows, there are many different colors that are normal for nipples and areola, a woman's nipple should be only slightly darker than the areola around it. It should also be even in color. In the breastfeeding woman, a white stripe, either vertical or horizontal, signals a poor latch-on. (See Chapter 6 for details on latch-on.)

Other Nipple Variations

Nipple protrusion, and elasticity should be carefully assessed. This was discussed in Chapter 7.

Nipple/Areola Size/Shape

Usually, the nipple is round, and located in the center of the areola. However, this is not always the case. In **Figure 206**, both the nipple and the areola have a somewhat oval shape. The nipple is not centered top-to-bottom. Predictably, this mother was able to breastfeed her infant using the cradle hold, but not the football hold. To grasp an oval-shaped nipple/areola complex, positioning must be such that it allows, as Wilson-Clay and Hoover explain in *The Breastfeeding Atlas*, "the widest span of the nipple [to be] between the corners of the baby's mouth" (page 75). An unusual nipple/areola shape might generate an interesting item on the IBLCE exam; remember that an unusual nipple shape does not preclude breastfeeding, but may well need a special management technique.

Small, short, and flat nipples were described in Chapter 7. Wide, long, or elongated nipples will be discussed in Chapter 10.

Note and document these and other observations in the record. In most cases, you can remain optimistic that these variations will require little or no special breastfeeding management.

"Extra" Nipples

I have seen multiple terms for "extra" nipples. Any of these are correct, and might be used by health care providers you encounter:

- *Accessory* nipples or accessory tissue – meaning extra, supplementary or subsidiary to the primary; this is the term preferred by *The Breastfeeding Atlas*
- *Ectopic* nipples – meaning arising from or produced at a site where it would not usually be
- *Hyperthelia* – from *hyper-* meaning excessive or above normal and *thelia* meaning nipple
- *Polythelia* – from *poly-* meaning many and *thelia* meaning nipple tissue
- *Supernumerary* nipples—from *super-* meaning above or beyond, and *numerary* meaning number

The presence of one or more accessory nipples is a congenital condition. Although they could be anywhere on the mother's body, most accessory nipples develop along the milk line—that is, in the underarm area, above the nipples, at the bra band, or along the waistband. **Figure 187** shows one at the bra band, and **Figure 189** shows it at anatomical right. Typically, an accessory nipple looks like a big mole (**Figure 187**), and it may have been mistakenly identified as a mole. In most cases, such nipples appear on one side only, but they can be on both sides, as in **Figure 188** and **Figure 189**. Sometimes, the accessory nipple is surrounded by an areola (**Figure 188, Figure 189**). I don't know of any official statistics on accessory nipples, but in light of clinical experience, I estimate that about half of the mothers who have supernumerary nipples experience leaking.

Although one could make the case that they are technically the same, I would argue that *double nipples* (**Figure 207**) are different from isolated accessory nipples. First, they are in close proximity to one another, and each nipple looks very much like the other in terms of size, shape, and so forth. I think it's fair to say that many double nipples secrete milk. Management of a double nipple differs from the more commonly-seen extra nipples in that the aim is to get the infant to latch by grasping the areola and both nipples. A wide gape (as described in Chapter 6) while important for all newborns, is critical for the infant who is trying to latch in this situation.

Complete Learning Exercise 9-3 to help you recognize how congenital variations might lactation.

Surgery and Related Issues

Mammoplasty (also called *mammaplasty* or *mastoplasty*) is the term for surgery on the breast to modify its shape or appearance. It may be either for augmentation or reduction, for reconstructive or cosmetic purposes. It may also be done for therapeutic purposes. An increasing number of articles have been written about adolescents who seek mammoplasty, so anticipatory guidance is becoming increasingly critical for patients (or their guardians) before consenting to surgery.

In past decades, breast surgery was a death knell for future breastfeeding. More recent literature has shown that it is possible, in some cases, to have surgery and go on to experience successful lactation. It depends on the type of surgical incision used, and the details of the surgery. The specifics of mammoplasty are outside the scope of this publication. In general, whether the incision interrupts innervation to the nipple is a critical determinant of whether women can successfully breastfeed at a future date. West's book[9] has drawings of several different types of incisions, with detailed explanations of each.

Breast Augmentation

Traditionally, breast implants can be inserted in the axilla, under the breast (called *submammary* or *infrasubmammary*), or *periareolar* (along the edge of the areola) regions (**Figure 198**). More recently, implants have been inserted through an incision in the umbilicus. Breast augmentation is frequently accomplished through a periareolar incision.

In counseling a mother who has had breast augmentation, you will want to ask what type of incision was used and how the surgery has affected her sensation of the nipple, areola, and breast. The primary innervation for breastfeeding is at the fourth, fifth, and sixth intercostal nerves.

The woman in **Figure 198** breastfed her first child successfully, and then had breast augmentation surgery. After the surgery, she had decreased nipple sensation. When she began breastfeeding another child some years later, she was unable to sense a poor latch, which resulted in damage to her nipple tissue.

Interestingly, the woman in **Figure 199** also had a periareolar incision with silicone implants. However, her surgeon was careful to avoid interrupting the primary nerves to the nipple. As seen in the photo, she had a spontaneous milk ejection reflex. She breastfed her child successfully, and even donated milk to a local milk bank!

Breastfeeding mothers with breast implants should be made aware of the possibility of rupture of the implant. Should this happen, an abscess can form, as shown in **Figure 200**. As explained in *The Breastfeeding Atlas*, the mother in **Figure 200** received unhelpful advice—including the recommendation that she abruptly wean her infant from breastfeeding. Thankfully, the lactation consultant offered several alternatives, including unilateral breastfeeding.

Breast Reduction

Typically, breast reduction surgery is done with the so-called *keyhole* incision or technique, as shown in a YouTube video from the Bergman Clinics [https://www.youtube.com/watch?v=PjwJE2wi18U] Here, a woman with macromastia (**Figure 201**) had reduction mammoplasty, and the incision is indicative of the usual surgery (**Figure 202**).

Diagnostic and Therapeutic Surgical Procedures

Surgery on the breast may also be done for diagnostic or therapeutic purposes. For example, the mother in **Figure 203** had a cancerous lump removed. Note the bronze color of her skin that results from the radiation therapy. There are a few published anecdotal reports about lactation success after radiation, but most lactation consultants have found that women are unable to exclusively breastfeed post-radiation treatment, perhaps due to changes in the breast tissue. A substantial decrease in milk volume in this population has been proven[10] and that implies that exclusive breastfeeding is unlikely.

To minimize the effects on future lactation, any incision for a biopsy should be made away from the areola. Note that the breast in **Figure 204** has a somewhat "empty" look, since this woman recently weaned a six-year old child. With time, she will regain the tissue she has lost, and will likely have a more normal appearance.

Various types of surgery and trauma can affect breastfeeding. **Figure 212** shows a mother with a scar from open-heart surgery that occurred during her early childhood; her ability to lactate was impaired, presumably due to interruption of the breast and related tissue. In my role as a nurse caring for critically ill infants, I assisted with insertion of chest tubes. There, I saw first-hand that even with deliberate attempts to avoid the breast and nipple area, inserting a chest tube in a small or premature newborn can affect these areas; the structures are all close to one another. It may be that lactation is affected by such early-life procedures.

Figure 213 shows a scar in a mother's axilla, which resulted from the treatment for hidradenitis (inflammation of sweat gland) by removing some of her axillary lymph glands. The woman's surgery was performed nine years prior to the photograph. Although she experienced minor problems, she had excellent management suggestions, and continued to breastfeed.

Cosmetic breast procedures

Nipple piercings have grown in popularity in recent years (**Figure 208**). **Figure 209** shows a nipple that had been pierced, but in which the jewelry was later removed. The nipple had only partial healing, as shown by the *granulation* tissue, consisting of connective tissue cells and ingrowing young vessels. Here, the mother is 9 months postpartum, and milk is leaking through the site where the tissue was pierced; otherwise, lactation was unremarkable. Interestingly, I recall a case that was seemingly the opposite; the woman was still breastfeeding a three-year old, and had removed her jewelry immediately after the birth of her infant; 3 years later, she still had some thick scarring in its place. It's difficult to tell how these things will work out.

A tattoo (**Figure 215**) consists of ink that goes into the dermis. Tattooing is a notoriously painful process, but, as Wilson-Clay and Hoover point out, tattoos do not affect breastfeeding and lactation. The biggest concern is the needles used to spread the ink. As with any procedure that uses needles, bloodborne diseases are a possible risk.

Looking Back, Looking Forward

In this chapter, we've talked about assessment of the corpus, the areola and areolar skin, the nipple and nipple skin, and finally, surgery and related issues. All were shown in photos in *The Breastfeeding* pages 179-181.

Evidence in the education field shows that writing your own summary helps your retention. The Summarize What You've Learned exercise helps you to do this, so take just a few minutes to complete that exercise now.

By now, if you have viewed the photos carefully, and if you've completed the written exercises, you should feel confident that you can recognize characteristics of multiple congenital and acquired nipple/breast variations and their implications for clinical breastfeeding management.

Recalling, Reinforcing, and Expanding Your Learning

Have you ever felt frustrated that you "learned" something, but later, can't recall it? That may be because you didn't reinforce the material you learned. And, perhaps what you originally learned isn't enough to get you through the next few decades of practice; sometimes you need to expand your learning. The exercises in this section are designed to help you recall, reinforce, and expand your learning.

What was your main motivation for reading this chapter?

- ❍ To study for the IBLCE exam, as a first-time candidate
- ❍ To review for the IBLCE exam, as a re-certificant
- ❍ To improve my clinical skills and clinical management

How soon do you think can use the information presented in this chapter?

- ❍ Immediately; within the next few days or so
- ❍ Soon; within the next month or so
- ❍ Later; sometime before I retire

Pro Tip! If you are preparing for the IBLCE exam, it would be wise to pace your studying. Set a target date for when you plan to complete the exercises, and check off them off as you go along.

Done!	Target Date	Learning Exercise
❑	________	Learning Exercise 9-1. Vocabulary for selected anatomical variations.
❑	________	Learning Exercise 9-2. The meaning of terms related to congenital variations in breasts/nipples.
❑	________	Learning Exercise 9-3. Impact of congenital variations on lactation.
❑	________	Explore What You've Learned in a Journal
❑	________	Summarize What You've Learned
❑	________	Quick Quiz

Master Your Vocabulary

Unless you know the meaning of a word, you cannot fully answer a question about it. There were many, many terms in this chapter; you might not need to know them all, but you never know which ones you'll need to know!

Instructions: Write the letter of the correct match next to each item. Answers are in the Appendix.

Learning Exercise 9-1. Vocabulary for selected anatomical variations.

F	1. axilla	A.	along the outline of the pigmented region surrounding the nipple
H	2. congenital	B.	discoloration due to bleeding beneath the skin
E	3. corpus mammae	C.	incision around the areola, with vertical downward scar to horizontal scar in the breast crease (underwire area.)
B	4. ecchymosis	D.	condition that is passed through the genes
D	5. genetic	E.	the body of the breast
I	6. granulation tissue	F.	space below the shoulder
C	7. keyhole incision	G.	stretch marks during pregnancy
L	8. mammoplasty	H.	condition is present at birth or appears shortly afterwards
J	9. Montgomery glands	I.	consisting of connective tissue cells and ingrowing young vessels
A	10. periareolar	J.	glands that are visible on the surface of the areola
G	11. striae gravidarum	K.	incision beneath the breast
K	12. submammary	L.	refers to either reduction or augmentation surgery

Learning Exercise 9-2. The meaning of terms related to congenital variations in breasts/nipples

Instructions: Make a simple line drawing to illustrate the meaning of each word below.

amastia mammary gland and possibly the nipple are absent
amazia (also amasia) breast is absent but nipple is present
athelia lack of nipple
hyperadenia, hypermastia extra mammary glands (observable)
hyperplasia, hyperplastic growth of cells within the ducts and/or lobules; this is internal can't be observed
hypomastia hypoplasia that affects the mammary glands
hypoplasia, hypoplastic any gland that is lacking in normal amount of tissue
macromastia large breasts with normal glandular tissue
symmastia web like appearance

Conquer Clinical Concepts

Learning Exercise 9-3. Impact of congenital variations on lactation.

Instructions: Hopefully, you are now able to recognize visual clues of congenital variations in breast tissue. Although recognition is important, the clinical question is, how does this affect breastfeeding, if at all?

This is a learning exercise, not a predictor of actual clinical outcomes! Exclusive or non-exclusive breastfeeding would depend on many factors, including whether one or both breasts were affected. However, to help yourself understand the relative impact of each condition, plot these terms along a continuum:

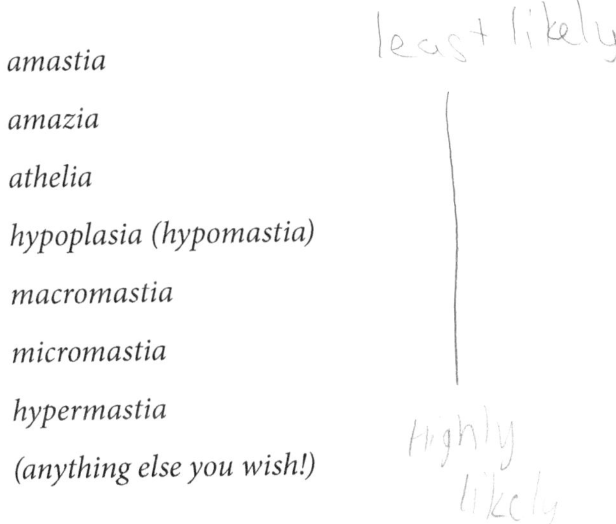

amastia

amazia

athelia

hypoplasia (hypomastia)

macromastia

micromastia

hypermastia

(anything else you wish!)

On the left, write conditions that are least likely to result in exclusive breastfeeding. In the middle, write the conditions that have a moderate likelihood. On right, name conditions that are most likely to result in exclusive breastfeeding.

Likelihood of Exclusive Breastfeeding

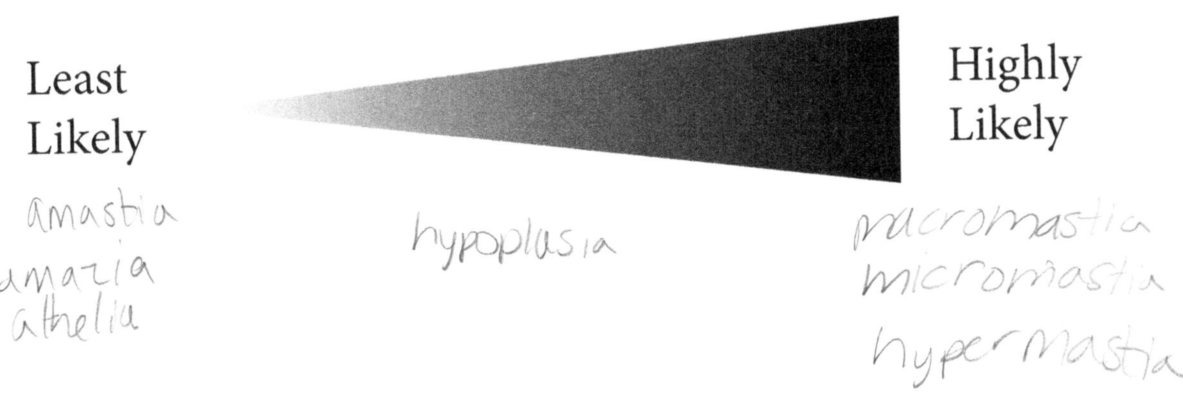

Explore What You've Learned in a Journal

Multiple studies have shown the benefits of using a learning journal. Among them are greater assimilation and integration of new information, better long-term retention of course concepts, increasing test and exam grades, and a means by which to have continuous feedback about one's own learning.

- Name at least three things you learned from this chapter.

- List at least three things you still need to learn, or more fully master, in this chapter.

- Briefly describe how this information fits (or doesn't fit) with what you've seen in clinical practice, what you learned in basic or college courses, or what you've observed in your own experience breastfeeding. (In some cases, you might want to include how the information fits or doesn't fit with what "experts" say, what the media says, or whatever.)

- Describe how you will use any or all of this information. How might it be related to problems and potential solutions that occur in real life or in clinical situations?

- If you wish, include how you felt about learning this information. Were you overwhelmed? Enlightened? Worried? Something else?

Summarize What You've Learned

Instructions: Write your own summary of what you just learned in this chapter.

The purpose of this chapter was to help you recognize characteristics of multiple congenital and acquired nipple/breast variations and their implications for clinical breastfeeding management.

Sometimes, the type of information in this chapter can seem much more theoretical than clinical. Take a moment to summarize: How can you arrange the most salient points into a few bullet points? How will you use this information for individual clients in your clinical practice? How might this information be important in the bigger world of system-level changes (e.g., procedures, standing orders, etc.) or issues with populations of clients (e.g., writing patient education materials.) How might you use this information on an exam?

Main Points

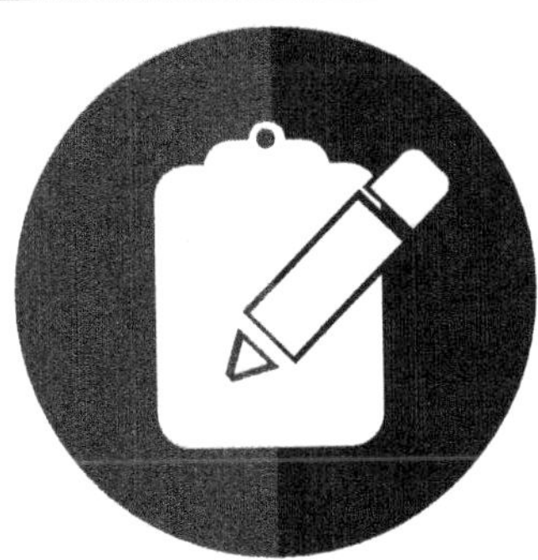

On the test

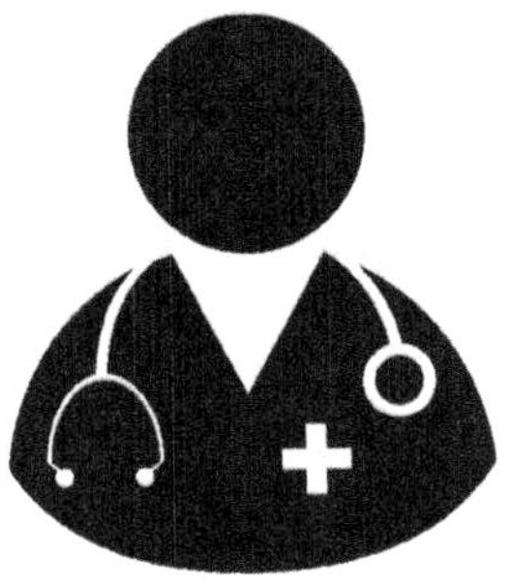

On the job

Self-Assessment

People often dive into a test before they have thoughtfully reflected on how well they have prepared for it. Instead, it would be helpful if they would take a few moments to give their alter-ego (their "other self") a chance to reflect on how confident they feel about mastering the stated objectives.

Instructions: Take a moment to review the chapter(below). Then rate yourself. How confident are you that you have achieved each objective below?

Objective	Highly Confident	Somewhat Confident	Somewhat Unsure	Completely Unsure
State the definition for at least 25 terms related to structural variations of the breasts.	❍	❍	❍	❍
Recognize visual clues of multiple congenital or acquired breast tissue variations and how (or if) they will affect breastfeeding and lactation.	❍	❍	❍	❍
Distinguish between anatomical breast variations that have similar appearances but are in fact different in terms of their underlying causes and implications for breastfeeding and lactation.	❍	❍	❍	❍
Suggest techniques to ensure optimal milk transfer with selected anatomic variations.	❍	❍	❍	❍

On the next page, you will some simple recall questions pertaining to this chapter. These are *not* the application-type questions you will find in the IBLCE exam. However, you cannot *apply* information unless you can fully *recall* that information! You should do these without looking up the answers.

When you finish with the quiz, look up the answers in the Appendix. Then, score your answers, using the Appendix. Finally, you should analyze the results of your quiz. It's not enough to just know what you got right or wrong; you must look at why you got the answers right.

Quick Quiz Chapter 9

Instructions: Circle the correct response. For a better understanding of how well you are mastering the material, try answering without looking it up. If you are really stuck, questions come from this workbook and from The Breastfeeding Atlas so go back and review the appropriate material. Answers are in the appendix.

1. The correct term for large breasts is:

   A. amastia

   B. amazia

   C. hypermastia

   D. hyperthelia

   E. macromastia

2. Of these, the observation that is LEAST likely to confirm the diagnosis of hypoplastic breasts is:

   A. asymmetrical

   B. fit into an A-cup

   C. have little tissue beneath the areola

   D. shaped like a tube or cylinder

   E. widely spaced

3. The suffix, *plasis* is from the Greek term meaning:

   A. aberration

   B. formation

   C. mutation

   D. striation

4. In counseling the mother in **Figure 206** about how to ensure good milk transfer, the aim would be for the infant to get:

   A. the widest part of the nipple at the corners of his mouth

   B. a latch-on in the straddle position

   C. a well-fitting shield to ensure milk transfer

   D. the entire areola into his mouth

5. When documenting in the client's record the lesion shown in **Figure 190**, description would be:

   A. birthmark

   B. bruise from poor latch-on

   C. herpes lesion

   D. sign of abuse

Analyze Your Own Quiz

- What percentage of the questions did you answer correctly?

- If you got 100% of them right, to what do you attribute your success?

- If you did not get all the questions right, can you identify your learning gap? (Example: Didn't know the information, knew the information but could not remember, knew some information but confused it with similar information, other.)

- Would you have been able to answer the questions as well if you had not read this chapter?

- What do you need to do next? (If you got them all right, what you need to do next is celebrate! Even a high-five with your child, a YESSS and a fist-pump in the air, or anything else is good! A small acknowledgement of your success is better than no acknowledgement!)

Additional Resources

1. Committee Opinion No. 658 Summary: Optimizing Support For Breastfeeding As Part Of Obstetric Practice. *Obstet Gynecol.* 2016;127(2):420-421.
2. Lawrence R, Lawrence, RM. *Breastfeeding: A guide for the medical profession.* 8 ed 2016.
3. Zucca-Matthes G, et al. Anatomy of the nipple and breast ducts. *Gland Surgery.* 2016;5(1):32-36.
4. Neifert MR, et al. Lactation failure due to insufficient glandular development of the breast. *Pediatrics.* 1985;76(5):823-828.
5. Neifert M. Breastfeeding after breast surgical procedure or breast cancer. *NAACOGS Clin Issu Perinat Womens Health Nurs.* 1992;3(4):673-682.
6. Geddes DT. Ultrasound imaging of the lactating breast: methodology and application. *Int Breastfeed J.* 2009;4:4.
7. Engstrom JL, et al. Comparison of milk output from the right and left breasts during simultaneous pumping in mothers of very low birthweight infants. *Breastfeed Med.* 2007;2(2):83-91.
8. Kent JC, et al. Volume and frequency of breastfeedings and fat content of breast milk throughout the day. *Pediatrics.* 2006;117(3):e387-395.
9. West D. *Defining your own success: Breastfeeding after breast reduction surgery.* . Chicago: La Leche League International; 2001.
10. Leal SC, et al. Breast irradiation and lactation: a review. *Expert Rev Anticancer Ther.* 2013;13(2):159-164.

Chapter 10
Impact of Breast/Nipple Anatomy on Clinical Management

Sometimes, the mother is motivated to breastfeed, but her infant is having some difficulty, and breastfeeding isn't going well. Maybe the infant is having trouble latching onto her nipples or areola. Maybe he's gagging. Maybe there's a different problem that doesn't involve the infant directly, such as a mother's difficulty with finding a breast pump flange that is both comfortable and effective at removing her milk. A visual assessment shows that the mother's nipples aren't quite what you think of as "normal," but how do you convey that to the mother without sending the message that her anatomy is not "normal" or isn't "right" for breastfeeding? These are some big questions.

In truth, the "not normal" is likely to be a variation of normal. Knowing how wide a "normal" nipple is, and other nipple/areola features can inform how you support the mother in breastfeeding her infant or expressing her milk for him.

This chapter will point you to not only photos, but also illustrations that will help you see subtle differences in breast anatomy. Like the other chapters of this workbook, this one also includes several written exercises to help you not only learn the material, but remember it for both your IBLCE exam and clinical practice.

I promise that when we finish this chapter, you will be able to recognize how variations in the size, shape, and elasticity of nipple tissue can affect breastfeeding management, as it pertains to optimal milk transfer, either when the mother is breastfeeding directly or expressing her milk.

Objectives

Given a clinical photo or drawing, you will be able to:

- Name, in millimeters, normal parameters for the diameter of the breast nipple.
- Recognize nipple shapes, lengths, and diameters that are outside the range of normal and their likely consequences for latch-on or pumping.
- Recognize at least five factors that alter a nipple's length and/or diameter.
- Recognize indicators and consequences of especially long or wide nipples.
- Recognize indicators that a flange is too small to accommodate a long or very large-diameter nipple.

Key Words

- connector
- diameter
- flange
- flare
- length
- rim
- shaft
- tunnel

Breast Size and Shape

A more thorough explanation of breast size, shape, and symmetry can be found in Chapter 9 of this workbook. Similarly, Chapter 6 dealt with positioning, latch, and milk transfer. Certainly, there is some overlap between those topics and this chapter's focus on the areola and nipple area of the breast. After all, breastfeeding doesn't happen in pieces! Sometimes, though, focusing on specific area helps us develop our communication techniques and assessment skills. This enables us to help mothers feel better about their ability to nourish and nurture their infants at breast.

Areolar Size and Shape

Many mothers are told to make sure the infant "gets all of the areola" when breastfeeding. For women with especially large areolae (**Figure 219**), that's just not possible. A better suggestion would be for her to help the infant take in "as much of the areola" as he can.

Some women have small nipples and small areolae (**Figure 220**). This might be ideal for a woman who is breastfeeding a premature infant. Often, a small nipple is found on a small areola, but not always! The woman in **Figure 221** has a small areola, and a large nipple.

Nipple Length, Diameter, and Shape

When assessing the size of the nipple, it's important to look at two factors: the *diameter*—that is, how far it measures across or how wide it is—and the length. *Length* means how far it measures from the base to the tip of the nipple. Length and diameter at the base and the tip can also affect the shape of the nipple.

How to Measure Nipples

In *The Breastfeeding Atlas,* Wilson-Clay and Hoover describe several studies of nipple measurement which applied different approaches to measuring women's nipples. Stark used calipers, Wilson-Clay used an engineer's circle template (**Figure 222**), and Hoover used a ruler. A less accurate but convenient way to measure (or at least estimate) either length or diameter is with coins.

- U.S. dime is 17.91 mm in diameter.
- U.S. nickel is 21.21 mm in diameter
- U.S. quarter is 24.26 mm in diameter

Elasticity, as discussed in Chapter 9, affects both the length and diameter. Wilson-Clay and Hoover point out that nipple size is also affected by:

- changes in pregnancy (typically, increases in midpregnancy)[1, 2]
- engorgement (especially during the postpartum period)
- location (the right is usually larger)[3]
- activity (at rest vs. feeding or pumping)
- ethnicity[4]
- duration of lactation[5]

Nipple Diameter and Shape

Early studies showed the average nipple diameter to be about 15 mm[6] or 16 mm.[7] Most full-term, healthy newborns have an oral cavity that can accommodate this without any problems. The problems begin when there is a disproportion between the infant's mouth and the mother's nipple. Using data provided by Wilson-Clay and Hoover in *The Breastfeeding Atlas* (page 79), below is a summary of four studies of nipple diameter. (All studies were small, and all used different study methods and different equipment to measure the nipples.) See page 79 in *The Breastfeeding Atlas* for details.

	# Women	# Nipples Measured	Method	Small < 12 mm	Medium 12-15 mm
Stark Thesis	59	118	Calipers	14	62
Stark - Lact Inst	86	172	Calipers	8	47
Wilson-Clay	34	68	Engineer's Circle Template	3	15
Hoover1	100	100	Ruler	14	17

Table 10-1. Summary of studies that measured diameters of nipples of breastfeeding mothers.

Some nipples have a fairly wide diameter, such as shown in **Figure 223**, where a nipple has the diameter of a U.S. quarter. Because this nipple is also inverted, effective latch-on and suckling will be difficult.

Some nipples have both a large diameter and a long length. **Figure 227** shows a nipple that is 2 cm in length when at rest. It is somewhat narrower at its base (20.6 mm) and wider at its tip (22.3 mm). This woman's infant, born at 36 weeks' gestation, had no stools in two days, became jaundiced, and lost 9% of his weight by six days after birth, likely because his small mouth could not accommodate her large nipple (**Figure 228**).

Some nipples are shaped like a door knob (**Figure 230**); note the shadow that accentuates this shape. This type of nipple is often difficult for the infant to grasp. The nipple on **Figure 230,** like that in **Figure 227**, is slightly narrower at the base and wider at the tip.

The nipple in **Figure 231** is 30 mm in diameter. Fortunately, all infants "grow into" these nipples, and breastfeeding becomes easier over time.[8]

Nipple Length

We have no data on the "normal" length of the nipple. (We do have some data that suggest a nipple of at least 7 mm facilitates successful breastfeeding.[9]) Some nipples seem very long, even at rest. **Figure 224** shows a nipple that is 17 mm long, which could certainly be considered a long nipple. **Figure 226** shows a nipple that is even longer, at 20 mm.

After seeing the very short nipples in Chapter 9, one might assume that long nipples are a good thing! True, a long nipple can stimulate the palate, while the short nipple usually does not. But the long nipple can go beyond the palate, stimulate the soft palate or posterior pharynx, and thereby cause the infant to gag.

Other consequences of long nipples can include poor milk transfer, a dwindling milk supply, and skin damage to the nipple. More serious consequences can include dehydration[10], failure to thrive, and possibly skin infection (**Figure 225**).

Choosing the Right Size Flange

In general, a flange is often described as a projecting rim, on a shaft, to provide a place for the attachment of another object. That's a good explanation of a flange that is attached to a breast pump and held against the mother's breast. Figure 10-1 shows such a flange. The part that goes on the woman's breast is the *rim* (**A**), which is at the end of the *flare* (**B**), or the widened part. The flare is at the end of the *shaft* (**C**), or *tunnel*, which is the long, narrow section between the flare and the *connector* (**D**). The connector attaches to both the vessel that will hold the mother's pumped milk and to the pump.

Choosing the right size flange for the mother's breast can be extremely difficult in the hospital setting, since often only one or two flange sizes are stocked. However, using the right size flange is important for the mother's milk supply, and getting the right one often depends on good measurements, good observations, and experience.

Many professionals assume that the size of the flange (in millimeters, often 24 mm or 25 mm) refers to the diameter at the rim. That is incorrect. Actually, it refers to the amount of space at the junction of the flare and the flange. This is important, because the only the nipple should be drawn into this space during pumping. Ideally, no more than about 6 mm (roughly ¼ inch) of areola should be drawn into this space.

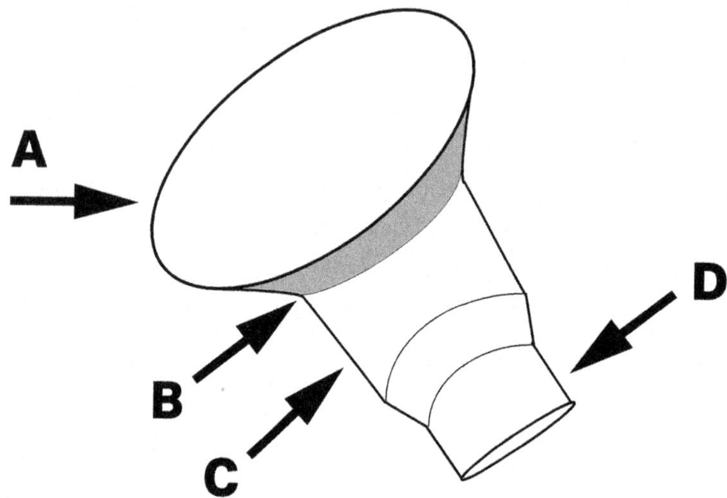

Figure 10-1. Parts of breast pump flange

Until you observe a pumping session, you cannot be sure that the flange fits correctly. You'll also want to consider the mother's comfort, as well as how effective the pump is when that flange size is used.

Changes in Diameter and Length While Pumping

Pump flanges are like shoes: You can't be sure of your actual size until you "wear" them. Just as feet fit into shoes differently when the wearer is sitting versus standing, so too do nipples "fit" into flanges differently when at rest versus pumping. Realizing that the nipple will be drawn to a larger size due to the pump's vacuum pressure, it's helpful to start out with a flange that is visibly larger than the nipple at rest. But until pumping begins, it is impossible to determine whether it fits.

While pumping, the nipple can increase in length—sometimes substantially. A pair of photos in *The Breastfeeding Atlas* show one nipple to be 2 cm long at rest (**Figure 227**) and about 4 cm long while pumping (**Figure 229**). That means the nipple has *doubled* in length!

The diameter can increase, too. In **Figure 235**, the diameter of a nipple is 20.64 mm at rest. After pumping the diameter is 23.81 mm **(Figure 236).**

One main principle that should guide the sizing decision is this: The nipple should move freely in and out of the shaft. Notice that the nipple is somewhat "stuck" in the shaft of a 25 mm flange in **Figure 232**; the next larger size would be a better fit. Discomfort, redness, cracks at the base (**Figure 233**) or abrasions (**Figure 234**) are all indicators of a flange that fits too tightly. Getting the right flange doesn't just affect the mother's comfort; she would be able to get a better volume of milk with a flange that fits properly.

Figure 237 demonstrates many points made in this chapter, as well as Chapter 9. As is typical of women with polycystic ovarian syndrome (PCOS), this woman has breasts that are spaced widely apart; each breast appears hypoplastic, and she has large diameter nipples. She is using a 30 mm flange in **Figure 238**. Do you notice how this is a rather tight fit? In this case, a 36 mm flange would likely offer better comfort and a better fit.

When fitting a flange, keep in mind that it's okay to use one size for one breast, and a different size for the other breast. Sometimes, no flange fits well. In that case, be prepared to convince the mother to try hand expression. (Many mothers are reluctant!) She might be surprised to find that hand expression is more comfortable and even more effective than using a pump.

Looking Back, Looking Forward

In this chapter, we've talked about breast size and shape as well as nipple length, diameter, and shape. Then, we looked at how to choose a flange size that would fit comfortably and perform effectively.

Evidence in the education field shows that writing your own summary helps your retention. The Summarize What You've Learned exercise helps you to do this, so take just a few minutes to complete that exercise.

By now, if you have viewed the photos carefully, and if you've completed the written exercises, you should feel confident that you can recognize how variations in size, shape, and elasticity of nipple tissue can affect breastfeeding management, as it pertains to optimal milk transfer, either when the mother is breastfeeding directly or expressing her milk.

Recalling, Reinforcing, and Expanding Your Learning

Have you ever felt frustrated that you "learned" something, but later, can't recall it? That may be because you didn't reinforce the material you learned. And, perhaps what you originally learned isn't enough to get you through the next few decades of practice; sometimes you need to expand your learning. The exercises in this section are designed to help you recall, reinforce, and expand your learning.

What was your main motivation for reading this chapter?

❍ To study for the IBLCE exam, as a first-time candidate

❍ To review for the IBLCE exam, as a re-certificant

❍ To improve my clinical skills and clinical management

How soon do you think can use the information presented in this chapter?

❍ Immediately; within the next few days or so

❍ Soon; within the next month or so

❍ Later; sometime before I retire

Pro Tip! If you are preparing for the IBLCE exam, it would be wise to pace your studying. Set a target date for when you plan to complete the exercises, and check off them off as you go along.

Done!	Target Date	Learning Exercise
❑	________________	Learning Exercise 10-1. Recognizing photos of nipple and flange issues.
❑	________________	Learning Exercise 10-2. Using correct terminology for parts of a flange.
❑	________________	Learning Exercise 10-3. Recognizing and labeling parts of a flange.
❑	________________	Learning Exercise 10-4. Nipple length and diameter and their clinical indicators and implications.
❑	________________	Explore What You've Learned in a Journal
❑	________________	Summarize What You've Learned
❑	________________	Quick Quiz

Learning Exercise 10-1. Recognizing photos of nipple and flange issues.

Instructions: View the photos in The Breastfeeding Atlas to page 182-183 (And ideally, you should cover up the caption beneath each photo!) Write the letter of the correct match next to each item. Answers are in the Appendix.

E	1. Figure 223	A. Too-tight fit of nipple in the shaft
B	2. Figure 224	B. A long nipple
C	3. Figure 230	C. Nipple is narrower at base, wider at tip
I	4. Figure 231	D. Abrasions from a too-tight flange
A	5. Figure 232	E. A wide-diameter, inverted nipple
G	6. Figure 233	F. Nipple has increased in diameter while pumping
D	7. Figure 234	G. Discomfort, redness, cracks at the base
J	8. Figure 229	H. Mother with PCOS and large diameter nipples
F	9. Figure 236	I. A very wide-diameter nipple
H	10. Figure 237	J. Nipple as doubled in length while pumping

Vocabulary

Learning Exercise 10-2. Using correct terminology for parts of a flange.

Instructions: Write the letter of the correct match next to each item. Answers are in the Appendix.

E	1. connector	A. edge of the flare
F	2. flange	B. becomes wider at one end
B	3. flare	C. also called the "shaft"
A	4. rim	D. long, narrow vertical section
D	5. shaft	E. attaches to the pump
C	6. tunnel	F. consists of the connector, flare, rim, and shaft.

Learning Exercise 10-3.

Instructions: Give a name to each of the flange parts that are marked with an arrow. Answers are in the appendix.

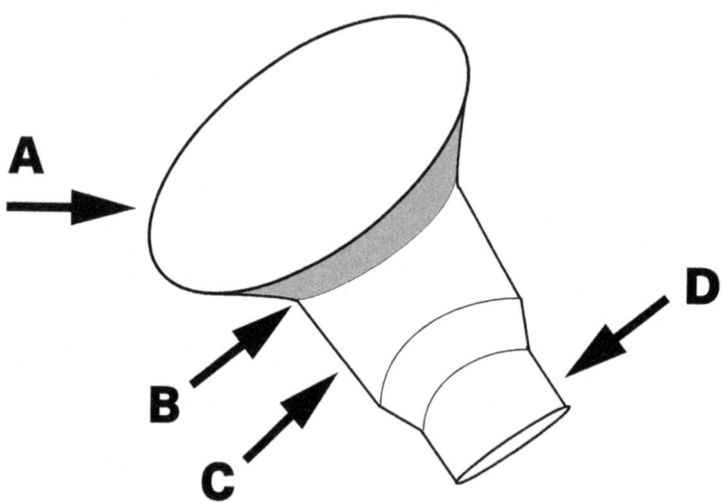

A. Rim

B. Flare

C. tunnel/shaft

D. Connector

Learning Exercise 10-4. Nipple length and diameter and their clinical indicators and implications.

Instructions: Complete the following table with information you've learned from this chapter.

Nipple length: What are possible consequences of an especially long nipple?	infant gag Poor milk transfer dwindling milk supply dehydration failure to thrive skin infection
Nipple diameter: What are three ways that nipple diameter be measured, or estimated?	calipers template ruler coins
Nipple diameter: What is considered the diameter of most nipples?	About 15-16mm Range 23-40mm
Nipple diameter: What five or six factors affect nipple size and diameter?	Δ in pregnancy engorgement location activity ethnicity duration of lactation
Nipple diameter: How do large-diameter nipples impact latch?	Disproportion between nipple and mouth can make it difficult for infant to latch
What indicators suggest that the flange size is incorrect, and how can you tell for sure?	Discomfort, redness cracks @ base of nipple abrasions
Compare nipples at rest to nipples during a pumping session. What happens?	increase in length

Summarize What You've Learned

The goal of this chapter was to help you recognize how variations in the size, shape, and elasticity of nipple tissue can affect breastfeeding management, as it pertains to optimal milk transfer, either when the mother is breastfeeding directly or expressing her milk.

Sometimes, the type of information in this chapter can seem much more theoretical than clinical. Take a moment to summarize: How can you arrange the most salient points into a few bullet points? How will you use this information for individual clients in your clinical practice? How might this information be important in the bigger world of system-level changes (e.g., procedures, standing orders, etc.) or issues with populations of clients (e.g., writing patient education materials.)

Main Points

On the test

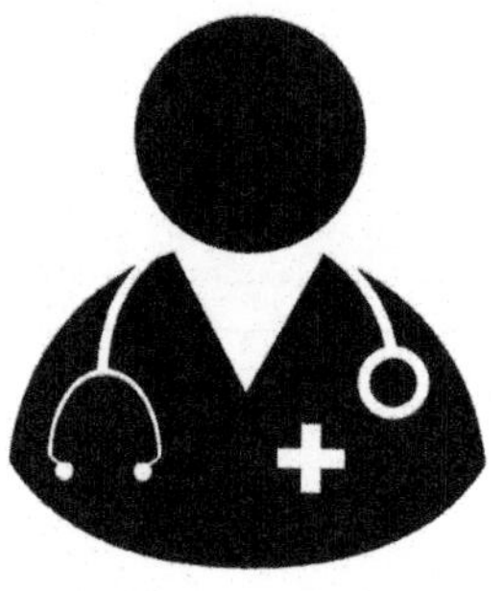

On the job

Explore Your Learning in a Journal

- Name at least three things you learned from this chapter.

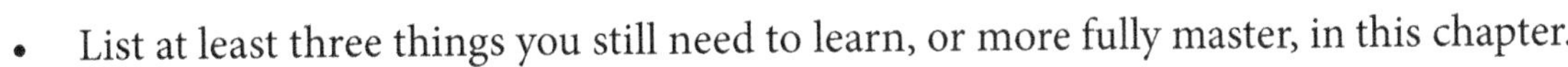

- List at least three things you still need to learn, or more fully master, in this chapter.

- Briefly describe how this information fits (or doesn't fit) with what you've seen in clinical practice, what you learned in basic or college courses, or what you've observed in your own experience breastfeeding. (In some cases, you might want to include how the information fits or doesn't fit with what "experts" say, what the media says, or whatever.)

- Describe how you will use any or all of this information. How might it be related to problems and potential solutions that occur in real life or in clinical situations?

- If you wish, include how you felt about learning this information. Were you bored? Overwhelmed? Enlightened? Frustrated? Worried? Something else?

Self-Assessment

People often dive into a test before they have thoughtfully reflected on how well they have prepared for it. Instead, it would be helpful if they would take a few moments to give their alter-ego (their "other self") a chance to reflect on how confident they feel about mastering the stated objectives.

Instructions: Take a moment to review the chapter objectives (below). Then rate yourself. How confident are you that you have achieved each objective below?

Objective	Highly Confident	Somewhat Confident	Somewhat Unsure	Completely Unsure
Name, in millimeters, normal parameters for the diameter of the breast nipple.	❍	❍	❍	❍
Recognize nipple shapes, lengths, and diameters that are outside the range of normal and their likely consequences for latch-on or pumping.	❍	❍	❍	❍
Recognize at least five factors that alter a nipple's length and/or diameter.	❍	❍	❍	❍
Recognize indicators and consequences of especially long or wide nipples.	❍	❍	❍	❍
Recognize indicators that a flange is too small to accommodate a long or very large-diameter nipple.	❍	❍	❍	❍

On the next page, you will some simple recall questions pertaining to this chapter. These are *not* the application-type questions you will find in the IBLCE exam. However, you cannot *apply* information unless you can fully *recall* that information! You should do these without looking up the answers.

When you finish with the quiz, look up the answers in the Appendix. Then, score your answers, using the Appendix. Finally, you should analyze the results of your quiz. It's not enough to just know what you got right or wrong; you must look at why you got the answers right.

Quick Quiz Chapter 10

1. Which action is MOST important to assure optimal milk expression while pumping?
   A. making sure that the nipple fills the flange's tunnel
   B. putting water on the inside of the flange
   C. warming the flange to improve duct expansion
   D. watching the mother pump for several minutes

2. When at rest, most women will be likely to have a nipple diameter of about:
   A. < 12 mm
   B. 12-23 mm
   C. 23-40 mm
   D. > 40 mm

3. You are explaining to a new lactation professional how to estimate the diameter of the average mother's nipple. You point out that the average diameter of a lactating mother's nipple (at rest) is slightly less than the diameter of which U.S. coin?
   A. dime
   B. nickel
   C. quarter

4. If the mother's nipple is especially long, a likely consequence for her newborn is:
   A. difficulty coping with a forceful let-down
   B. increased fatigue of the orofacial muscles
   C. increased likelihood of gagging

5. If a mother is pumping with a flange that is too small, which is the LEAST likely outcome?
   A. a large volume of milk outflow
   B. abrasions on the tip of the nipple
   C. cracks at the base of the nipple
   D. full and lumpy breasts after pumping

Analyze Your Own Quiz

- What percentage of the questions did you answer correctly?

- If you got 100% of them right, to what do you attribute your success?

- If you did not get all the questions right, can you identify your learning gap? (Example: Didn't know the information, knew the information but could not remember, knew some information but confused it with similar information, other.)

- Would you have been able to answer the questions as well if you had not read this chapter?

- What do you need to do next? (If you got them all right, what you need to do next is celebrate! Even a high-five with your child, a YESSS and a fist-pump in the air, or anything else is good! A small acknowledgement of your success is better than no acknowledgement!)

Additional Resources

1. Rohn RD. Nipple (papilla) development in girls: III. The effects of pregnancy. *J Adolesc Health Care.* 1989;10(1):39-40.

2. Cox DB, et al. Breast growth and the urinary excretion of lactose during human pregnancy and early lactation: endocrine relationships. *Exp Physiol.* 1999;84(2):421-434.

3. Thanaboonyawat I, et al. Pilot study of normal development of nipples during pregnancy. *J Hum Lact.* 2013;29(4):480-483.

4. Park IY, et al. Association of the nipple-areola complexes with age, parity, and breastfeeding in Korean premenopausal women. *J Hum Lact.* 2014;30(4):474-479.

5. Park IH, et al. High volumetric breast density predicts risk for breast cancer in postmenopausal, but not premenopausal, Korean Women. *Annals of surgical oncology.* 2014;21(13):4124-4132.

6. Ziemer MM, Pigeon JG. Skin changes and pain in the nipple during the 1st week of lactation [see comments]. *J Obstet Gynecol Neonatal Nurs.* 1993;22(3):247-256.

7. Ziemer MM, et al. Evaluation of a dressing to reduce nipple pain and improve nipple skin condition in breast-feeding women. *Nurs-Res.* 1995;44(6):347-351.

8. Sakalidis VS, et al. Longitudinal changes in suck-swallow-breathe, oxygen saturation, and heart rate patterns in term breastfeeding infants. *J Hum Lact.* 2013;29(2):236-245.

9. Puapornpong P, et al. Nipple length and its relation to success in breastfeeding. *J Med Assoc Thai.* 2013;96 Suppl 1:S1-4.

10. Caglar MK, et al. Risk factors for excess weight loss and hypernatremia in exclusively breast-fed infants. *Brazilian journal of medical and biological research = Revista brasileira de pesquisas medicas e biologicas / Sociedade Brasileira de Biofisica ... [et al.].* 2006;39(4):539-544.

Chapter 11
Engorgement, Oversupply and Mastitis

Milk stasis is a serious problem; so is milk overproduction. Such conditions can result in a variety of problems for mothers and infants, including forceful letdown, mastitis, gagging, and more.

You'll need to deal with these possibly unexpected, but nevertheless relatively common conditions. You'll need to help mothers who are basically healthy, but wish to persevere through some mild or transient discomfort. You'll also need to know when to refer mothers who need medical help.

And—if you're like me—you'll need to know when to question the "diagnosis" of the mother who reports on the telephone. Often, the mother has had no medical care and has self-diagnosed one of these common problems. (I call these the "Dr. Google" diagnoses!)

I promise that when we finish this chapter, you will be able to recognize signs, clinical course, and treatment options for infectious and noninfectious conditions associated with oversupply and milk stasis.

Objectives

Given a clinical photo, you will be able to:

- Compare and contrast signs of physiologic and pathologic engorgement, including possible patterns of onset and resolution.
- Recognize possible indications of overactive milk ejection reflex (MER), consequences, and techniques to help the infant cope during a feeding.
- Recognize signs of milk stasis that indicate the need for medical referral.
- Recognize characteristics (e.g., milk color, milk texture, milk volume) often associated with mastitis and/or breast abscess.
- Recognize characteristics of breast abscess in terms of formation and location, clinical course, treatment options, consequences of non-treatment, and techniques for breastfeeding during (or shortly after) treatment.
- Distinguish between visible indicators of mastitis and cellulitis.

Key Words

- afebrile
- asymptomatic
- block feeding
- breast abscess
- cellulitis
- coagulase
- engorgement, pathologic
- engorgement, physiologic
- erythematous, erythema
- febrile
- galactocele
- hypergalactia
- hyperlactation
- induration
- mastitis
- multilocular
- peau d'orange
- percutaneous
- proinflammatory cytokines
- prolactinoma
- reverse pressure softening
- Staphylococcus aureus
- Streptococcus lactarius
- subareolar abscess
- subclinical mastitis
- symptomatic
- unilocular

Engorgement

When I talk to parents, I use the phrase "breasts filling with milk" because so many people—parents and professionals as well—misunderstand the word "engorgement." To delineate the types of engorgement, I use the classic nomenclature used by Dr. Ruth Lawrence and Dr. Robert Lawrence,[1] specifically physiologic engorgement and pathologic engorgement.

Physiologic Engorgement

As discussed in Chapter 5, the onset of a copious supply of milk is normal. This is called *physiologic engorgement.*

Engorgement of the normal, healthy breast is always bilateral. This is an important observation, because it can help the observer to distinguish engorgement from some other conditions of the breast.

With physiologic engorgement, both breasts feel tender and are swollen with milk. This is different from the fluid edema that a mother may experience early in the postpartum period, which is associated with intravenous fluid given during labor. To distinguish between engorgement with milk and fluid edema, look for edema elsewhere in the body (e.g., the hands and fingers). This almost always accompanies fluid edema of the breasts, but not necessarily milk engorgement.

Sometimes, physiologically engorged mothers have a slight elevation in body temperature. In addition to filling with milk (and possibly leaking), the breasts feel firm but not hard. The mother may describe feelings of tenderness or discomfort, but she should not be in pain. While her nipples may seem to become somewhat shortened, they can often be grasped by a healthy, vigorously-suckling infant.

The onset and experience of engorgement varies between women. Wilson-Clay and Hoover point out studies by Hill & Humenick[2] and Humenick & Hill[3] in which researchers identified four distinct patterns of engorgement:

- One episode of very firm, tender breasts followed by a rapid decline in signs and symptoms.
- Multiple peaks of engorgement, each followed by a rapid decline in signs and symptoms.
- Intense episode of engorgement, in which signs and symptoms persist for 2 weeks or longer. Note engorgement in this mother at six days postpartum (**Figure 241**) and again at eight days postpartum (**Figure 240**).
- Slight breast changes with little or no perceptible engorgement.

Often, those who experience the discomforts of engorgement look for a way to relieve it. Unfortunately, a recent Cochrane review[4] could not establish any of the following common practices as an effective intervention for engorgement:

- acupuncture
- acupressure
- cabbage leaves
- hot/cold gel packs
- scraping therapy (Gua-Sha)
- pharmacological treatments
- ultrasound

Interestingly, this Cochrane review did not look at three interventions that are frequently used here in the United States. No mention was made of the efficacy of breast shells, or expressing milk from the breasts. Although the review does briefly address "massage" it did not specifically address *reverse pressure softening* (**Figure 242**), which is technically not massage. Reverse pressure softening is a technique developed by experienced nurse and lactation consultant Jean Cotterman[5] that has been used successfully by many clinical experts.

While the review is interesting reading, the authors acknowledge that they were limited to small studies with a limited number of participants. They caution that the existing evidence does not justify widespread implementation. Yet, their findings do not mean you should tell mothers to "do nothing". Remember, many clinicians have successfully recommended the application of warm or cold compresses for relief, an intervention which has been encouraged by the World Health Organization.

Pathologic Engorgement

Pathologic engorgement presents differently than physiologic engorgement. Mothers who are pathologically engorged experience painful, rock-hard breasts. Nipples are also rock-hard, and they are too short for the infant to grasp. Most especially, the skin is shiny and taut, and the breasts are typically positioned at a sharp angle out from chest (**Figure 239**). Rather than being the result of normal "filling" with milk, pathologic engorgement is brought on by severe stasis of milk.

It has long been established that pathologic engorgement is related to delay of feedings.[6] Pathologic engorgement creates a situation that is difficult to manage. Areolar distention may be so extreme that the nipple is shortened and may virtually disappear. This can create a snowball effect: the infant is unable to latch on and effectively transfer milk out of the breast; milk accumulates, and engorgement becomes more severe and more painful. The mother may become reluctant to offer her breast. You can see how this becomes a self-perpetuating problem.

It will be important for you to recognize the difference between physiologic engorgement and pathologic engorgement, and, later in the chapter, the difference between engorgement and mastitis.

Complete Learning Exercise 11-3 about the similarities and differences between physiologic and pathologic engorgement.

Overactive Milk Ejection Reflex, Oversupply

It's critical to remember that women who have an oversupply of milk often have an overactive milk ejection reflex. However, that's not always the case. Let's discuss each separately.

Overactive Milk Ejection Reflex

There appears to be no quantifiable description for an "overactive" milk ejection reflex (MER) or "let-down." However, the onlooker might describe this event as a particularly fast or powerful or high-volume spray of milk (**Figure 246**).

Mothers sometimes describe it as painful. Some mothers—who have nothing else to compare it to—may find it simply annoying or otherwise undesirable. They may experience substantial leaking of milk between feedings, which has sometimes been identified as a reason for weaning.[7]

A forceful MER could begin any time. If it occurs (and for some mothers, it never occurs), it is more likely to be noticed at about 3-4 weeks postpartum. The signs and symptoms are easy to identify. The mother or the onlooker can see that the infant simply cannot cope with the speed, the force, or the volume of the milk coming towards him. Initially, he may come off the nipple entirely, leaving his mother entirely bewildered. This should not be misinterpreted as a sign that he doesn't want to continue feeding. In fact, shortly after the big "gusher," he may be eager to try again. (However, whereas many infants like to nurse for comfort, this infant might not be interested in doing so since he may expect that he would have to contend with the forceful MER.)

During the feeding, the infant may emit coughing, squeaking, squealing, gasping, or gulping sounds. He may clamp down on the nipple in attempt to stop the fast flow. He may pull away from the breast each time there is a MER. Long after the feeding is over, the infant may exhibit colic-like symptoms because he has consumed the milk too fast.

In a phone conversation, I find a question that works well is: "Does it seem as if he is drowning when you have a let-down?" This visual image seems to work in such instances, eliciting an emphatic "Yes" from the mother.

It can be difficult for mothers to know how to cope with this. Fortunately, there are a number of actions that can be helpful. Wilson-Clay and Hoover offer several suggestions in *The Breastfeeding Atlas*. I will summarize these below, and add a few of my own.

From the maternal aspect, the goal is to reduce the speed, force and volume of the milk ejection. The "stop technique" works well. When the mother begins to feel the sensation of MER, she can apply direct pressure to her nipple with her fingers or hands, or by crossing her arms over her breasts to apply direct pressure to the nipple. Alternatively, she can anticipate that an overactive MER will occur, and she can control it proactively. She can manually stimulate her nipple and allow the big "gusher" of milk to go into a thick towel or even a disposable diaper. (Unless you have a clear indication that she has an undersupply, don't worry about discarding the milk. In all likelihood, she has plenty more!) She could also try briefly using a nipple shield as a barrier to block the milk spray, and then removing the shield once the "gusher" has subsided.[8]

Some mothers with overactive MER are instructed to pump off some of the milk before she feeds her infant. Unless there is some serious reason to do so, I don't follow this approach. It seems to me that this directive not only implies that the mother needs some piece of external equipment for breastfeeding, it also forces her to add one more step to the feeding process—a step that may seem complex, if she has no prior breast pump experience. From getting the pump and fitting the flange to handling the milk and cleaning the pump afterwards, pumping can seem like a big hassle to a new mother! Whenever possible, I favor a simple approach for the mother who is already overwhelmed, and likely sleep-deprived.

Mothers who experience significant leaking as a result of overactive MER may find that breast pads and other devices help to keep her comfortable. (I distinctly remember one woman who routinely used five breast pads to control her leaking; as soon as they were moist, she applied another five!)

From the infant aspect, the goal is to help the infant cope with the flow of milk. Many helpful techniques are easy to learn and require no extra equipment.

For example, positioning might be critical for helping the infant to cope with the milk flow. The prone position (**Figure 247**), or even a semi-prone position (Figure 85), are good first steps. These positions can help since they ensure the gravitational pull of the milk is towards the mother, rather the infant. The side-lying (**Figure 99**) or upright position (**Figure 103**) may also help.

Oversupply

While many mothers may worry about not having enough milk, some mothers have an oversupply of milk. It is not helpful to tell such a mother she is "blessed"; she may feel that her condition is more of a curse!

Oversupply of milk in healthy women is known by several medical terms, including *hypergalactia*, *hyperlactation*, and *increased lactation*. Eglash points out these terms are nearly synonymous or interchangeable, and they appear in *The 10th International Classification of Diseases*. The term that is most consistently found in dictionaries to describe excessive milk is *hypergalactia*. [9]

Why might hypergalactia occur? It's possible that the cause is a pathologic condition known as *prolactinoma*. As its name implies, "-oma" means tumor. A prolactinoma is a benign tumor on the pituitary gland that produces hormones, increasing the levels of prolactin.

More often, it might be difficult—or pointless—to explain. Just as some women have thicker hair or longer toes, some women have a greater milk supply.

It may also be that some women inadvertently create oversupply. It seems that an increasing number of women are being instructed to pump their milk when there is little or no reason to do so. Since breastfeeding is a "supply and demand" enterprise, they build up a huge supply of milk. This oversupply is not always a good thing. Oversupply opens the door for blocked ducts and related issues. And, if the mother has an oversupply of milk, the infant will likely have explosive, frothy, green stools.

This woman's resolution of engorgement was spontaneous (**Figure 243**). However, there are several method to down-regulate supply. Pharmacologic preparations are one such method. For example, the common decongestant pseudoephedrine appears to reduce milk volume by as much as 24 percent.[10]

Another method of down-regulation is so-called *block feeding*. Van Veldhuizen-Staas[11] describes this technique as "full removal of milk followed by unilateral breastfeeding *ad lib* with the same breast offered at every breastfeed in a certain time block." I agree with the authors that this can be a very effective means by which to reduce the mother's supply of milk. However, using just one breast at a time creates a possible risk of stasis in the other breast, so this technique should be used with caution.

Mastitis

Mastitis can be defined as "inflammation of the breast, which may or may not involve an infection."[1 p. 567] Mastitis includes "fever of 38.5° C (101° F) or more, chills, flulike aching, systemic illness and a pink, tender, hot, swollen, wedge-shaped area of the breast." [1 p. 567]

For many cases of mastitis, the etiology (causative pathogen) is *Staphylococcus aureus*. Although *S. aureus* resides as normal flora on our skin, it can cause infection if it gets into the milk ducts. Other staphylococcus species, such as the recently-identified *S. lactarius*,[12] may also cause mastitis. In the laboratory, *coagulase* (a protein enzyme) makes it possible to distinguish between different types of staphylococcus strains. This can be an important step in ensuring that the prescribed antibiotic covers the identified organism. The onset of mastitis can be either sudden, or gradual. Several studies have shown that women who have cracked nipples are more at risk for mastitis, and a recent study has also shown pacifier use to be associated with mastitis.[13] Often, mastitis will follow an unresolved blocked milk duct. However, the condition does not necessarily have any identifiable warning signs.

The mastitic lesion is a hot, hard, *erythematous* (reddened) lump. Note the erythema from 4 o'clock to 12 o'clock on the breast of the mother who is only 4 days postpartum in **Figure 248**. Often, parents or providers assume that mastitis occurs later in the postpartum period—and it's true that mastitis can occur any time during lactation, or even after weaning. Still, most episodes that occur during the first 12 weeks happen in the first week postpartum.[14]

Mastitis may be anywhere on the breast, but it is frequently found in the upper, outer quadrant.[1] Often, it is located near a surgical incision, or in a spot where a tight-fitting bra has cut into the tissue (**Figure 248**). Almost always, mastitis is unilateral. In rare cases, mastitis is bilateral (**Figure 249** and **250**). In cases of bilateral mastitis, the etiologic agent is often *Streptococcus pyogenes.*[1]

Although the lesion is localized, the signs and symptoms are generalized. Women usually report flu-like symptoms, such as fever, aches and pains, in addition to warmth of the site and discomfort of the affected breast.

Mastitis is typically caused by *Staphylococcus*, and some cases are resistant to treatment with methicillin-based drugs These are methicillin-resistant Staphylococcus aureus (MRSA) cases (**Figure 260**). They do not respond to a methicillin-based drug, such as the dicloxicillin, which is often the drug of choice for treatment of mastitis.

How does mastitis affect the milk? Generally, the volume of milk is decreased in the breast that is affected with mastitis. If the infant continues to suckle directly at the breast, we might never know what the mother's milk looks like. If the mother expressed her milk, we may observe that it is congealed (**Figure 266**, **Figure 267**) or that it forms "clumps" (**Figure 259**). The infant may still consume such milk, although it likely to be too thick to put through an artificial nipple.

We may find that it appears as white as uninfected milk, or it might be yellow (**Figure 261**), orange (**Figure 262**), or red (**Figure 264**). However, the presence of yellow or orange milk doesn't necessarily point to the presence of a MRSA infection. Often, colored milk might be explained by the mother's consumption of food or drugs; carrots, pumpkins, or sweet potatoes are likely explanations for yellow or orange milk.

Mastitis can cause damage to the connective tissue and skin (**Figure 263**), and milk can leak through broken skin (**Figure 265**). Healing can vary (**Figure 269**), but women should be able to start to feel better within 48 hours of starting antibiotics. **Figure 270** shows a woman one year after a bout with mastitis.

Some women with mastitis choose to breastfeed only on the unaffected side (**Figure 268**).

Figure 244 shows a woman with *peau d'orange*, French for "skin of the orange," a condition in which the skin has the appearance and dimpled texture of an orange peel. Peau d'orange is caused by cutaneous lymphatic edema, which causes swelling. Some might argue that this image is not a true peau d'orange, since it does not have a distinct discoloration, but the dimpled texture is very apparent. The mother in (**Figure 245**) has peau d'orange, with the characteristic discoloring, during a bout of mastitis.

The Breastfeeding Atlas mentions subclinical mastitis. An infection that is *subclinical* is one that exists, but the client is asymptomatic (i.e., does not experience symptoms). Yet, it has implications for care, so readers are urged to see the discussion on Page 87 of *The Breastfeeding Atlas.*

Abscess

An *abscess* is a localized collection of pus in bodily tissues, often accompanied by swelling and inflammation; frequently, it is caused by bacteria. A breast abscess is caused by a pathogen (in the breast, usually *Staphylococcus*) and is a pus-filled space located in the fatty or connective tissue. (This should not be confused with a cancerous lesion or a *galactocele*, either of which can also be related to blockages. A galactocele is a milk-filled cyst located within a milk duct.)

Very often, a breast abscess occurs when mastitis is untreated or incompletely treated. Among lactating women worldwide, about 11% experience a breast abscess at some time during lactation.[14, 15]

Factors that increase the risk for developing a breast abscess include:

- Obstetrical factors: Primipara, giving birth after 41 weeks' gestation[16, 17]
- Lactational factors: the first 3 months of lactation, and abrupt weaning
- Lifestyle issues: smoking,[18] obesity[18]
- Medical therapy: wrong antibiotic, delayed prescription or incomplete prescription.

You may have seen a boil or a furuncle; both are types of abscesses in the cutaneous (skin) tissue. A breast abscess is similar, but located deeper within the tissue. Pressure within the abscess tends to come to a head or a point; the infectious debris is inside, and it may spread to other parts of the body. Usually antibiotic therapy alone is insufficient. The pressure inside the abscess must be released.

Abscesses can develop anywhere in the body. A lactating woman might experience a *subareolar* abscess, which occurs on the areolar gland, under or below the areola **(Figure 253, Figure 255)**. A subareolar abscess is caused by a blockage of the small glands below the skin of the areola.

Typically, an abscess looks like a tender, soft-tissue mass with erythema and surrounding induration (**Figure 251**). *Induration* is a hardening of normally soft tissue. (Although induration can occur in an abscess, it is also typical of a cancerous lesion.)

In the initial stages, the abscess feels solid. Later, when the pus has formed within it and it is "ripe", it has a wave-like motion when palpated, because it is not solid. (By comparison, a galactocele is always a solid mass.)

However, some abscesses are much deeper in the breast tissue. An *intramammary abscess* is a collection of pus within the mammary gland. It may be either *unilocular* (affecting a single small cavity) or, more frequently,[19] *multilocular* (affecting multiple small cavities, as shown in **Figure 257**).

Abscesses are usually diagnosed by culture and sensitivity tests. However, while this type of test is accurate for infections in other body parts, it may not be accurate in the breast, because the mammary gland consists of many lobes. The lobe with the infectious organism may not have been tested.

Very often, we assume that a mother will be *febrile* (have a fever) if she has a breast abscess. While some do, many do not.[20] The case study in Chapter 11 of *The Breastfeeding Atlas* demonstrates this, as the mother was *afebrile* (i.e., does not have a fever).

The Breastfeeding Atlas (page 185) shows photos of "ripe" abscesses (**Figure 251**, **252**). Ripening is an important concept in the management of an abscess. In the initial stages, the cyst is filled with inflammatory debris, and it presents as a solid mass. Later, there is a collection of pus.

By allowing it to ripen, the exact location of the abscess can be more easily identified, and the abscess can then be drained; a smaller incision can be made in an exact location, and the pus can be drained. Attempting to drain a solid mass of inflamed tissue is pointless.

Abscesses must be drained. There are three approaches to draining the abscess:

- Incision and drainage ("I and D")
- Ultrasound-guided needle aspiration percutaneous drain (**Figure 256**), which is thought to be less invasive, more conservative, and having a shorter recovery time
- Mini periareolar incision with drain tube held in place by a suture, which provides continuous negative pressure draining[21]

Incision and drainage has been used for abscesses for many years. In this procedure, the abscess is lanced with a scalpel. After the abscess is opened and the pus drained, the wound is usually irrigated with saline. Then, if the abscess is not too large or too deep, an *antiseptic wick* (**Figure 253**) may be inserted for 24-48 hours to absorb the pus and discharge. The antiseptic wick is generally ribbon gauze soaked in a special antiseptic (e.g., betadine) and packed into the wound. (Note: A common misconception is that the antiseptic property of the wick aids in healing; it does not. The wick aids in healing because it prevents the skin edges of the abscess from re-sealing.)

For larger lesions, a drainage tube (**Figure 258**) may be inserted after the irrigation, a few stitches made to close the incision and a sterile dressing (**Figure 254**) applied over the wound. The abscess must be allowed to drain for several days to prevent re-formation of the abscess. The infant can continue breastfeeding, even with the tube. After several days, the tube is removed, but antibiotic therapy continues. Healing can take several weeks.

Image-guided needle aspiration with a percutaneous drain.[16, 22] This technique uses imaging guidance (usually CT scan, ultrasound or fluoroscopy) to accurately determine the best placement of a thin needle into the abscess. Then a *percutaneous* drain (from the Latin *per cutem*, meaning "through the skin") is left in place (**Figure 256**) for several days.

Occasionally, abscesses that cannot be treated by percutaneous drainage may require surgical drainage in the operating room. This procedure requires only a small nick in the skin—not a true incision—and therefore there are no stitches. It is minimally invasive, and the recovery period is usually faster than if the client had had a traditional incision.

A *mini periareolar incision* might be made. Like the traditional incision-and-drainage technique, the surgeon makes an incision and places a drain. However, a tube is inserted into the abscess, connected to a negative pressure bottle, and then secured to the skin with a suture. This tube continually drains exudate from the abscess until it is no longer detectable on ultrasound.[21]

Without prompt, effective treatment of an abscess, the consequences can be severe (**Figure 271**).

The question, however, is what treatments are effective. A Cochrane review reported, "There is insufficient evidence to determine whether needle aspiration is a more effective option to I&D for lactational breast abscesses, or whether an antibiotic should be routinely added to women undergoing I&D for lactational breast abscesses."[23] In a small study, 32 mothers received the traditional I&D treatment, and 30 mothers received the newer approach found no difference in terms of treatment effectiveness.[21]

Complete Learning Exercise 11-1 and 11-2 about terms related to milk stasis, oversupply, mastitis, and abscess.

Cellulitis

Cellulitis, shown in **Figure 292**, should not be confused with mastitis. Cellulitis is a bacterial infection of the connective and/or fatty tissue in the dermis and hypodermis (subcutaneous) layers. Like mastitis, cellulitis has a red appearance. However, the borders of the lesion are not well-defined (**Figure 263**) and it worsens when milk leaks through the broken tissue (**Figure 365**). Furthermore, mastitis and cellulitis can coexist.

Cellulitis is treated with antibiotic therapy. Cellulitis can also be mistaken for an abscess, and vice versa. If a fluctuation in the tissue can be felt, it is suggestive of an abscess, rather than cellulitis. However, if the abscess if deep, it may be impossible to feel the tissue fluctuating. Further, sometimes an abscess can have a cellulitis component.

Diagnosis often must be confirmed by ultrasound.

An accurate medical diagnosis is critical, because the treatment for cellulitis is different than for an abscess. An abscess must be drained; antibiotics are often prescribed, but antibiotics alone will not resolve the abscess. However, antibiotics alone are a sufficient treatment for cellulitis, unless there is some serious underlying factor (e.g., the patient is immunocompromised).

Looking Back, Looking Forward

In this chapter, we've talked about commonly-encountered conditions—including physiologic and pathologic engorgement, oversupply, overactive milk ejection reflex, abscess and other conditions associated with milk stasis.

Educational research shows that writing your own summary helps your retention. The Summarize What You've Learned exercise helps you to do this, so take a few minutes to complete it.

By now, if you have viewed the photos carefully, and if you've completed the written exercises, you should feel confident that you can recognize signs, clinical course, and treatment options for infectious and noninfectious conditions associated with oversupply and milk stasis.

Recalling, Reinforcing, and Expanding Your Learning

Have you ever felt frustrated that you "learned" something, but later, can't recall it? That may be because you didn't reinforce the material you learned. And, perhaps what you originally learned isn't enough to get you through the next few decades of practice; sometimes you need to expand your learning. The exercises in this section are designed to help you recall, reinforce, and expand your learning.

What was your main motivation for reading this chapter?

- ❍ To study for the IBLCE exam, as a first-time candidate
- ❍ To review for the IBLCE exam, as a re-certificant
- ❍ To improve my clinical skills and clinical management

How soon do you think can use the information presented in this chapter?

- ❍ Immediately; within the next few days or so
- ❍ Soon; within the next month or so
- ❍ Later; sometime before I retire

Pro Tip! If you are preparing for the IBLCE exam, it would be wise to pace your studying. Set a target date for when you plan to complete the exercises, and check off them off as you go along.

Done!	Target Date	Learning Exercise
❑	____________	Learning Exercise 11-1. Terms related to milk stasis and milk overproduction.
❑	____________	Learning Exercise 11-2. Terms related to lactational mastitis
❑	____________	Learning Exercise 11-3. Comparison of physiologic and pathologic engorgement.
❑	____________	Explore What You've Learned in a Journal
❑	____________	Summarize What You've Learned
❑	____________	Quick Quiz

Master Your Vocabulary

Unless you know the meaning of a word, you cannot fully answer a question about it. There were many, many terms in this chapter; you might not need to know them all, but you never know which ones you'll need to know!

Learning Exercise 11-1. Terms related to milk stasis and milk overproduction.

Instructions: Write the letter of the correct match next to each item. Answers are in the Appendix.

E	1. block feeding	A. caused by a severe milk stasis
D	2. breast abscess	B. tiny sac anywhere in the body that contains a liquid, gaseous, or semi-solid substance
L	3. cellulitis	C. caused by normal change of lactogenesis
B	4. cyst	D. a localized collection of pus in connective and fatty tissue of the breast, often accompanied by swelling and inflammation
M	5. erythema	E. unilateral breastfeeding ad lib with the same breast offered at every breastfeed in a certain time block
O	6. galactocele	F. excessive maternal milk
F	7. hypergalactia	G. an inflammation or infection of the breast tissue
K	8. induration	H. a technique to shift some interstitial fluid away from the edematous nipple-areola complex
G	9. mastitis	I. having or comprising several small cavities or compartments
I	10. multilocular	J. an abscess that occurs in the tissue beneath the areola
A	11. pathologic engorgement	K. hardening of a normally soft skin (or other tissue) due to inflammation, infiltration of a neoplasm, or accumulation of blood
N	12. peau d'orange	L. common bacterial infection of the skin and the soft tissues underneath
C	13. physiologic engorgement	M. superficial reddening of the skin (and dilation of blood capillaries) usually in patches due to injury or irritation
H	14. reverse pressure softening	N. thickened, dimpled skin that resembles the rind of an orange
J	15. subareolar abscess	O. cyst containing milk or a milky substance that is usually located in the mammary glands

Learning Exercise 11-2. Terms related to lactational mastitis.

Instructions: Write the letter of the correct match next to each item. Answers are in the Appendix.

Answer	Term	Match
E	1. afebrile	A. having a single small cavity that is infected
M	2. asymptomatic	B. protein enzyme that enables the conversion of fibrinogen to fibrin
I	3. block feeding	C. indicator that a disease process is present
B	4. coagulase	D. common cause of mastitis
L	5. febrile	E. normal body temperature
F	6. multilocular	F. having multiple small cavities that are infected
K	7. proinflammatory cytokines	G. recently-identified organism that is the cause of mastitis
H	8. prolactinoma	H. benign tumor of the pituitary gland
D	9. Staphylococcus aureus	I. using one breast for each feeding over a several-hour period of time
G	10. Streptococcus lactarius	J. a disease that has no recognizable clinical findings
J	11. subclinical	K. small secretions that have a specific effect on interactions and communications between cells
C	12. symptomatic	L. elevated body temperature
A	13. unilocular	M. without symptoms

Conquering Clinical Concepts

Learning Exercise 11-3. Comparison of physiologic and pathologic engorgement.

Instructions: Give a description of the characteristics for each of these conditions.

	Physiologic Engorgement	Pathologic Engorgement
Likely maternal perception	tender uncomfortable	very painful
Breast is soft, firm or hard?	firm (chin)	Hard (forehead)
Appearance of skin	veins visible skin normal color	taut shiny Redness or red streaking
Other?	resolves spontaneously	usually progresses to mastitis or plugged duct

Summarize What You've Learned

The goal of this chapter was for you to be able to recognize signs, clinical course, and treatment options for infectious and noninfectious conditions associated with oversupply and milk stasis.

Sometimes, the type of information in this chapter can seem much more theoretical than clinical. Take a moment to summarize: How can you arrange the most salient points into a few bullet points? How will you use this information for individual clients in your clinical practice? How might this information be important in the bigger world of system-level changes (e.g., procedures, standing orders, etc.) or issues with populations of clients (e.g., writing patient education materials.)

Main Points

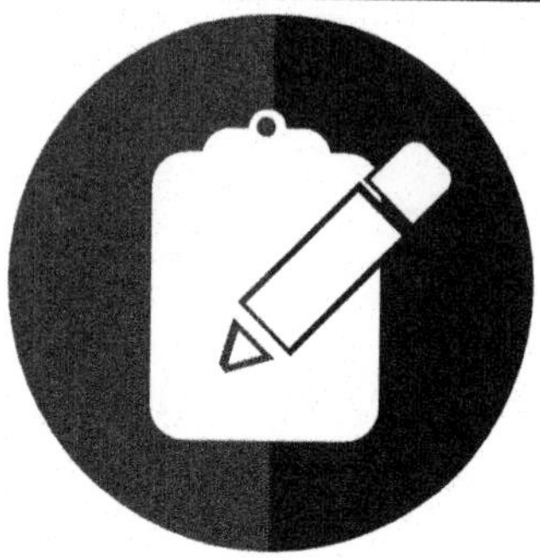

On the test

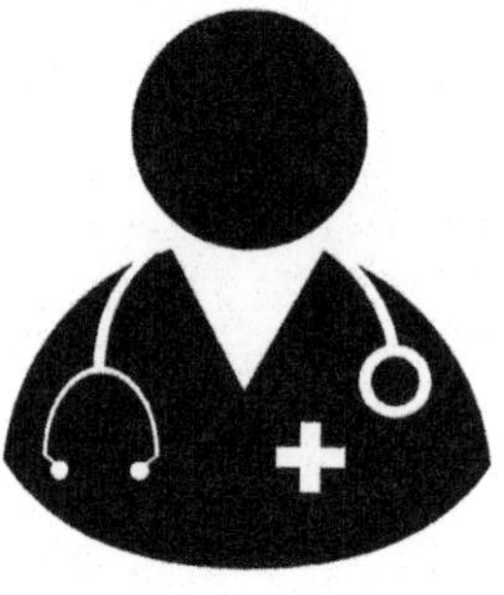

On the job

Explore What You've Learned With a Journal

Multiple studies have shown the benefits of using a learning journal. Among them are greater assimilation and integration of new information, better long-term retention of course concepts, increasing test and exam grades, and a means by which to have continuous feedback about one's own learning.

- Name at least three things you learned from this chapter.

- List at least three things you still need to learn, or more fully master, in this chapter.

- Briefly describe how this information fits (or doesn't fit) with what you've seen in clinical practice, what you learned in basic or college courses, or what you've observed in your own experience breastfeeding. (In some cases, you might want to include how the information fits or doesn't fit with what "experts" say, what the media says, or whatever.)

- Describe how you will use any or all of this information. How might it be related to problems and potential solutions that occur in real life or in clinical situations?

- If you wish, include how you felt about learning this information. Were you overwhelmed? Enlightened? Worried? Something else?

Self Assessment

People often dive into a test before they have thoughtfully reflected on how well they have prepared for it. Instead, it would be helpful if they would take a few moments to give their alter-ego (their "other self") a chance to reflect on how confident they feel about mastering the stated objectives.

Instructions: Take a moment to review the chapter objectives (below). Then rate yourself. How confident are you that you have achieved each objective below?

Objective	Highly Confident	Somewhat Confident	Somewhat Unsure	Completely Unsure
Compare and contrast signs of physiologic and pathologic engorgement, including possible patterns of onset and resolution.	❍	❍	❍	❍
Recognize possible indications of overactive milk ejection reflex (MER), consequences, and techniques to help the infant cope during a feeding.	❍	❍	❍	❍
Recognize signs of milk stasis that indicate the need for medical referral.	❍	❍	❍	❍
Recognize characteristics (e.g., milk color, milk texture, milk volume) often associated with mastitis and/or breast abscess.	❍	❍	❍	❍
Recognize characteristics of breast abscess in terms of formation and location, clinical course, treatment options, consequences of non-treatment, and techniques for breastfeeding during (or shortly after) treatment.	❍	❍	❍	❍
Distinguish between visible indicators of mastitis and cellulitis.	❍	❍	❍	❍

On the next page, you will some simple recall questions pertaining to this chapter. These are *not* the application-type questions you will find in the IBLCE exam. However, you cannot *apply* information unless you can fully *recall* that information! You should do these without looking up the answers.

When you finish with the quiz, look up the answers in the Appendix. Then, score your answers, using the Appendix. Finally, you should analyze the results of your quiz. It's not enough to just know what you got right or wrong; you must look at why you got the answers right.

Quick Quiz Chapter 11

Instructions: Circle the correct response. For a better understanding of how well you are mastering the material, try answering without looking it up. If you are really stuck, questions come from this workbook and from The Breastfeeding Atlas so go back and review the appropriate material. Answers are in the appendix.

1. Which of these words is frequently used to describe mastitis, but not engorgement?
   - A. distended
   - B. febrile
   - C. painful
   - D. unilateral

2. For the woman in **Figure 241**, which treatment option is LEAST indicated?
   - A. antibiotic therapy
   - B. cold/heat therapy
   - C. reverse pressure softening
   - D. use of cabbage leaves

3. Three of these descriptions are highly likely to be used for physiologic engorgement. Which one is not?
   - A. breasts full or leaking
   - B. discomfort
   - C. shiny, taut skin
   - D. shortened nipples

4. An infant is feeding in a prone feeding position. Of these, the most likely reason the mother chose this position to help the infant:
   - A. avoid congealed milk from mastitis
   - B. cope with an overactive MER
   - C. improve nipple grasp during engorgement
   - D. obtain hindmilk

5. Which treatment for a breast abscess does not require an incision with a scalpel?
   - A. antiseptic wick
   - B. drainage tubes
   - C. gauze packing
   - D. percutaneous drain

Analyze Your Own Quiz

- What percentage of the questions did you answer correctly?

- If you got 100% of them right, to what do you attribute your success?

- If you did not get all the questions right, can you identify your learning gap? (Example: Didn't know the information, knew the information but could not remember, knew some information but confused it with similar information, other.)

- Would you have been able to answer the questions as well if you had not read this chapter?

- What do you need to do next? (If you got them all right, what you need to do next is celebrate! Even a high-five with your child, a YESSS and a fist-pump in the air, or anything else is good! A small acknowledgement of your success is better than no acknowledgement!)

Additional Resources

1. Lawrence R, Lawrence, RM. *Breastfeeding: A guide for the medical profession.* 8 ed 2016.
2. Hill PD, Humenick SS. The occurrence of breast engorgement. *J Hum Lact.* 1994;10(2):79-86.
3. Humenick SS, et al. Breast engorgement: patterns and selected outcomes. *J Hum Lact.* 1994;10(2):87-93.
4. Mangesi L, Zakarija-Grkovic I. Treatments for breast engorgement during lactation. *Cochrane Database Syst Rev.* 2016(6):Cd006946.
5. Cotterman KJ. Reverse pressure softening: a simple tool to prepare areola for easier latching during engorgement. *J Hum Lact.* 2004;20(2):227-237.
6. Moon JL, Humenick SS. Breast engorgement: contributing variables and variables amenable to nursing intervention. *J-Obstet-Gynecol-Neonatal-Nurs.* 1989;18(4):309-315.
7. Cooke M, et al. A description of the relationship between breastfeeding experiences, breastfeeding satisfaction, and weaning in the first 3 months after birth. *J Hum Lact.* 2003;19(2):145-156.
8. Wilson-Clay B. Milk oversupply. *J Hum Lact.* 2006;22(2):218-220.
9. Eglash A. Treatment of maternal hypergalactia. *Breastfeed Med.* 2014;9:423-425.
10. Aljazaf K, et al. Pseudoephedrine: effects on milk production in women and estimation of infant exposure via breastmilk. *Br J Clin Pharmacol.* 2003;56(1):18-24.
11. van Veldhuizen-Staas CG. Overabundant milk supply: an alternative way to intervene by full drainage and block feeding. *Int Breastfeed J.* 2007;2:11.
12. Tena D, et al. Lactational mastitis caused by Streptococcus lactarius. *Diagnostic microbiology and infectious disease.* 2016;85(4):490-492.
13. Zarshenas M, et al. Incidence and Risk Factors of Mastitis in Shiraz, Iran: Results of a Cohort Study. *Breastfeed Med.* 2017;12:290-296.
14. Foxman B, et al. Lactation Mastitis: Occurrence and Medical Management among 946 Breastfeeding Women in the United States. *Am J Epidemiol.* 2002;155(2):103-114.
15. Kataria K, et al. Management of lactational mastitis and breast abscesses: review of current knowledge and practice. *The Indian journal of surgery.* 2013;75(6):430-435.
16. Ulitzsch D, et al. Breast abscess in lactating women: US-guided treatment. *Radiology.* 2004;232(3):904-909.
17. Kvist LJ, Rydhstroem H. Factors related to breast abscess after delivery: a population-based study. *Bjog.* 2005;112(8):1070-1074.

18. Bharat A, et al. Predictors of primary breast abscesses and recurrence. *World journal of surgery.* 2009;33(12):2582-2586.

19. Burtis WJ, et al. Immunochemical characterization of circulating parathyroid hormone-related protein in patients with humoral hypercalcemia of cancer [see comments]. *N Engl J Med.* 1990;322(16):1106-1112.

20. Amir LH, et al. An audit of mastitis in the emergency department. *J Hum Lact.* 1999;15(3):221-224.

21. Wei J, et al. Negative Suction Drain Through a Mini Periareolar Incision for the Treatment of Lactational Breast Abscess Shortens Hospital Stay and Increases Breastfeeding Rates. *Breastfeed Med.* 2016;11:259-260.

22. Sun HD, et al. Combination of ultrasound-guided drainage and antibiotics therapy provides a cosmetic advantage for women with methicillin-resistant Staphylococcus aureus breast abscess. *Taiwan J Obstet Gynecol.* 2014;53(1):115-117.

23. Irusen H, et al. Treatments for breast abscesses in breastfeeding women. *Cochrane Database Syst Rev.* 2015;8:Cd010490.

Chapter 12
Breast Cancer, Issues for Lactation

Breast cancer can and does happen during the childbearing years, even during lactation. Some changes in the breast that may initially seem abnormal or worrisome aren't; pregnancy and lactation often cause breasts to look or feel different than they did before. The problem is that some abnormalities are entirely unrelated to lactation. This raises many questions: How can women tell the difference? How can they get accurate information and follow-up for breast conditions? How can lactation consultants determine when what they see warrants better management of lactation, and when it is a pathologic condition that needs referral to a doctor? Just as importantly, when should they help women figure out when they need a second opinion?

In this chapter, you'll learn how to recognize "red flags" that suggest a breast condition is unrelated to lactation and how to inform and educate women about care before and after diagnostic and therapeutic procedures. You'll also gain practical guidance for how the condition or procedures will impact the woman's current or future experience of lactation—if at all.

If you've devoted much of your career to lactation, you might feel that issues related to cancer are "foreign territory" and outside of your domain. Remember, you don't need to become an oncologist! You just need to know how to help the lactating woman. With the many exercises that are provided in this chapter, you'll soon be well on your way to doing exactly that.

I promise that when we finish this chapter, you will be able to recognize the effects and the teaching implications of selected conditions, diagnostic tests, and therapeutic interventions associated with breast cancer during lactation.

Objectives

Given a clinical photo, you will be able to:

- Describe selected diagnostic tests in terms of indications for use, anticipatory guidance (including appropriate preparation, technology and equipment, and typical procedure and post-procedure events), scope of information it can provide, and implications for breastfeeding.
- Relate the scars or visible consequences from diagnostic or therapeutic interventions for suspected or confirmed breast cancer to their impact (if any) on current or future ability to lactate.
- Recognize suspicious signs/symptoms in the breast that warrant prompt medical follow-up with one or more physicians.
- State the definition of at least 15 terms that are related to the diagnosis and management of cancer of the breast.

Key Words

- biopsy
- core needle biopsy
- erosive adenomatosis
- excisional biopsy
- fine aspiration needle
- incisional biopsy
- induration
- lumpectomy
- mammogram
- mastectomy
- MRI
- needle aspiration
- Paget disease
- punch biopsy
- tumor
- ultrasound scan

Brief Overview of Breast Cancer as Related to Lactation

Breast cancer is the term for any of several diseases that affect breast tissue. It is the second most common cancer among women in the U.S., after skin cancer. Some women are at higher risk of breast cancer, due to family history, medical history, or behavioral factors—including not breastfeeding. Studies show that breastfeeding—especially for longer than a year—can lower the risk of developing breast cancer.

Women can experience breast cancer during their childbearing years or even while they are actively lactating. While there are several non-cancer reasons a woman may have a lump in her breast or other worrisome symptom, sometimes cancer is the cause.

Quite apart from any concerns about cancer, it's important to observe breasts and nipples in a systematic way. Always look at size and symmetry, color, retraction, texture, and general appearance. Also, look for the presence of characteristics such as lesions or discharge. Remember to check supernumerary nipples (discussed in chapter 9) or other "extra" tissue too, since it can become cancerous.[1, 2]

The tricky part for providers looking at lactating breasts is that observations that might be within normal parameters—lumpy breasts, for example—could also be pathologic. Using the model suggested above, here are some very simple guidelines to help distinguish between what is probably within normal parameters and what needs prompt referral. Keep in mind that this is an oversimplified set of guidelines, and evaluation by a physician is never inappropriate.

Size and symmetry: Nearly all women have one breast that is a little larger than the other. Marked asymmetry might be congenital, or it might be a sign that the lactating mother has more milk in one breast than in another. However, unilateral enlargement of the breast has been shown to occur with inflammatory breast cancer.[3]

Color: Reddened areas might be worrisome. If the woman has mastitis, redness of the breast is typical. However, with mastitis, she is also likely to have a fever. If there is redness but no fever, prompt medical follow-up is warranted. The literature includes a detailed case study[3] of a woman who had no fever, yet had warmth of the breast with edema, and mottled erythema over more than one-third of her breast. No lump was palpable, but breast cancer was present.

Retraction and texture: An unusual skin texture, or changes in the texture of the skin, can be worrisome. *Peau d'orange*, a dimpling of the skin (**Figure 244** and **245**), may or may not be accompanied by edema (swelling) or exaggerated hair follicle pits (**Figure 244**). *Induration* (**Figure 280**) of the skin is not necessarily a sign of cancer—it could occur with an abscess (**Figure 251**, as described in Chapter 11)—but it often is, so it requires prompt medical evaluation.

Discharge: Especially during the early days, if the infant is not well-latched, it is common to see a little blood come from the nipples. However, a bloody, oozing discharge—especially if it is unilateral—is a worrisome sign that warrants follow-up.

Lumps and general appearance: Lumps are not uncommon in the lactating breast. However, milk-related lumps typically feel similar to one another, are regularly-shaped, and are fluid-filled. A solid mass that is fixed and is irregularly-shaped is worrisome, Any mass that persists for more than 2 weeks should be evaluated with ultrasound.[4]

Other: What might appear to be a routine case of mastitis might instead be cancer. Because it is frequently misdiagnosed,[5] patients and health care professionals alike need to seek follow-up care for cases of mastitis that aren't typical. Dahlbeck and colleagues differentiate these, [6] recommending that when "mastitis" does not respond to antibiotic treatment, an ultrasound is the next important step.

Learning Exercise 12-2. Comparing lactation observations that may be pre-cancerous conditions.

Diagnostic Tests

Much of the time, lumps occur due to an abundance of milk. Other times, lumps appear for a more serious reason. To determine whether lumps are lactation-related, physicians frequently order diagnostic tests such as mammograms, ultrasound scans, MRIs, and/or biopsies.

Mammograms

Mammograms rely on x-rays (i.e., electromagnetic radiation). Mammograms are more frequently referred to as a "screening" tool, rather than a diagnostic tool, and for good reason. It's often difficult to "diagnose" breast cancer from a mammogram alone. Some argue that an ultrasound is the only way to go for the lactating woman,[7] whereas others suggest a combination approach.[8]

Although they pose no threat to the lactating breast or the mother's milk, they are often difficult to interpret. Accurate interpretation is most likely if the woman drains her breasts shortly before the mammogram, and if the radiologist is experienced in interpreting mammograms for lactating breasts. However, if a woman has a problem area, or if the results of the mammogram are unclear, she will likely be asked to get an ultrasound of the breast.

Ultrasound Scans

Ultrasound scans, also called sonograms, use high-frequency sound waves to visualize internal body parts. Ultrasound scans of the fetus during pregnancy have become popular as a safe and easy technique for internal visualization. However, ultrasounds are also performed to detect abnormalities in other body parts, including breasts.

Although initially used only for the non-lactating breast, ultrasound technology is now used for visualizing the lactating breast too. Ultrasound can detect normal functions in the lactating breast (e.g., milk ejection) or fairly simple problems (e.g., plugged duct) or more serious problems (e.g., cancer).[9] With ultrasound, it's possible to distinguish between lesions that have cancerous characteristics and those that are benign. Fluid-filled cysts (whether a milk-filled galactocele or a pus-filled abscess, as described in chapter 8) are characteristic of benign lesions, whereas solid lesions are more likely to be cancerous. By definition, tumors are solid lesions (see chapter 8), but not all solid tumors are cancerous.

While pregnant or lactating women normally have a rather nodular texture to their breasts, a mass that persists for more than 2 weeks should be evaluated with ultrasound.[4] Vashi and colleagues explain that "[s]onography is the first-line modality in the workup of a palpable breast mass in a pregnant or lactating patient."[10 p. 321]

It is easy for breastfeeding women to prepare for ultrasound scans. No lotion or powder should be applied to the upper body on the day of the exam, not even deodorant. Fasting is not required. Emptying her breast shortly before the procedure is ideal. The test is simple and painless, and there is no sedation. The client, dressed in a hospital gown, is asked to lie face up on an exam table (**Figure 272**) and to raise her arm while the breast is exposed. A transducer—a device that sometimes looks a bit like a microphone—is moved over the breast, gliding due to the use of a lubricating jelly. Generally, the procedure takes less than 30 minutes. The test poses no threat to the lactating breast or the mother's milk, and she can nurse her child as soon as after the procedure as she wishes.

Complete Learning Exercise 12-3 to see the similarities and differences in mammograms and ultrasounds.

MRIs

Electromagnetic resonating imaging (MRI) may be a necessary next step after a woman has had a mammogram or an ultrasound. An MRI provides a different, clearer sort of picture. Generally, it is less comfortable than an ultrasound, as it requires the woman to lie face-down on an exam table that moves slowly through the MRI machine. However, it can help health care providers to distinguish between cancerous and noncancerous conditions and determine whether more invasive testing is necessary.

Biopsies

A *biopsy* is a diagnostic procedure that allows the physician to examine sample cells to determine the presence or the extent of a disease process. Biopsies of the breast are usually done when a lump or lesion is suspected of being cancerous.

While there are variances in how the procedures may be performed, there are basically two types of biopsies. One uses aspiration, while the other uses a surgical technique. OncoLink[11] describes some of the sub-types.

- A *fine needle aspiration* (FNA), as the name suggests, uses a very small needle to remove a sample of the cells in question.
- A *core needle (CN) biopsy* uses a larger, hollow needle (**Figure 283**) to remove cells, as well as a small amount of surrounding tissue.
- An *incisional biopsy* takes out more—but not all—of the surrounding tissue. The incision is made with a scalpel. Skin lesions are done with a special circular blade (punch biopsy).
- An *excisional biopsy* removes the entire lesion.

Some use the term *lumpectomy* synonymously with excisional biopsy, but technically they are different. The goal of an excisional biopsy is diagnosis; a *lumpectomy* (**Figure 276**) is a treatment that is performed to have "clean margins" after the lesion is removed.

The woman in **Figure 273** initially had a biopsy. She breastfed her children. Eight years later, she had a lumpectomy. Both scars can be seen in **Figure 273**.

Prior to pregnancy, a different woman underwent a lumpectomy of her left breast, as well as chemotherapy and radiation. Later, she became a newly postpartum mother (**Figure 276**). Although she has not experienced any breast changes during this pregnancy or the postpartum period, she planned to breastfeed using only her right breast.

Paget disease of the nipple (PDN) is a rare but serious condition. In most cases, it is initially present on the nipple, and then spreads to the areola. (Paget disease of the breast/nipple should not be confused with a different and unrelated condition, Paget disease of the bone.) PDN can and does occur in lactating mothers. The prognosis for complete recovery is good—if the lesion is caught early and therapeutic measures are taken. However, stories abound about women who have been misdiagnosed with nipple eczema when they had Paget disease. See page 105 of *The Breastfeeding Atlas* for one such case.

Paget disease is also mistaken for *erosive adenomatosis of the nipple* (EAN),[12, 13] a rare, benign neoplasm of the breast's lactiferous ducts. We need to be aware of these misdiagnoses, and urge women to get prompt help for worrisome symptoms—sometimes to talk with a second or even third provider. The woman in the case study on page 105 met with four providers before she received the diagnosis and treatment she truly needed.

The primary technique for diagnosing skin lesions is the so-called *punch biopsy*. This allows full-thickness skin specimens—a disc-shaped piece of tissue—to be obtained.

The punch tool (**Figure 282**) has a circular blade, about 3-4 mm in diameter, attached to a pencil-like handle. A punch biopsy is a relatively painless procedure; numbing cream is applied to the nipple skin, and then a local anesthetic is injected (**Figure 281**). The client perceives some pulling and tugging, but usually no pain.

Mastectomy

A *mastectomy* is the removal of a breast (**Figure 278**). There are several different types of mastectomies:

- The simple (also called "total") mastectomy involves only the breast tissue of the affected side. This is usually performed if the woman has multiple or large areas of ductal carcinoma in situ (DCIS). It might also be performed prophylactically, such as when the woman's family history and genetic profile indicate a high risk of breast cancer.
- The radical mastectomy involves removal of the breast and all surrounding tissue, including the lymph nodes and chest muscles. This is usually performed if the woman has invasive breast cancer.
- The modified radical mastectomy includes the breast tissue plus the lymph nodes on the affected side and is the most common type of mastectomy.
- The partial mastectomy is the removal of part of the breast. Although similar to a lumpectomy, it removes more of the breast tissue.
- The subcutaneous (nipple-sparing) mastectomy is the removal of all of the breast tissue, although the nipple remains.

Complete Exercise 12-1 so you can master several terms related to breast cancer diagnostics and treatments.

Interventions and Their Implications

Women often wonder about how breast conditions or surgery will affect their ability to breastfeed—even if years have passed since they needed treatment.

For various reasons—the impossibility of conducting randomized controlled trials, low incidence in a younger maternal population, frequency of initial misdiagnosis, and more—research is limited about the long-term breastfeeding implications for many of these conditions and their treatments.

What we do know is that radiation is the most serious non-surgical procedure (although it often follows on the heels of surgery); unfortunately, it can significantly reduce the likelihood of a full milk supply, by as much as half.[14] Mothers should be counseled about the benefit of any breastfeeding, and perhaps the availability of donor milk.

The most severe surgical procedure is the mastectomy. A woman who has had a mastectomy prior to pregnancy may wish to breastfeed using her one remaining breast. As professionals, it's important for us to promote unilateral breastfeeding (**Figure 278**). This is unlikely to pose a problem for milk supply. Be careful, though, to remember that any "routine" problem on one breast is magnified in importance for the mother who is relying on only one breast. For example, a sore nipple due to suboptimal latch and positioning (**Figure 277**) may require extra attention when that is the mother's only breastfeeding nipple. It is good practice to encourage her to seek support for even "minor" breastfeeding problems, so you can help her with any problems as they arise.

Complete Learning Exercise 12-4, 12-5, 12-6, 12-7 to see how individual cases often play out in a way we might not anticipate.

Looking Back, Looking Forward

In this chapter, we've looked at signs and symptoms that are common in lactation, but can also be pathologic. We've also talked about many aspects of the equipment and procedures related to diagnostic or therapeutic intervention, and matched those with their likely origins, as well as implications that they may (or may not!) have for breastfeeding and lactation.

By now, if you have carefully viewed the images on page 187 of *The Breastfeeding Atlas* and completed the written exercises here, you should feel confident that you can recognize the effects and the teaching implications of selected conditions, diagnostic tests, and therapeutic interventions associated with breast cancer.

Recalling, Reinforcing, and Expanding Your Learning

Have you ever felt frustrated that you "learned" something, but later, can't recall it? That may be because you didn't reinforce the material you learned. And, perhaps what you originally learned isn't enough to get you through the next few decades of practice; sometimes you need to expand your learning. The exercises in this section are designed to help you recall, reinforce, and expand your learning.

What was your main motivation for reading this chapter?

- ❍ To study for the IBLCE exam, as a first-time candidate
- ❍ To review for the IBLCE exam, as a re-certificant
- ❍ To improve my clinical skills and clinical management

How soon do you think can use the information presented in this chapter?

- ❍ Immediately; within the next few days or so
- ❍ Soon; within the next month or so
- ❍ Later; sometime before I retire

Pro Tip! If you are preparing for the IBLCE exam, it would be wise to pace your studying. Set a target date for when you plan to complete the exercises, and check off them off as you go along.

Done!	Target Date	Learning Exercise
❑	______	Learning Exercise 12-1. Terms related to breast cancer diagnostics and treatments.
❑	______	Learning Exercise 12-2. Comparing lactation observations that may be pre-cancerous conditions.
❑	______	Learning Exercise 12-3. How implications for ultrasounds are both similar and different.
❑	______	Learning Exercise 12-4. Case Study A (Figures 273-275)
❑	______	Learning Exercise 12-5. Case Study B (Figure 277)
❑	______	Learning Exercise 12-6. Case Study C (Figures 278-280)
❑	______	Learning Exercise 12-7. Case Study D. (Figures 281-283)
❑	______	Explore What You've Learned in a Journal
❑	______	Summarize What You've Learned
❑	______	Quick Quiz

Master Your Vocabulary

Learning Exercise 12-1. Terms related to breast cancer diagnostics and treatments.

Instructions: Write the letter of the correct match next to each item. Answers are in the Appendix.

__P__ 1. biopsy

__K__ 2. core needle biopsy

__O__ 3. erosive adenomatosis

__H__ 4. excisional biopsy

__Q__ 5. fine aspiration needle

__L__ 6. incisional biopsy

__J__ 7. induration

__G__ 8. lumpectomy

__A__ 9. mammogram

__C__ 10. mastectomy

__M__ 11. MRI

__D__ 12. needle aspiration

__F__ 13. Paget disease of the nipple

__E__ 14. peau d'orange

__N__ 15. punch biopsy

__B__ 16. tumor

__I__ 17. ultrasound scan

A. uses lower dose x-rays to check the breast for lesions

B. solid mass

C. complete removal of the breast

D. removes cells to determine if they are cancerous without making an incision

E. dimpled texture of the skin

F. rare disease of the nipple that is frequently mistaken for eczema or other condition

G. lesion is removed with the goal of having "clean margins"

H. diagnostic test that aims to remove the entire lesion

I. also called a sonogram

J. hardening of normally soft tissue

K. uses a larger, hollow needle to remove cells and a small amount of surrounding tissue

L. removes a substantial amount of surrounding tissue

M. uses electromagnetic waves to check for breast lesions

N. uses a tool with a round blade to obtain full-thickness skin cell samples

O. rare, benign neoplasm of the mammary lactiferous ducts

P. diagnostic test to sample cells for presence or extent of disease process

Q. a very small needle used to remove a sample of cells

Conquer Clinical Concepts

Learning Exercise 12-2. Comparing lactation observations that may be pre-cancerous conditions.

Instructions: Compare the observations that are commonly associated with lactation to those that need prompt medical follow-up as a possible cancerous condition. Mark each observation as "likely lactation-related" or "worrisome". Answers are in the appendix.

Observation	Commonly-observed in lactating mothers	Needs follow-up
Breast Size	enlarged bilaterally w/ milk one may be fuller then other	enlargement not explained by milk supply
Breast symmetry	approx. equal	unequal not explained by diff in milk supply
Color	normal skin color reddened area can be easily explained	Red in one area
Edema	Present esp. in early days after anasthesia	edema heat & reddness not mastitis
Induration	possible w/ abscess	NO Abscess
Peau d'orange	possible w/ abscess	possible
Nipple discharge	a little blood usually bilateral explained by poor latch	copious & spontaneous
Mastitis	may recur but responds to antibiotics	mastitis like symptoms DOES NOT respond to abx
Lumps	fluid filled decrease within weeks	persist solid irregular shape

Learning Exercise 12-3. Similarities and differences between implications for mammograms and ultrasounds.

Instructions: It's not unusual for women to say, "What's the difference between..." By using a Venn diagram, you can compare and contrast points that apply to one thing, another thing, or both things; for example, points related to a mammogram or ultrasound. Diagraming is probably a little out of your comfort zone! But try it! You may quickly see how writing those similarities and difference on a Venn diagram can make it easier to explain them to others. (If you are stuck the answers are in the Appendix.)

Put details related to mammogram only on the left, details for ultrasound only on the right, and details for both in the center. To streamline your responses, answer these questions:

- *Technology: By what means does this equipment work?*
- *Patient Preparation: What must the woman do or not do the morning of the test?*
- *Patient Preparation: What should she do to improve readability of the test?*
- *Notification: Is it necessary to notify the technician that she is lactating?*
- *Safety: Is it okay to nurse the baby after the test?*
- *Results: What can the test detect?*

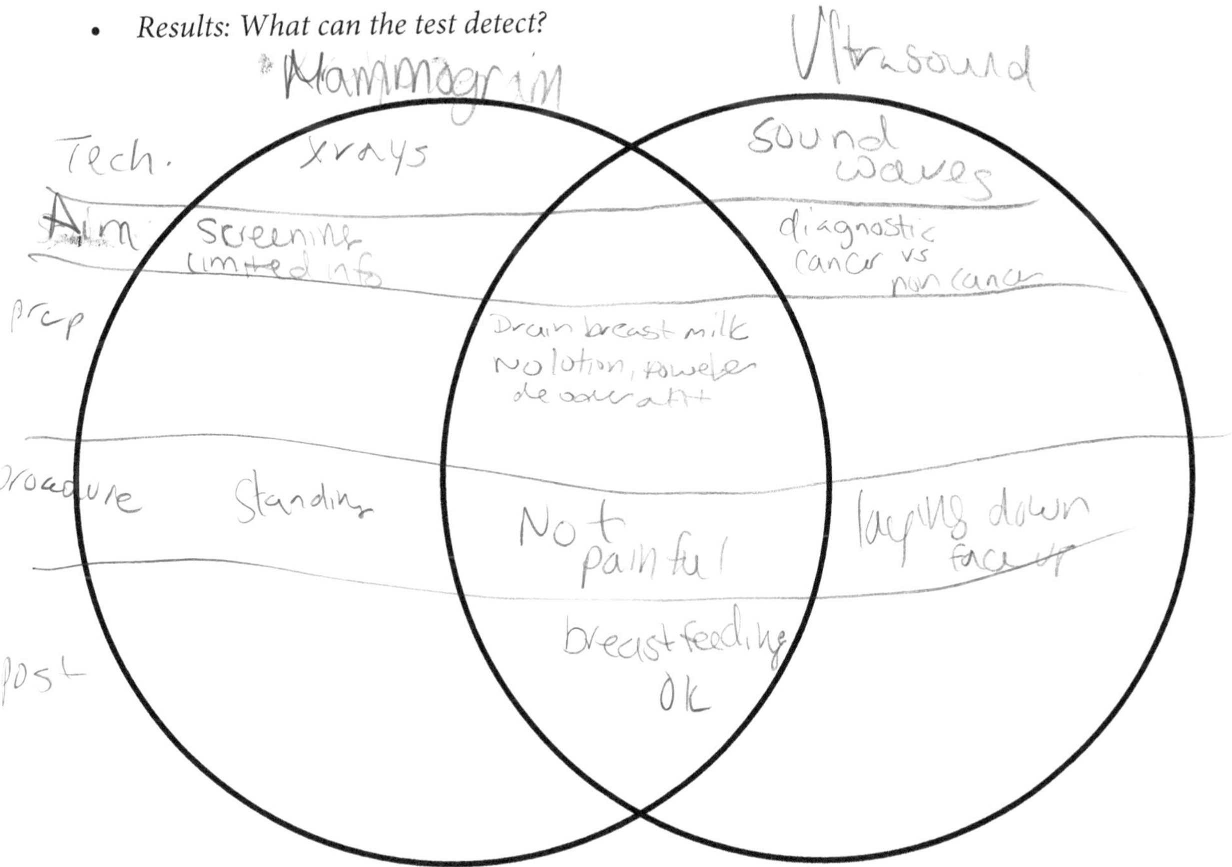

Learning Exercise 12-4. Case Study A (*Figures 273-275.*)

Instructions: Use page 104 and the accompanying images in The Breastfeeding Atlas *to answer the questions below.*

During her childbearing years, the woman described in these images found a lump in her breast after she finished lactating.

- At that time, what did the biopsy confirm?

- At that time, what type of incision was made? (**Figure 273**). Clearly describe the characteristics of the scar.

Years later, at age 48, she had a lumpectomy.

- What type of incision was used? (**Figure 273**). Where was this scar in relation to the previous scar from the biopsy?

- At this time, what condition was confirmed?

She was then treated with radiation therapy and developed the characteristic bronzed skin on her breast (**Figure 274**). (Routine skin-care for the "bronzed" skin has been well-studied[15,16] and is addressed in detail in *The Breastfeeding Atlas.*) A subsequent biopsy was performed in her axillary region (**Figure 275**) to determine if the cancer had spread.

- What is the main goal of the lumpectomy?

- Is it okay to wash radiation-bronzed skin?

- On the diagram below, draw the two scars of the woman in **Figure 273**, and see if you can label them correctly.

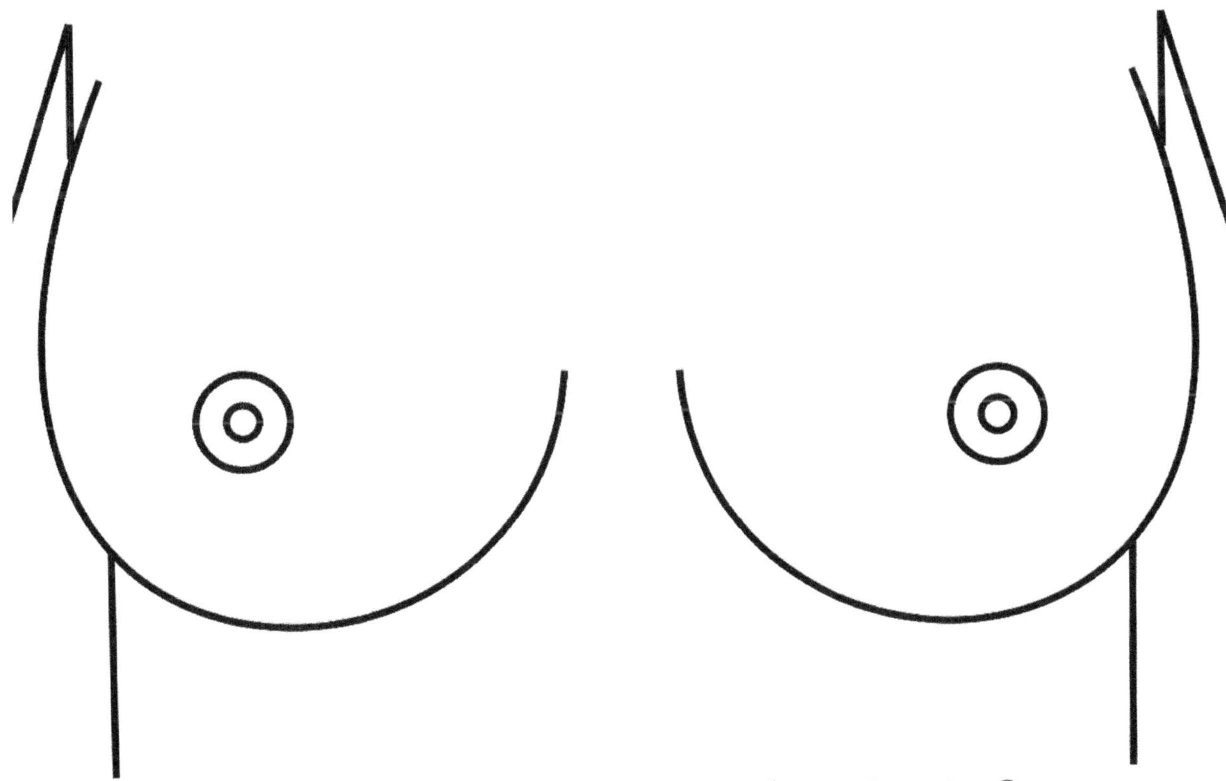

Reprinted with permission from Marie Biancuzzo's Comprehensive Lactation Course.

Learning Exercise 12-5. Case Study B (Figure 277).

Instructions: Use page 105-106 and the accompanying image in The Breastfeeding Atlas *to answer the questions below.*

A 32-year old woman had three children at the time she was diagnosed with breast cancer. She underwent a mastectomy (**Figure 277**). Then, four months after her breast was removed, she became pregnant with her fourth child. She decided to do unilateral breastfeeding for her newborn. She developed a lesion on her breast so severe that she pumped her milk for five days to give the nipple a chance to heal, and the infant was given her milk in a bottle.

- Would you have hesitated to recommend "resting" the nipple for five days? Are you concerned about nursing after having had the bottle for five days?

- Was this nipple lesion related to her previous bout with cancer?

Learning Exercise 12-6. Case Study C (Figures 278-280).

Instructions: Answer the questions below. Some of the answers are on page 105; some you will need to figure out yourself!

This 28-year-woman was breastfeeding her second child (a two-year old toddler) when her husband discovered a lump in her left breast.

- Imagine the breast is a clock viewed from the front. Describe the location of the needle biopsy.

- What can be seen in **Figure 279?** (See page 105.)

- What did the biopsy detect? (See page 105.)

- The surgeon recommended two actions. What were they? (See page 105.)

Wilson-Clay assisted with emergency weaning of the toddler.

- Although the authors do not say, you should know. What was MOST likely reason for the emergency weaning of the toddler?

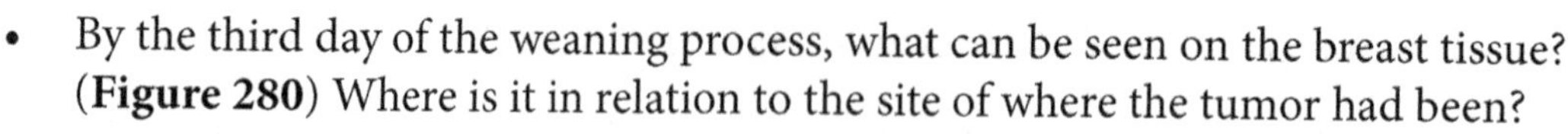

- By the third day of the weaning process, what can be seen on the breast tissue? (**Figure 280**) Where is it in relation to the site of where the tumor had been?

- What does *induration* mean? What could it indicate? (Explanation is in Chapter 11.)

After the toddler was weaned, the mastectomy was performed to remove the left breast and axillary lymph nodes. The mother then underwent chemotherapy and radiation treatment; she became pregnant while undergoing the radiation treatment. In **Figure 278**, the mother is unilaterally breastfeeding her 18-day-old infant.

- In what way did the radiation treatment affect the woman's pregnancy? (Page 105)

- How long did she breastfeed the infant? (Page 105)

Learning Exercise 12-7. Case Study D. (*Figures 281-283*).

Instructions. In this case study, fill in the blanks. The answers are on page 105 of The Breastfeeding Atlas.

This 32-year-old mother breastfed her firstborn for 15 months; history was unremarkable. With her second infant, she experienced an "oozing, crusty" lesion on the left nipple, as well as bleeding and cracking on the right nipple. The lactation consultant offered help with positioning, but the woman became febrile, so her primary care provider prescribed antibiotics. The problem persisted. Over the course of about six months, the mother consulted four different dermatologists.

The first dermatologist advised the mother to apply _______________. As a result, the healing of the lesion on her nipple _____________ .

Thereafter, the mother was treated for three different conditions, including ____________________, _________________________, and ________________. She was prescribed six medications plus Vaseline. Cultures of the wound were negative. She pumped her milk for six months, but her nipples did not completely heal, and in fact they _____________ as soon as she resumed any amount of breastfeeding.

At six months postpartum, the left nipple again became _________ and _________ . Finally, she consulted a fourth dermatologist, who recommended a punch biopsy to rule out Paget disease of the nipple.

This is not the first—and probably not the last—story of a woman who has a cancerous lesion that is mistaken for a different condition.

The take-home message for the lactation professional is ______________ .

Explore What You've Learned in a Journal

Multiple studies have shown the benefits of using a learning journal. Among them are greater assimilation and integration of new information, better long-term retention of course concepts, increasing test and exam grades, and a means by which to have continuous feedback about one's own learning.

- Name at least three things you learned from this chapter.

- List at least three things you still need to learn, or more fully master, in this chapter.

- Briefly describe how this information fits (or doesn't fit) with what you've seen in clinical practice, what you learned in basic or college courses, or what you've observed in your own experience breastfeeding. (In some cases, you might want to include how the information fits or doesn't fit with what "experts" say, what the media says, or whatever.)

- Describe how you will use any or all of this information. How might it be related to problems and potential solutions that occur in real life or in clinical situations?

- If you wish, include how you felt about learning this information. Were you overwhelmed? Enlightened? Worried? Something else?

Summarize What You've Learned

The goal of this chapter was for you to be able to recognize the effects and the teaching implications of selected conditions, diagnostic tests, and therapeutic interventions associated with breast cancer.

Instructions: Write your own summary of what you just learned in this chapter.

- When you think about a lactating mother who is about to undergo or has recently undergone clinical evaluation through a mammogram, ultrasound, MRI, or biopsy, what are the most important points you would want to remember?

- The scars or other visible remnants of diagnostic or therapeutic interventions for cancerous lesions can sometimes have an impact on lactation. How can you best help the lactating woman?

- What signs/symptoms would you consider suspicious on the breasts/nipples/areolar or accessory tissue of a lactating woman?

- Which terms were entirely new to you that you feel would be especially important for you to remember in the future?

Self-Assessment

People often dive into a test before they have thoughtfully reflected on how well they have prepared for it. Instead, it would be helpful if they would take a few moments to give their alter-ego (their "other self") at chance to reflect on how confident they feel about mastering the stated objectives.

Instructions: Take a moment to review the chapter objectives (below). Then, on a scale of 1 to 4, rate yourself, in writing. How confident are you that you have achieved each objective below?

Objective	Highly Confident	Somewhat Confident	Somewhat Unsure	Completely Unsure
Describe selected diagnostic tests in terms of indications for use, anticipatory guidance (including appropriate preparation, technology and equipment, and typical procedure and post-procedure events), scope of information it can provide, and implications for breastfeeding.	❍	❍	❍	❍
Relate the scars or visible consequences from diagnostic or therapeutic interventions for suspected or confirmed breast cancer to their impact (if any) on current or future ability to lactate.	❍	❍	❍	❍
Recognize suspicious signs/symptoms in the breast that warrant prompt medical follow-up with one or more physicians.	❍	❍	❍	❍
State the definition of at least 15 terms that are related to the diagnosis and management of cancer of the breast.	❍	❍	❍	❍

On the next page, you will find some simple recall questions pertaining to this chapter. These are *not* the application-type questions you will find in the IBLCE exam. However, you cannot *apply* information unless you can fully *recall* that information! You should do these without looking up the answers.

When you finish with the quiz, look up the answers in the Appendix. Then, score your answers, using the Appendix. Finally, you should analyze the results of your quiz. It's not enough to just know what you got right or wrong; you must look at why you got the answers right or wrong.

Quick Quiz Chapter 12

Instructions: Circle the correct response. For a better understanding of how well you are mastering the material, try answering independently, without flipping back or looking at the source material. If you are really stuck, questions come from this workbook and from The Breastfeeding Atlas, so go back and review the appropriate material. Answers are in the Appendix.

1. A lactating mother who has been diagnosed with breast cancer will be undergoing chemotherapy. She will be MOST likely to need help learning techniques for:

   A. emergency weaning

   B. maintaining good hydration

   C. preventing plugged ducts

   D. pumping and dumping

2. A lesion on skin that is normally soft and pliable but later becomes thick and fibrous would be described accurately as:

   A. abirritation

   B. ablation

   C. incretion

   D. induration

3. During and after radiation treatment, the skin on the affected breast is MOST likely to appear:

   A. bronzed

   B. bruised

   C. freckled

   D. pale

4. After radiation of the breast occurs, the change in later milk production[14] is MOST likely to be:

   A. increased

   B. decreased

   C. negligible

5. By viewing **Figure 273**, you realize that a scar from an incisional biopsy is MOST likely to be:

   A. a short, thin line

   B. a short, thin, round spot

   C. a long, keloid line

   D. invisible

Analyze Your Own Quiz

- What percentage of the questions did you answer correctly?

- If you got 100% of them right, to what do you attribute your success?

- If you did not get all the questions right, can you identify your learning gap? (Example: Didn't know the information, knew the information but could not remember, knew some information but confused it with similar information, other.)

- Would you have been able to answer the questions as well if you had not read this chapter?

- What do you need to do next? (If you got them all right, what you need to do next is celebrate! Even a high-five with your child, a YESSS and a fist-pump in the air, or anything else is good! A small acknowledgement of your success is better than no acknowledgement!))

Additional Resources

1. Sanguinetti A, et al. Invasive ductal carcinoma arising in ectopic breast tissue of the axilla. Case report and review of the literature. *Il Giornale di chirurgia.* 2010;31(8-9):383-386.

2. Shukla S, et al. Carcinoma in ectopic breast: a cytological diagnosis. *Breast disease.* 2015;35(3):217-219.

3. Molckovsky A, et al. Approach to inflammatory breast cancer. *Can Fam Physician.* 2009;55(1):25-31.

4. Woo JC, et al. Breast cancer in pregnancy: a literature review. *Arch Surg.* 2003;138(1):91-98; discussion 99.

5. Cristofanilli M. Inflammatory breast cancer: a new approach. *The Lancet. Oncology.* 2016;17(5):544-546.

6. Dahlbeck SW, et al. Differentiating inflammatory breast cancer from acute mastitis. *Am Fam Physician.* 1995;52(3):929-934.

7. Prasad SN, Houserkova D. A comparison of mammography and ultrasonography in the evaluation of breast masses. (1213-8118 (Print)).

8. Cong J, et al. A Selective Ensemble Classification Method Combining Mammography Images with Ultrasound Images for Breast Cancer Diagnosis. *Computational and Mathematical Methods in Medicine.* 2017;2017:4896386.

9. Geddes DT. Ultrasound imaging of the lactating breast: methodology and application. *Int Breastfeed J.* 2009;4:4.

10. Vashi R, et al. Breast imaging of the pregnant and lactating patient: imaging modalities and pregnancy-associated breast cancer. *AJR Am J Roentgenol.* 2013;200(2):321-328.

11. Oncolink. Incisional and excisional biopsy. ***https://www.oncolink.org/cancer-treatment/procedures-diagnostic-tests/biopsy-procedures/incisional-excisional-biopsy*** Accessed June 21, 2017.

12. Miller L, et al. Erosive adenomatosis of the nipple: a benign imitator of malignant breast disease. *Cutis.* 1997;59(2):91-92.

13. Spohn GP, et al. Nipple adenoma in a female patient presenting with persistent erythema of the right nipple skin: case report, review of the literature, clinical implications, and relevancy to health care providers who evaluate and treat patients with dermatologic conditions of the breast skin. *BMC dermatology.* 2016;16(1):4.

14. Leal SC, et al. Breast irradiation and lactation: a review. *Expert Rev Anticancer Ther.* 2013;13(2):159-164.

15. Chan RJ, et al. Prevention and treatment of acute radiation-induced skin reactions: a systematic review and meta-analysis of randomized controlled trials. *BMC cancer.* 2014;14:53.

16. Roy I, et al. The impact of skin washing with water and soap during breast irradiation: a randomized study. *Radiother Oncol.* 2001;58(3):333-339.

17. Chirappapha P, et al. Nipple sparing mastectomy: does breast morphological factor related to necrotic complications? *Plastic and reconstructive surgery. Global open.* 2014;2(1):e99.

18. Higgins S, Haffty BG. Pregnancy and lactation after breast-conserving therapy for early stage breast cancer. *Cancer.* 1994;73(8):2175-2180.

19. Martin RM, et al. Breast-feeding and cancer: the Boyd Orr cohort and a systematic review with meta-analysis. *J Natl Cancer Inst.* 2005;97(19):1446-1457.

20. Moran MS, et al. Effects of breast-conserving therapy on lactation after pregnancy. *Cancer journal (Sudbury, Mass.).* 2005;11(5):399-403.

21. Zhou Y, et al. Association Between Breastfeeding and Breast Cancer Risk: Evidence from a Meta-analysis. *Breastfeed Med.* 2015.

22. Cristofanilli M, et al. Update on the management of inflammatory breast cancer. *The oncologist.* 2003;8(2):141-148.

23. National Cancer Institute. Paget Disease of the Breast. ***https://www.cancer.gov/types/breast/paget-breast-fact-sheet*** Accessed June 25, 2017.

Chapter 13
Twins, Triplets and Tandem Nursing

In 2014, the rate of twin births in the U.S. reached a record high of 33.9 births out of every 1,000 deliveries. Although the rates for triplet and higher-order births were lower than previous years, the twin birth rate was slightly higher than 2013's rate of 33.7 out of every 1,000 births. Given that more than 135,336 U.S. births that year resulted from a twin pregnancy, and that the rate has been increasing for the past few decades, it's highly likely that you will soon find yourself helping a mother with twins or other higher-order multiples (HOMs).

More than half of twin pregnancies result in preterm births, presenting a number of feeding obstacles that must be overcome. Mothers' and infants' experiences will differ, but all will benefit from breastfeeding support.

Tandem breastfeeding—feeding two siblings of different ages—is entirely different from feeding twins. However, mothers and infants in both cases can benefit from several different positions. Both topics will be discussed in this chapter.

Some mothers of twins perceive themselves to be unable to produce enough milk for their infants. Worse still, some are told by others—including health care providers—that they should not even try because it will be impossible. This chapter will provide a few simple principles, many age-appropriate techniques, and essential information about the pros and cons of various breastfeeding positions, for mothers with twins, triplets, and more.

I promise that when we finish this chapter, you will be able to suggest optimal positioning and simple techniques to improve breastfeeding initiation and continuation for mothers of twins or tandem-nursing siblings.

By using photos in *The Breastfeeding Atlas* with the text and exercises of this workbook, you will soon gain the insights and skills to help mothers of twins or triplets, and those who wish to tandem nurse.

Objectives

Given a clinical photo, you will be able to:

- Recognize signs that twins are being held in suboptimal positions and suggest corrective strategies.
- Identify postural support as a priority for newborn twins, along with specific suggestions for how to achieve it.
- Recognize multiple age-appropriate techniques for optimizing weight gain for twins, higher-order multiples, and tandem breastfeeders.
- Briefly discuss how mothers of children two years and older may perceive pros and cons of breastfeeding older children, including tandem.
- State the definition of at least five terms related to breastfeeding twins, higher-order multiples, and tandem breastfeeding.

Key Words

- discordant twins
- *en face* position
- higher-order multiples
- low birth weight
- sequential breastfeeding
- simultaneous breastfeeding
- small for gestational age (SGA)
- tandem breastfeeding

Using Correct Terminology

Twins (two infants from one pregnancy) are often born before they reach full-term, so we classify them as preterm or premature. However, apart from their gestational maturity, we also classify them according to weight. Infants who weigh 1501 to 2500 grams are considered *low birth* weight. Those infants who are smaller than other infants at the same number of weeks of pregnancy are considered *small for gestational age* (SGA). SGA babies usually have birthweights below the 10th percentile for babies of the same gestational age. Do not confuse these two very different terms.

Sometimes, in a pair of twins, one infant is substantially larger than the other. These are called *discordant twins* (**Figure 284**). Sometimes, this happens as the result of twin-to-twin transfusion syndrome, a condition that can happen with monozygotic (identical) twins with a shared placenta. The birth weight of the smaller twin may be as much as 20 percent less than that of the larger twin.

Positioning Newborn Twins

Just as with breastfeeding singletons, optimal positioning and latch are the keys to achieving optimal milk transfer for mothers breastfeeding twins.

For some reason—often "to save time" or "so the mother can sleep", or worry that one infant will "go without" while the other feeds—mothers of twins are often urged to try to breastfeed both at the same time. But consider: Many new mothers of singletons need substantial help with positioning in the early days! Breastfeeding both infants at once—*simultaneous breastfeeding*—is a skill many mothers of twins will master, eventually. But, in the early days after birth, very few can manage it.

Postural support for the newborn is a priority. As discussed in Chapter 6, successful milk transfer depends upon good head-to-toe alignment.

Consider the twins in **Figure 285**. The infant in the foreground is being held in the football position; the infant in the background is lying in the cradle position. Observe factors that could interfere with successful milk transfer:

- the infant in the background appears to be falling asleep
- head-to-toe alignment is questionable, or poor
- suboptimal alignment could block the infant's nose and interfere with breathing
- After assistance from *The Breastfeeding Atlas*' Wilson-Clay and Hoover, (**Figure 286**):

- The mother uses the pillow appropriately. Rather than laying her infant on the pillow, she uses it to support her arm, so that her hands and arms are free to support her.
- The mother and infant have the benefit of the *en face position*. In this position, the infant is directly facing the mother, eye-to-eye.
- The newborn's chin indents the breast, which is essential for good milk transfer (see Chapter 6).
- The newborn's nose is less likely to be occluded.

Preterm infants are often hypotonic and sleepy. They might be assisted to achieve good alignment, but often cannot *sustain* it for the duration of the feeding. Postural support is a priority, and attention must be given so it is sustained for the duration of the feeding.

Beware of professionals who push for simultaneous feedings early in the postpartum period—often, during the hospital stay! They seem unaware that postural support and good milk transfer must be the priority, and that most mothers do not have the coordination to achieve that until they are more comfortable handling their twins.

At first, most mothers of twins need to breastfed one twin, and then the other. That's called *sequential breastfeeding* (**Figure 287**). The mother should continue sequential feedings until each has optimal postural support and evidence of successful milk transfer. For some mothers, this may be several weeks.

When the mother does opt to do simultaneous feedings, it will be imperative for her to have help from someone else for positioning the infants at the beginning of the feeding. As she becomes more adept at simultaneous feedings, she will be able to do it herself.

Techniques to Optimize Milk Transfer and Weight Gain

There are several techniques that can help to optimize milk production and transfer. Skin-to-skin contact provides many physiologic and psychologic benefits for infants and mothers. For infants who are unable to obtain a full feeding at the breast, cup feeding the mother's expressed milk is a good strategy. Compressing the breast (**Figure 287**) to express the milk into the infant's mouth, if necessary, can also help with milk transfer.

I cannot emphasize enough: Postural support remains a priority for breastfeeding. With time (and their infants' development), nearly all mothers of twins can provide simultaneous feedings. They become more comfortable and more coordinated with holding and feeding two infants simultaneously, and the infants grow stronger and require less postural support. (Not all mothers will switch to simultaneous feeding. Some will elect to continue sequential feedings.)

If milk transfer is confirmed, simultaneous feedings can be initiated in a variety of ways. (All options listed here are variations of those discussed in Chapter 6; they may work for twins in early infancy.)

The cradle-cradle hold positions the twin infants in a "V" (**Figure 288**). While this is often used, it opens the door for poor alignment because newborns, especially preterm newborns, need substantial postural support that a double cradle-hold cannot reliably provide.

Figure 289 shows seven-day-old near-term infants who appear to be on a nursing pillow. Using the principles discussed in this chapter and Chapter 6, you will note that positioning is not optimal.

For mothers who want to begin simultaneous feedings of twins, a dual football hold (**Figure 290**) can be helpful, at least initially. The football position allows the mother to provide good head, neck, and shoulder support for each twin while keeping both in the *en face* position. In situations where one twin is stronger, that twin might be placed in a cradle hold, while the other is positioned in a football hold (**Figure 293**).

Exclusive or nearly exclusive breastfeeding is possible not only for twins, but for higher-order multiples (HOMs) as well (**Figure 296**). Feeding three—or more!—infants with two breasts requires some rotation. When all infants want to eat at the same time, the mother can offer one breast to Baby A and one to Baby B while Baby C waits (perhaps in another caregiver's arms, or in an infant bouncer, as recommended by expert Karen Kerkhoff Gromada, on the 11/11/2013 episode of "Born to be Breastfed") Baby C can be offered both breasts after his siblings have been fed. Rotation occurs at the next feeding.

Developmental changes that occur during the first months of the twins' life—such as being able to hold their own heads up, sit up assisted, or sit up independently—create opportunities for different positions in simultaneous feeding. Five-month-old twins can kneel (**Figure 291**) to breastfeed. The mother of eight-month-old twins in **Figure 292** feeds them in a twin carrier. For those twins who are on the go, standing while breastfeeding works (as demonstrated by a pair in **Figure 295**)! And, when it's time for everyone to relax, toddlers can breastfeed in a side-lying position while the mother reclines (**Figure 294**). (Note that while this position would be a suffocation hazard for young infants, these children are old enough to pull away to breathe, if necessary.)

In my experience, young twins tend to start exhibiting feeding cues at about the same time. Ironically, when they are older and more physically able to support themselves during simultaneous feedings, twins may not show feeding cues at the same time. It will be important for the mother to watch for feeding cues from each of her infants. They soon begin to develop separate personalities and preferences.

To solidify your understanding of terms and techniques, complete Learning Exercises 13-1, 13-2, 13-3, 13-4.

Perceptions, Risks and Realities About Tandem Breastfeeding

Tandem breastfeeding is the breastfeeding of two different-aged siblings at the same time. (Often, the term *tandem* is used incorrectly to refer to twins who are feeding at the same time; it should be reserved only for situations where siblings of different ages are breastfed by the same mother.) Breastfeeding a child while pregnant is also not "tandem nursing" but the concept is the same, and certainly the mother who breastfeeds throughout her pregnancy is more likely to tandem breastfeed afterwards than a mother who weans prior to or during her pregnancy.

The mother shown feeding her two-year-old in **Figure 297** is pregnant with twins; she also breastfeeds her four-year-old, who is not shown in the picture. This pregnancy went well, but twin gestation put the mother at higher risk for a preterm delivery for two reasons: (1) twin gestation, and (2) breastfeeding during pregnancy increases the levels of circulating oxytocin, thereby raising the risk for the onset of labor contractions.

Many mothers assume that they cannot continue breastfeeding a toddler if they are pregnant or have a newborn, and they wean the older child. Some mothers do continue to nurse during or after pregnancy, but they do not want others to know about it, out of concern about expected criticism.

Unquestionably, the newborn must have priority at the breast to avoid cases of failure to thrive.

As the photos in *The Breastfeeding Atlas* show, tandem nursing is entirely possible. We see mothers nursing a four-year-old and a 16-month-old (**Figure 298**), a four-year-old and a 19-month-old (**Figure 299**), and a four-year-old and a two-year old (**Figure 300**). Mothers who tandem nurse tend to find that the older child requires less support and can be positioned in any way that is mutually comfortable.

In the United States, health care professionals often discourage breastfeeding of toddlers or preschoolers, such as the three-year-old in **Figure 301**. However, mothers can determine for themselves whether nursing an older child (either in tandem or alone) is right for them. See page 113 of *The Breastfeeding Atlas* for discussion of positive and negative perceptions that the mother breastfeeding an older child might have.

Looking Back, Looking Forward

In this chapter, we've talked about how to position more than one infant or child at the breast, techniques to help optimize milk transfer and weight gain, and the perceptions, risks, and realities about tandem breastfeeding. By now, if you have carefully viewed the images on pages 188-189 of *The Breastfeeding Atlas*, and if you've completed the written exercises here, you should feel confident that you can suggest optimal positioning and simple techniques to improve breastfeeding initiation and continuation for mothers of twins or tandem-nursing siblings.

Recalling, Reinforcing, and Expanding Your Learning

Have you ever felt frustrated that you "learned" something, but later, can't recall it? That may be because you didn't reinforce the material you learned. And, perhaps what you originally learned isn't enough to get you through the next few decades of practice; sometimes you need to expand your learning. The exercises in this section are designed to help you recall, reinforce, and expand your learning.

What was your main motivation for reading this chapter?

❍ To study for the IBLCE exam, as a first-time candidate

❍ To review for the IBLCE exam, as a re-certificant

❍ To improve my clinical skills and clinical management

How soon do you think can use the information presented in this chapter?

❍ Immediately; within the next few days or so

❍ Soon; within the next month or so

❍ Later; sometime before I retire

Pro Tip! If you are preparing for the IBLCE exam, it would be wise to pace your studying. Set a target date for when you plan to complete the exercises, and check off them off as you go along.

Done!	Target Date	Learning Exercise
❑	____________	Learning Exercise 13-1. Basic vocabulary related to twins, triplets, and tandem nursing.
❑	____________	Learning Exercise 13-2. Recognizing feeding strategies in photos.
❑	____________	Learning Exercise 13-3. Techniques for sequential or simultaneous feedings.
❑	____________	Learning Exercise 13-4. Recognizing key indicators of positioning.
❑	____________	Explore What You've Learned in a Journal
❑	____________	Summarize What You've Learned
❑	____________	Quick Quiz

Master Your Vocabulary

Unless you know the meaning of a word, you cannot fully answer a question about it. There were several terms in this chapter; you might not need to know them all, but you never know which ones you'll need to know!

Learning Exercise 13-1. Basic vocabulary related to twins, triplets, and tandem nursing.

Instructions: Write the letter of the correct match next to each item. Answers are in the Appendix.

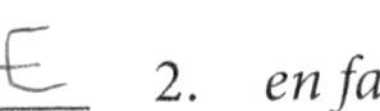

___ 1.	discordant twins	A.	feeding two infants at the same time
___ 2.	*en face*	B.	significant size or weight different between twins
___ 3.	low birth weight	C.	breastfeeding two children of different ages
___ 4.	sequential feeding	D.	smaller in size than normal for the gestational age
___ 5.	simultaneous feeding	E.	facing the mother
___ 6.	SGA	F.	weighing less than 2500 grams
___ 7.	tandem breastfeeding	G.	feeding one at one time and the other one later

Learning Exercise 13-2. Recognizing feeding techniques in photos.

Instructions: Match the phrase on the left to the photo listed on the right. Answers are in the Appendix.

___ 1.	discordant twins	A.	#298
___ 2.	*en face*	B.	#284
___ 3.	sequential feeding	C.	#288
___ 4.	simultaneous feeding	D.	#287
___ 5.	tandem breastfeeding	E.	#286

Conquer Clinical Concepts

Learning Exercise 13-3. Techniques for sequential or simultaneous feedings.

Instructions: Given an individual situation or a specific age, which techniques work well, and which ones don't? Why so? Write some simple answers to help you review later.

Sequential	
Simultaneous	
Cradle/Cradle	
Football/football	
Side-lying	
Standing	
Use of pillows	

Learning Exercise 13-4. Learning Exercise 4. Recognizing key indicators of positioning.

Instructions: Write short answers for each situation.

Figure 289. The infant was born near term and is now seven days old. Using the photo, name at least three indicators for postural/positional changes needed.

-
-
-
-

Figure 290. Name at least two indicators that should help to achieve good milk transfer.

-
-
-

Figure 297. If you were counseling the mother shown in this photo, you might want to praise her for doing such a good job, but offer her a gentle caution of what?

Explore What You've Learned in a Journal

Multiple studies have shown the benefits of using a learning journal. Among them are greater assimilation and integration of new information, better long-term retention of course concepts, increasing test and exam grades, and a means by which to have continuous feedback about one's own learning.

- Name at least three things you learned from this chapter.

- List at least three things you still need to learn, or more fully master, in this chapter.

- Briefly describe how this information fits (or doesn't fit) with what you've seen in clinical practice, what you learned in basic or college courses, or what you've observed in your own experience breastfeeding. (In some cases, you might want to include how the information fits or doesn't fit with what "experts" say, what the media says, or whatever.)

- Describe how you will use any or all of this information. How might it be related to problems and potential solutions that occur in real life or in clinical situations?

- If you wish, include how you felt about learning this information. Were you overwhelmed? Enlightened? Worried? Something else?

Summarize What You've Learned

The goal of this chapter was for you to be able suggest optimal positioning and simple techniques to improve breastfeeding initiation and continuation for mothers of twins or tandem-nursing siblings.

Instructions: Write some simple notes to yourself to help you review later.

- What is the MOST important principle to keep in mind when helping a breastfeeding mother of multiples during the early days?

- Techniques to facilitate breastfeeding for newborn twins, or higher-order multiples: What is the priority during the first month of life (or beyond)? Why so?

- What benefits and risks are associated with tandem nursing?

- What positive perception(s) might mothers have about tandem nursing? (*The Breastfeeding Atlas*, page 113.)

- What negative perception(s) might mothers have about tandem nursing? (*The Breastfeeding Atlas*, page 113.)

Self-Assessment

People often dive into a test before they have thoughtfully reflected on how well they have prepared for it. Instead, it would be helpful if they would take a few moments to give their alter-ego (their "other self") at chance to reflect on how confident they feel about mastering the stated objectives.

Instructions: Take a moment to review the chapter objectives (below). Then rate yourself. How confident are you that you have achieved each objective below?

Objective	Highly Confident	Somewhat Confident	Somewhat Unsure	Completely Unsure
Recognize signs that twins are being held in suboptimal positions and suggest corrective strategies.	❍	❍	❍	❍
Identify postural support as a priority for newborn twins, along with specific suggestions for how to achieve it.	❍	❍	❍	❍
Recognize multiple age-appropriate techniques for optimizing weight gain for twins, higher-order multiples, and tandem breastfeeders.	❍	❍	❍	❍
Briefly discuss how mothers of children two years and older may perceive pros and cons of breastfeeding older children, including tandem.	❍	❍	❍	❍
State the definition of at least five terms related to breastfeeding twins, higher-order multiples, and tandem breastfeeding.	❍	❍	❍	❍

On the next page, you will some simple recall questions pertaining to this chapter. These are *not* the application-type questions you will find in the IBLCE exam. However, you cannot *apply* information unless you can fully *recall* that information! You should do these without looking up the answers.

When you finish with the quiz, look up the answers in the Appendix. Then, score your answers, using the Appendix. Finally, you should analyze the results of your quiz. It's not enough to just know what you got right or wrong; you must look at why you got the answers right or wrong.

Quick Quiz Chapter 13

Instructions: Circle the correct response. For a better understanding of how well you are mastering the material, try answering independently, without flipping back or looking at the source material. If you are really stuck, questions come from this workbook and from *The Breastfeeding Atlas*, so go back and review the appropriate material. Answers are in the Appendix.

1. Whether for singletons, twins, or multiples, which factor is MOST important for effective breastfeeding?

   A. eye-to-eye contact

   B. frequent burping

   C. postural support

2. When assisting the mother of twins during the first month of life, the aim is to make sure which outcome is achieved?

   A. milk transfer to newborn

   B. 10-minute-minimum feeding

   C. sequential feeding

   D. simultaneous feeding

3. When determining whether the twins in **Figure 285** have postural support for effective latch, you should notice that the:

   A. hips of the twin in the background are not aligned with his head

   B. lips of both infants are not adequately flanged

   C. **nose of the twin in the foreground is buried in the breast**

4. If a preterm twin is not getting enough milk for optimal weight gain, which technique is LEAST appropriate to suggest to the mother?

   A. breast compression during the feeding

   B. cup-feeding supplemental formula

   C. skin-to-skin care when not feeding

   D. finger-feeding a friend's unpasteurized breast milk

5. If a mother is breastfeeding her newborn and a toddler, the highest priority for care is:

   A. encouraging her to ignore disapproving remarks from others.

   B. helping her to explore her feelings about this arrangement.

   C. suggesting birth control methods with minimal impact on milk supply.

   D. teaching her that her newborn is given preference for breast access.

Analyze Your Own Quiz

- What percentage of the questions did you answer correctly?

- If you got 100% of them right, to what do you attribute your success?

- If you did not get all the questions right, can you identify your learning gap? (Example: Didn't know the information, knew the information but could not remember, knew some information but confused it with similar information, other.)

- Would you have been to able answer the questions as well if you had not read this chapter?

- What do you need to do next? (If you got them all right, what you need to do next is celebrate! Even a high-five with your child, a YESSS and a fist-pump in the air, or anything else is good! A small acknowledgement of your success is better than no acknowledgement!)

Additional Resources

1. Flower H. Adventures in Tandem Nursing: Breastfeeding During Pregnancy and Beyond. Chicago: La Leche League International, 2003.

2. Gromada KK. "Breastfeeding Twins, Triplets or More!" Born to be Breastfed, with Marie Biancuzzo. November 11, 2013. Available ***http://www.voiceamerica.com/episode/73969/breastfeeding-twins-tripletsor-more***

3. Gromada, KK. Mothering Multiples: Breastfeeding and Caring for Twins or More! Chicago: La Leche League International, 2007.

4. Kuhnly JE, Juliano M, McLarney PS. The Development and Implementation of a Prenatal Education Program for Expectant Parents of Multiples. J Perinat Educ. 2015;24(2):110-8.

5. McGovern T. The challenges of breastfeeding twins. Nurs N Z. 2014 Dec-2015 Jan;20(11):26-7, 44.

6. Mikami FC, de Lourdes Brizot M, Tase TH, Saccuman E, Vieira Francisco RP, Zugaib M. Effect of Prenatal Counseling on Breastfeeding Rates in Mothers of Twins. J Obstet Gynecol Neonatal Nurs. 2017 Jan 5. pii: S0884-2175(16)30429-4.

7. Whitford HM, Wallis SK, Dowswell T, West HM, Renfrew MJ. Breastfeeding education and support for women with twins or higher order multiples. Cochrane Database Syst Rev. 2017 Feb 28;2:CD012003.

Chapter 14
Alternative Feeding Methods

Although we know that early supplementation negatively affects duration and exclusivity of breastfeeding, formula supplementation without a medical indication happens to as many as 87 percent of newborns during their hospital stay.[1] Most commonly, bottles are used when supplements are given, but this has not been shown to be the best practice, when compared with cup-feeding or other methods.[2]

The implication for breastfeeding advocates is clear: Until exclusive breastfeeding is established as the norm, supplementation is likely to happen. (For some infants, supplementation will be necessary even when breastfeeding is desired.) When supplementation does occur, it will be given by an *alternative feeding method*, which includes any non-breastfeeding device, such as a bottle, syringe, or cup, etc. We should be prepared to help parents to choose a method that works for their infant and to teach them how to use it appropriately until breastfeeding can be initiated or resumed.

Understandably, some of this content might sound a little foreign—or even distasteful to you! But by viewing the photos on Pages 190-192 of *The Breastfeeding Atlas*, following along with my commentary, viewing the videos, and completing the exercises throughout this chapter, you'll sail right through the quick quiz at the end!

I promise, by the time you finish this chapter, you will be able to facilitate the correct use of an alternative feeding method in specific situations and minimize interruption of the breastfeeding relationship.

Objectives

Given a photo, you will be able to:

- List indications or contraindications for using an alternative feeding device to help maintain the breastfeeding relationship when an infant cannot fully feed at the breast.
- Recognize techniques that help or hinder the use of an alternative feeding method.
- Discuss pros and cons of alternative feeding methods in terms of ease of use, efficacy, and other factors.
- Briefly describe the use of nasogastric and orogastric feeding tubes and their possible impact on breastfeeding.
- Recognize stress cues an infant may exhibit while bottle-feeding.
- Describe paced bottle feeding in terms of its indications, benefits, and techniques for use.
- State the definition for at least five terms related to alternative feeding methods and bottle feeding.

Key Words

- alternative feeding methods
- cup feeding
- finger feeding
- Lact-Aid™
- nasogastric (NG) tube
- nursing supplementer
- oral aversion
- oral-tactile hypersensitivity
- orogastric (OG) tube
- paced feeding, paced bottle-feeding
- paladai
- periodontal syringe
- spoon feeding
- supplementary feeding
- Supplemental Nurser System™
- syringe feeding
- tube feeding

Supplementation

We often talk about the negative effects of "supplementation" or about breastfeeding management when supplementation cannot be avoided. However, before any discussion of supplementation is meaningful, we need to become clear on the meaning of "supplementation."

In its protocol for supplementary feeding for healthy, term infants[3], the Academy of Breastfeeding Medicine (ABM) uses "supplementation" to refer to the giving of extra feedings in addition to or as a replacement for direct breastfeeding. Choices of supplement, in order of priority, are: expressed milk from the mother, donor human milk, and protein hydrolysate formula, although other fluids may be considered (e.g., cow's milk formulas, soy formulas).

To support mothers' confidence in their ability to meet their infants' nutritional needs, breastfeeding advocates should reserve the term "supplementation" for feeding fluids other than the mother's own milk[3], and use "breastfeeding" for "feeding only breastmilk (at the breast or own mothers' expressed breast milk), no food or water except vitamins, minerals, and medication." In this case, supplementation is used for additional fluids for a breastfed infant who is less than six months old, and these fluids "may include donor human milk, infant formula or other breast milk substitutes (e.g., glucose water)."[3]

This chapter focuses on the devices that deliver feedings, such as tube-feeding devices, spoons, cups, paladai, and bottles. The chapter does not address specific types of fluid in the feeding device.

Among the competencies for lactation consultants set forth by the International Board of Lactation Consultant Examiners (IBLCE) is the ability to "carefully choose a method of feeding when supplementation is unavoidable and use strategies to maintain breastfeeding to meet the parents' goal." I have my concerns about this statement, since it implies that the "choice" does not rest with the parent. It also implies that only one method can be used, and that such a choice is made only once. Often, especially in the early days, a short-term tactic can often support a long-term goal. Helping the mother to revisit her decision for the method by which her infant is fed should be encouraged.

Here, we will explore the devices that will deliver the feeding to the infant. In selecting among them, my personal rule is this: *Always play to the strengths of the family.*

Tube-Feeding Devices

Tube-feeding devices may be:

- commercially-made or homemade
- attached to another device (**Figure 312**), a finger, or a breast
- non-invasive or invasive (e.g., nasogastric tube)
- delivering the entire feeding (e.g., if mother has no milk, or if the infant cannot nurse) or "extra" milk (e.g., if the mother has a low supply, the infant tires too easily to complete the feeding, or the infant has limited ability to transfer milk).

Finger feeding, nursing supplementers, and even nasogastric tubes can be classified as alternative feeding methods that use a feeding tube. *The Breastfeeding Atlas* has covered these in more detail; so have I, elsewhere.[4] Here, we will look at basic principles for use, pros and cons, and helpful techniques.

Finger Feeding

Finger feeding is a means of feeding in which the infant sucks on the caregiver's finger. It may be done with a tube only, or with a tube and a syringe. A #5 French feeding tube is usually used for this purpose.

Finger feeding may be used in many situations in which a truly "full" feeding cannot be accomplished at the breast. One common situation is a lack of full milk production, such as when the mother has not given birth to the infant she is nursing (**Figure 316**). Another is that an infant is not efficiently transferring milk and is failing to thrive (**Figure 313**).

Finger feeding gives the infant the chance to develop the muscles used for sucking, while at the same time becoming familiar with his mother's scent. A word of caution, though: in my experience, some parents just don't like doing finger feeding. As with any of the methods we'll discuss, it's always good to check in later to see how the parent feels about the feeding method they are using. Note, this inquiry is not about whether the parent is capable of performing the task; it's about whether the parent likes or dislikes doing it. Often parents don't offer that information, so it's important to ask.

Finger-feeding can also be accomplished without being attached to any other device. The tube can be taped, so that the tip of the tube is at the tip of the feeder's largest finger. In **Figure 311**, the caregiver has the feeding tube along the side of her thumb. The thumb, being the largest digit is well-suited to this purpose because it encourages the wide gape that would be necessary for breastfeeding (see Chapter 6). Note that the mother has her finger pad side up in the photos (**Figures 311, 312, 313, and 315).**

Figure 311 demonstrates one of the disadvantages of finger feeding without a syringe. The infant is unlikely to transfer sufficient milk to himself because his lips have a poor seal around the caregiver's finger. In this situation, milk transfer is entirely dependent on the infant's ability to actively transfer the milk (with an adequate seal, adequate negative pressure, and adequate compression, as explained in chapter 6). Had the tube been attached to a syringe, the infant could have passively accepted what the parent actively delivered by pushing the plunger of the syringe.

Wilson-Clay and Hoover give many tips for how to finger feed. This directive on page 118 is especially important:

> *The feeder's hands should be clean and the nails clipped short. Health care providers should be gloved. Gentle massage around the lips encourages the baby to open and willingly draw in the finger. The fingertip is inserted pad side up, close to the hard/soft palate junction so that it triggers a sucking response. Inserting the fingertip beyond the hard/soft palate junction will trigger a gag reflex.*

Like all methods discussed in this chapter, the goal is not using it indefinitely; rather, the alternative feeding method is merely an interim step towards establishing or re-establishing breastfeeding. Finger feeding has several commonalities with breastfeeding:

- The jaw moves in a forward motion during the feeding.
- Within a few seconds of sucking, the infant has the reward of milk.
- The finger has skin that, presumably, smells like the mother.
- The infant makes sucking motions, rather than simply swallowing (as with other methods).
- The tongue protrudes over the lower alveolar ridge (gum).

Like other nurses,[5] I'm skeptical about the safety and convenience of finger feeding. Although some articles lay out "how to" do finger feeding with preterm newborns,[6,7] only one research study[8] has been published, and it failed to address either safety or convenience. Nevertheless, it's an option that should be presented to parents. As with all of the alternative methods discussed in this chapter, the parents should be taught how to use the technique, and required to demonstrate successful implementation of what they have learned, before being left unsupervised. Having to "teach back" the skill they were taught, sometimes called a *return demonstration or teach-back*, can help both parents and health care providers to identify gaps in knowledge and highlight opportunities for clarification.

Syringe Feeding

Milk can be delivered to the infant by using the syringe alone. **Figure 314** shows the infant suckling at the breast while the mother is putting a little milk into the corner of his mouth with a *periodontal* syringe. The curved tip of this type of syringe is used with the intention of inserting it into the corner of the infant's mouth while he is at breast (**Figure 310**). Some people might use a regular syringe.

In *The Breastfeeding Atlas*, Wilson-Clay and Hoover mention "anecdotal" reports of hospitals that use a periodontal syringe as a stand-alone method for supplementing, inserting the syringe directly into the infant's mouth, without a finger or a nipple. On page 119, they note that "there is no advantage to inserting a narrow, pointed device…

into the mouth of an infant," since "a pursed mouth configuration does not facilitate breastfeeding, and there is increased [risk of] aspiration when the milk is squirted into the mouth." Having worked at a hospital where this was common practice, I agree with their objections, and feel eager to add another: This approach requires a steady-handed adult with good hand-eye coordination and a very cooperative infant. It's easy to see why there is "no advantage" to this approach!

Nursing Supplementer

Nursing supplementer is the generic term for tube-feeding devices that are used at the breast. Like finger-feeding, the main objective of nursing supplementers is to deliver milk that the infant might not be able to obtain through breastfeeding.

The nursing supplementer offers two special advantages over other alternative feeding methods: it provides stimulation to the breast, and it gives the infant the opportunity to suckle. A disadvantage is that some parents find them awkward to assemble and hard to use. (One mother I worked with always referred to it as "that contraption.") Also, this method isn't feasible for an infant who cannot compress the breast, since he is likely to suck only on the tube, but not the breast.

In the United States, there are two popular brands, the Supplemental Nursing System (SNS) manufactured by Medela, and the LactAid.

Supplemental Nursing System™

The *Supplemental Nursing System*™ (SNS) is a commercially-sold nursing supplementer. It consists of a firm container attached to two tubes (**Figure 316**). Each of the tubes can be clamped off when it is not in use, and the SNS comes with different sized tubes. A larger tube allows the milk to flow faster than a smaller tube. The container is hung from the mother's neck, and it can be filled with human milk or artificial milk. A "Starter SNS" is also available, and is meant for short-term use.

The usual technique for using this device is to attach one tube to one side of the container and the other tube to the other side. One tube is directed to one breast; the other tube is directed to the other breast. Note that, according to the manufacturer, the tube should be positioned *above* the nipple, and its end extended about ¼ inch beyond the nipple. The tube then rests in the center of the infant's upper lip.

However, Wilson-Clay and Hoover suggest two special techniques. The first of these, *reverse positioning* of the feeding tube (**Figure 319** and **Figure 320**), may be more acceptable to an infant who has some feeding aversion.

Note how different this is from the usual technique. Here, the tube is placed at the side of the breast, and it nearly touches, but does not extend past the nipple (**Figure 319**). It is then taped in place. When the infant approaches, the lower lip and tongue are in contact with the tube (**Figure 320**).

Complete Learning Exercise 14-2 to compare standard and reverse positioning.

The second special technique is to use "double tubes." **Figure 317** shows that two tubes, attached to the same breast, can be used simultaneously to increase the flow rate to the infant. This idea was contributed to *The Breastfeeding Atlas* by nurse expert Kittie Frantz RN CPNP-PC.

LactAid

The LactAid Nursing Trainer System™ (**Figure 318)** has a collapsible bag, which is usually positioned so that its bottom is below the infant's chin. (The device may also, in special circumstances, be hung so that gravity assists in milk delivery.) With the collapsible bag, pressure is the same as atmospheric pressure; the infant can obtain milk without having to overcome the vacuum created by a rigid container. There is one tube coming from the container, and it is available in one size. It does not have to be positioned in the exact center of the infant's lower lip. Instructions are included for adjusting flow to accommodate artificial milk, which is thicker than human milk.

Homemade

A non-commercial tube-feeding device can also be constructed. The feeding tube can be attached to a bottle, the tube can be attached to the mother's finger, and the newborn can suck on the finger when feeding (**Figure 315**). While homemade devices aren't forbidden, I never encourage their use. Although I am sympathetic to the expense of the commercial products, I worry that homemade alternatives may carry risks that we don't know.

Nasogastric/Orogastric Feeding

Infants who are unable to suckle may be fed through a tube directly into their stomach. For newborns or young infants, this is a #5 French feeding tube. These tubes are inserted either through the nose (*nasogastric feeding*, as shown in **Figure 321**) or through the mouth (*orogastric feeding*.) Whether the tube is inserted through the mouth or the nose depends on how the physician has written the order.

Although this method of feeding an infant may seem invasive, it does offer one great advantage—namely, it eliminates concern that the infant will become "nipple confused." (While so-called "nipple confusion" has never been proven to exist, it remains a concern for many parents and providers.[9])

A major disadvantage is that infants (particularly preemies) who have been exposed to this type of tube feeding can exhibit oral aversion later. Oral aversion, also called *oral-tactile hypersensitivity*,[10] is when the infant has a strong negative response to having anything in or near his mouth. Everything—a breast, a pacifier, a teat on a bottle, a tube-feeding device, or even a finger—is rejected by the infant. The infant with oral-tactile hypersensitivity gives off unmistakable cues, such as tightly pursing his lips and/or turning his head away. For the mother, this can be a psychologically devastating behavior, causing her to feel rejected by the infant. Fortunately, such aversion typically subsides with time. In the meanwhile, it is important to not exacerbate the situation with more oral stimuli that the infant finds offensive. (Oddly, there is very little published on this topic with respect to feeding.)

Other Devices

Since ancient times, a variety of non-bottle devices have been used for feeding. In modern, bottle-centric societies, such devices are often looked upon with skepticism. Yet, there is little evidence to justify bottles as the 'best" or even the default method.

Why then, do we continue to use bottles? It's probably because they are familiar. Otherwise, we might be using spoons, cups, paladai, and more.

Spoon

While a spoon may seem more like a toddler-feeding utensil than an infant-feeding device, it can be especially useful during the colostral phase. It can be held next to the nipple as the mother expresses some milk onto it. Note that 0.6 ml (**Figure 305**) fits nicely into a spoon; that's about the amount needed to stimulate an infant's swallow response. Also, the infant can take the milk from the spoon. Since it does not need to be transferred from one device to another, less of the colostrum or milk is wasted with spoon-feeding.

Sometimes, infants are a little sleepy and disinterested in feeding. Offering the infant some colostrum or milk on a spoon (**Figure 306**) may rouse the infant (**Figure 307**).

Spoon-feeding can be used with infants of any age, and most of them will readily accept the milk. However, a disadvantage is that this method offers no opportunity for sucking.

Cup

Cup feeding (**Figure 308**) is the alternative feeding method recommended by the World Health Organization in the Baby-Friendly Hospital Initiative.

It may be used by full-term or preterm infants.[11-13] In underdeveloped countries, a "cup" is often an adult mug, but it can work well. In the United States, a 30-cc plastic medicine cup is typically used, because it is malleable and easy to handle. Preterm infants tend to "lap" the milk, whereas term infants tend to "sip" the milk,[13] but unless the infant has some serious structural defect, he is likely to do well with cup feeding. Details for creating a protocol for cup feeding[14] and techniques are covered elsewhere.[4] However, the most important step to ensure safe cup feeding is this: *Wait for the infant to swallow before offering more milk.*

There are many research studies that show the safety and efficacy of cup feeding.[15] As with other alternative feeding methods, experts often voice concern that newborns might aspirate during a cup-feeding, while ignoring the fact that bottle-fed newborns can and do aspirate, too.

Although one study identified spillage as a disadvantage of cup-feeding,[16] I question this. I have had extensive experience cup feeding, and have noted that skilled and coordinated caregivers don't spill. However, a big disadvantage is that cup feeding does not meet the newborn's inborn desire to suck.

Paladai

The paladai (sometimes called "palady") is a "shallow cup with a spout."[17](**Figure 309**) It has been used for centuries in India as alternative feeding device for infants who are unable to suckle at the breast. More recently, it has been used in the western world, for any infant who needs to use an alternative feeding method. The paladai has been used successfully with healthy infants born at term, as well as those who are low birthweight and those who have cleft defects.[17] Interestingly, one study found that infants who had orofacial clefts gained more weight when they were given supplemental feedings by paladai, as opposed to the bottle or the spoon.[18]

The paladai has several advantages over other alternative feeding devices. One study found that infants fed by paladai were able to achieve full oral feedings earlier than those who were fed by cup.[19] Another study found that infants took the maximum volume in the least amount of time (and kept quiet longest) when fed by paladai.[20] In addition, the device is lightweight, portable, and easy to clean.

One possible drawback of feeding with the paladai is more spilling.[21] However, with practice and dexterity, this risk may be reduced.

An online video[*] demonstrates good technique:

- How is the paladai used? An excellent video demonstrates this technique:
- Hold the infant semi-upright
- Gently rest the paladai on the infant's lower lip.
- Tip the paladai very slightly towards the infant so that she realizes the milk is there,
- Do not "pour" the milk! (There is a tendency for the caregiver to do this.[20] Instead, wait for the infant to swallow before offering more milk.)

Bottle-Feeding

In the United States, the vast majority of infants are bottle-fed sometime, whether the bottle is filled with formula or the mother's milk, whether they are otherwise breastfed or not.[22] Presumably, parents choose the bottle as a feeding method because it is common and familiar. For modern parents, bottles are a baby registry staple item.

Some parents may avoid bottles because they have been frightened by suggestions that "nipple confusion" will sabotage breastfeeding. Studies suggest such concern is overblown. The literature suggests there is no cause-and-effect relationship between the use of a bottle and "confusion" at the breast.[9,23]

* *https://www.youtube.com/watch?v=wkfksu9p5kY*

My experience as a nurse informs my thinking about the effects of bottle-feeding on infants (and, I believe, aligns with the perspective of Wilson-Clay and Hoover). Having observed and fed many newborns, I believe that *some* infants do have difficulty applying bottle-feeding skills to suckling a breast. This is different from nipple confusion, which has never been proven, and I do not mention "nipple confusion" to parents.

If parents are reluctant to use a bottle because they fear nipple confusion, or if they are fearful about re-trying breastfeeding after feeding with a bottle, I assure them that they may need help, but it's entirely possible for the infant to begin or resume breastfeeding. With so little science, and no proof of a cause-and-effect relationship, I feel free to speculate: I think it's likely that the fast flow of the bottled milk and the piston-like motion used to suck a teat (compared to the undulating motion used to suckle a breast[24,25]) are more likely explanations for any "confusion." Of course, any advertisements that claim a particular artificial nipple is "just like mother's" are entirely false. Furthermore, I agree with the argument made by Wilson-Clay and Hoover in Chapter 7 that nipple elasticity is a very plausible explanation.

Bottle-feeding Stress

Unquestionably, infants can experience stress due to bottle-feeding, as demonstrated in **Figure 322** and **Figure 323**. Note the angle of the bottle in **Figure 322**, **Figure 323**, and **Figure 325**. When the bottle is tilted too much, there is increased pressure on the nipple, which causes the milk to flow faster.

There are four major steps that may help mitigate this problem: using a feeding method other than a bottle, finding a teat (nipple) that is more acceptable to the infant, recognizing stress cues, and practicing external paced bottle feeding.

Non-bottle feeding methods

Consider a feeding method that does not involve a bottle; several have been suggested in this chapter. Remember that anyone on the healthcare team can suggest alternatives to the parent, it is ultimately the parent who must choose which method to use. In my experience, physicians tending to hospitalized infants are more likely to be leery of (or even forbid!) feedings with anything other than a bottle. After the infant is discharged to home, they seem to be more focused on the ends—getting food into the infant—and less concerned about the means by which that is accomplished.

Teat and bottle selection

It's common sense: different teats affect milk flow differently. Parents and providers should be open to trying more than one type, and more than one brand. The rate of flow delivered from the teat differs substantially from one brand to another.[26] Mathew[27] points out several determinants that affect the flow of bottles with teats:

- firmness of the teat material
- number and size of holes
- shape of the teat

- elevation of the bottle (Increased elevation of the bottle increases the force of gravity, and therefore, the flow of the milk. See discussion of paced feeding, below.)

The question is: What type of teat works best for the infant? I would urge readers to consider Wilson-Clay and Hoover's excellent observations about the shaft of the teat. Below, I have summarized their points about width and length, and added my observations about the material and cut of the teat.

- Width: A narrow-based teat is likely to help an infant whose lips have low tone (see Chapter 3) and who may not be able to get a good seal on a wider-based teat. A wide-based teat (although often advertised as "just like mother's nipple") can cause infants to latch on to the narrower part and avoid the wider part entirely.
- Length: A shorter teat is better for an infant who gags on a longer teat, including preterm infants and some term infants. Conversely, a longer teat may help an infant who needs extra stimulation to this tongue.
- Material: Most teats today are made from silicone. However, latex is softer and more flexible than silicone, and it may work better if an infant has low muscle tone.
- Cut: The cut is the hole, where the milk flows out. Given that cuts come in different shapes, different sizes, and different positions on the nipple, it may seem that some might be logically classified as "slow flow." However, there is wide variability in the flow rates of different nipples tested[26] and nipples marketed as "slow-flow" varied considerably in the flow rates delivered, with some having three times the flow rate of others.

Stress cue recognition

When feeding the infant, parents and caregivers must read their infant's signs, and be ready to respond to stress cues. This is true no matter what method of feeding they are using, and it cannot be overemphasized. The feeding is, quite literally, in the hands of the parent, as the infant works to consume the milk that moves from the bottle into their mouth.

Stress cues occur in term infants, but they are more frequent and more dramatic in preterm infants (**Figure 325**). The preterm infant has extreme difficulty coordinating the physiologic processes of sucking, swallowing, and breathing.[28] Infants who are transitioning to sucking, such as those who have been fed with a nasogastric or orogastric tube until now, often exhibit stress cues when faced with a flow of milk that is too fast.

Watch, too, for signs of respiratory instability. Those signs have been organized in the box, which have been drawn from *The Breastfeeding Atlas,* and my own experience.

- **Classic Signs of Physiologic Stress**
    - nasal flaring, grunting, sternal retracting
    - circumoral cyanosis (lips turn blue)
- **Defensiveness, Motor Cues**
    - stiffening of the extremities
    - pushing away from the feeding device
- **Disengaging, Sensory Cues**
    - furrowing of the brow
    - facial grimacing
    - eyes widening
    - spilling milk from the corners of the mouth
    - falling asleep

Figure 14-1. Signs of stress during infant feeding.

Suck-swallow-breathe and flow

Feeding is a complex activity for the infant, involving many different anatomical structures. To have a successful feeding, the infant must be efficient at coordinating the rhythmic processes of sucking, swallowing, and breathing.[28] Not only must he successfully coordinate these processes, he also must adapt to the bolus of fluid being offered, as well as any feeding conditions.[29] Some infants cannot do this successfully. Speed of flow is one such factor to which he must adapt.

In their now-classic study, Lau and colleagues[30] looked at the issue of speed according to three parameters: (1) proficiency (i.e., the percentage of milk volume transferred in the first 5 minutes, divided by the total volume ordered—what I call a feeding “quota”), (2) efficiency (i.e., the volume of milk transferred per unit of time) and (3) overall transfer (i.e., the percentage of milk transferred). They found that with a slower flow rate, infants were less likely to struggle with milk flow when they needed to pause for a breath. This ability to pause is essential to coordinated swallowing and breathing.[31] In essence, this means that when infants can consume milk at a slower rate, they can consume more milk.

Here’s an analogy: In baseball, a starting pitcher usually cannot throw a pitch as hard or as fast as a closing pitcher. However, he can pitch for several innings—perhaps the entire game—whereas the closing pitcher can pitch only an inning or two.

Paced Bottle-Feeding

Paced feeding is often referred to as "externally-paced bottle-feeding." It's a technique in which the parent aims to enable the infant to accept the milk in the amount and at the speed that works best for him. In other words, the caregiver attempts to return as much control to the infant as possible.[32] A major objective of paced feeding is reducing the force of gravity that propels the milk into the infant's mouth.

Paced feeding techniques (**Figure 324**) help slow the flow of milk to the infant, and they can be used for any feeding method. However, they tend to be discussed most often with regards to bottle-feeding, since that is currently the most common means of infant feeding.

Systematic pacing of feeding was introduced by speech pathologist and pediatric feeding specialist Marjorie Meyer Palmer, who has written extensively about it.[33] Paced bottle feeding enables the infant to better coordinate a rhythmic suck-swallow-breathe pattern, thus decreasing the likelihood he will become overwhelmed with fluid and experience psychological and physical consequences (e.g., frustration, lack of cooperation, gagging, choking, aspiration).

Paced feeding is especially helpful for infants who are having difficulty swallowing or breathing, or coordinating suck-swallow-breathe, such as those who are premature, or whose health is compromised in some way. However, Wilson-Clay and Hoover highlight a guiding principle of paced feeding that suggests its role for all infants: If the caregiver strives to partner with the infant, and attempts to return as much control as possible to the infant, stress cues during the feeding will be reduced.

How then, does the parent accomplish paced feeding? Presuming that the infant is stable, and the caregiver has performed proper hand hygiene and is situated in a comfortable spot, there are a few simple steps. (See the box.)

1. Select a teat that you think might work. (Keep in mind that you may need to try more than one.)
2. Move the infant into a comfortable position. A more upright position reduces the likelihood that gravity will pull the milk towards the infant. Ideally, he should be held in a position that is similar to breastfeeding (**Figure 327**).
3. Hold the bottle so that the fluid within the teat is horizontal with the infant's lips (**Figure 326**). DO NOT tilt the bottle so that it is "aimed" (**Figure 323** or **Figure 325)** at the infant, since that would cause a gravitation pull of milk towards the infant and defeat the purpose and benefit of paced feedings.
4. Observe and count the number of sucks and swallows. If the infant does not take a breath spontaneously after 3-5 sucks, stop the flow of fluid, rest the teat lightly on his upper lip (**Figure 324**), and WAIT for a few seconds, to allow the infant to take a breath.[34]

5. At all times, watch for stress cues. Avoid the temptation to pull the bottle completely out of the infant's mouth. Many "experienced" infants will respond by exerting more negative pressure on the teat, and the feeding interaction become a tug-of-war between infant and caregiver—hardly a "return of control" to the infant! Instead, move the bottom of the bottle towards the infant's chest.
6. Avoid having the teat completely filled with milk (**Figure 325**).
7. Reassure the parent that having air in the teat is not harmful. All infants take in air while feeding, and they burp later.

Anyone who is attempting to offer a paced bottle-feeding should view an excellent video* which demonstrates those steps.

Other Issues

Figure 328 shows how to bottle-feed an infant while he is facing away from the caregiver's body. The aim of this technique is to avoid contact with a stranger. Sometimes, infants will not accept a feeding from an unfamiliar caregiver because the amount of eye contact might feel too unfamiliar or intrusive.

Complete Learning Exercises 14-3, 14-4, and 14-5 now to strengthen your knowledge of alternative feeding devices.

Looking Back, Looking Forward

In this chapter, we've addressed several aspects of alternative feeding devices, including indications or contraindications for use, risks and benefits, and techniques for using them appropriately. We've also talked about stress cues and feeding aversion, and finally, the rationale and technique for paced bottle-feeding.

Evidence in the education field shows that writing your own summary helps your retention. The Summarize What You've Learned exercise helps you to do this, so take just a few minutes to complete that exercise.

By now, if you have viewed the photos and the videos carefully, and if you've completed the written exercises, you should feel confident that you can facilitate the correct use of an alternative feeding method in specific situations and minimize interruption to the breastfeeding relationship.

* *https://www.youtube.com/watch?v=TuZXD1hIW8Q*

Recalling, Reinforcing, and Expanding Your Learning

Have you ever felt frustrated that you "learned" something, but later, can't recall it? That may be because you didn't reinforce the material you learned. And, perhaps what you originally learned isn't enough to get you through the next few decades of practice; sometimes you need to expand your learning. The exercises in this section are designed to help you recall, reinforce, and expand your learning.

What was your main motivation for reading this chapter?

❍ To study for the IBLCE exam, as a first-time candidate

❍ To review for the IBLCE exam, as a re-certificant

❍ To improve my clinical skills and clinical management

How soon do you think can use the information presented in this chapter?

❍ Immediately; within the next few days or so

❍ Soon; within the next month or so

❍ Later; sometime before I retire

Pro Tip! If you are preparing for the IBLCE exam, it would be wise to pace your studying. Set a target date for when you plan to complete the exercises, and check off them off as you go along.

Done!	Target Date	Learning Exercise
❑	____________	Learning Exercise 14-1. Vocabulary related to alternative feeding methods
❑	____________	Learning Exercise 14-2. Comparison of the standard positioning and reverse positioning techniques
❑	____________	Learning Exercise 3. Recalling pertinent details on techniques for alternative feeding methods.
❑	____________	Learning Exercise 14-4. Indications and contraindications for alternative feeding devices.
❑	____________	Learning Exercise 14-5. Advantages and disadvantages of alternative feeding devices.
❑	____________	Explore What You've Learned in a Journal
❑	____________	Summarize What You've Learned
❑	____________	Quick Quiz

Master Your Vocabulary

Unless you know the meaning of a word, you cannot fully answer a question about it. There were many, many terms in this chapter; you might not need to know them all, but you never know which ones you'll be tested on, or which ones you'll find in the medical record!

Learning Exercise 14-1. Vocabulary related to alternative feeding methods.

Instructions: Write the letter of the correct match next to each item. Answers are in the Appendix.

______	1. finger feeding	A. curve-tipped device to deliver fluid
______	2. nasogastric tube	B. a means of feeding in which the infant sucks on the caregiver's finger
______	3. nursing supplementer	C. a technique in which the client shows a skill they were taught by a professional
______	4. oral aversion	D. infant has a strong negative response to anything being in or near his mouth or lips
______	5. orogastric tube	E. allowing the infant to be in "control" of the feeding process
______	6. paced feeding	F. tube device to help deliver milk at the breast
______	7. paladai	G. a flexible tube that is passed through the **nose** and down through the nasopharynx and esophagus into the stomach
______	8. periodontal syringe	H. a flexible tube passed through the **mouth** and down through the nasopharynx and esophagus into the stomach
______	9. return demonstration	I. a shallow cup with a spout

Conquering Clinical Concepts

Learning Exercise 14-2. Comparison of the standard positioning and reverse positioning techniques.

Instructions: Give a brief description of how to do each technique.

	Standard Positioning Technique	Reverse Positioning Technique
What is a likely reason for using the technique?		
How is the tube entering and contacting the tongue?		
Where is the tube positioned in relation to the breast/nipple?		
How far should the tube extend beyond the nipple?		

Learning Exercise 14-3. Recall pertinent details about techniques for alternative feeding methods.

Instructions: Fill in the blanks; the first 7 items require only a one-word answer.

1. When cup feeding, it is critical to wait for the infant to ______ before offering more milk.
2. Paced feeding can be used with ______ alternative feeding method.
3. When pacing the feeding, the caregiver should pause if the infant does not spontaneously breathe after ____ to ____ sucks.
4. In paced feeding, the fluid is held ______________ to the infant's lips.
5. Trying to completely withdraw the bottle from the infant's mouth may result in him exerting more _______ pressure on the nipple.
6. There is no need have milk _______ the teat when bottle-feeding an infant.
7. Finger-feeding should be done with the caregiver's finger pad-side ______ .
8. The purpose of paced feeding is to help the infant avoid coping with _________ .
9. Feeding with a syringe is best accomplished when the syringe is ______________________ .
10. An infant is not a candidate for using a nursing supplementer unless he can ________ .

Learning Exercise 14-4. Indications and contraindications for alternative feeding devices.

Instructions: Make a short list of indications and contraindications for each device.

Device	Indication(s)	Contraindication(s)
Bottle		
Spoon feeding		
Finger feeding		
Cup feeding		
Nursing supplementer		
Paladai		

Learning Exercise 14-5. Advantages and disadvantages of alternative feeding devices.

Instructions: Make a list of advantages and disadvantages for each device.

Device	Advantage(s) over other alternative methods	Disadvantages compared to other alternative methods
Bottle		
Spoon feeding		
Finger feeding		
Cup feeding		
Nursing supplementer		
Paladai		

Learning Journal

Multiple studies have shown the benefits of using a learning journal. Among them are greater assimilation and integration of new information, better long-term retention of course concepts, increasing test and exam grades, and a means by which to have continuous feedback about one's own learning.

- Name at least three things you learned from this chapter.

- List at least three things you still need to learn, or more fully master, in this chapter.

- Briefly describe how this information fits (or doesn't fit) with what you've seen in clinical practice, what you learned in basic or college courses, or what you've observed in your own experience breastfeeding. (In some cases, you might want to include how the information fits or doesn't fit with what "experts" say, what the media says, or whatever.)

- Describe how you will use any or all of this information. How might it be related to problems and potential solutions that occur in real life or in clinical situations?

- If you wish, include how you felt about learning this information. Were you overwhelmed? Enlightened? Worried? Something else?

Summarize What You've Learned

The purpose of this chapter was to facilitate the correct use of an alternative feeding method in specific situations and minimize interruption of the breastfeeding relationship.

Sometimes, the type of information in this chapter can seem much more theoretical than clinical. Take a moment to summarize: How can you arrange the most salient points into a few bullet points? How will you use this information for individual clients in your clinical practice? How might this information be important in the bigger world of system-level changes (e.g., procedures, standing orders, etc.) or issues with populations of clients (e.g., writing patient education materials.)

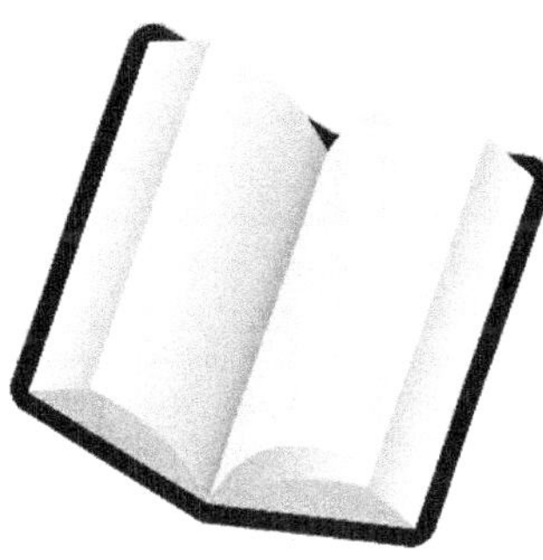

Main Points

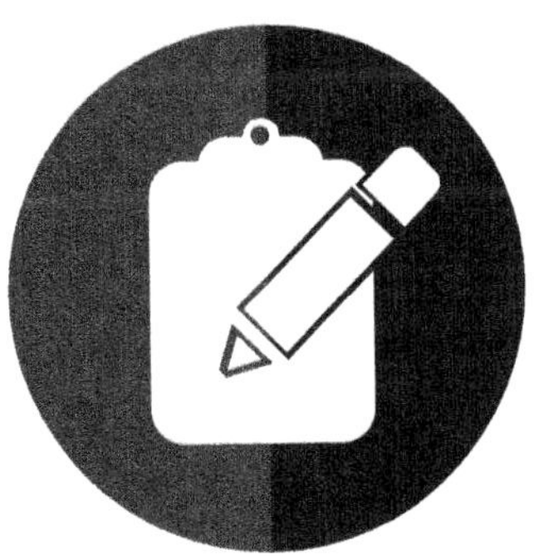

On the test

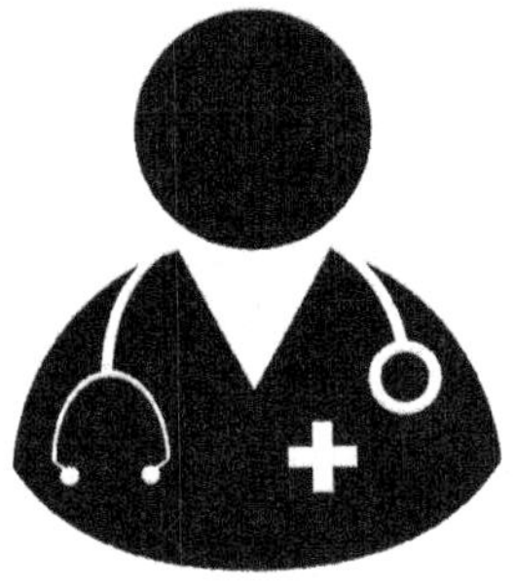

On the job

Self-Assessment

People often dive into a test before they have thoughtfully reflected on how well they have prepared for it. Instead, it would be helpful if they would take a few moments to give their alter-ego (their "other self") a chance to reflect on how confident they feel about mastering the stated objectives.

Instructions: Take a moment to review the chapter objectives (below). Then rate yourself. How confident are you that you have achieved each objective below?

Objective	Highly Confident	Somewhat Confident	Somewhat Unsure	Completely Unsure
List indications or contraindications for using an alternative feeding device to help maintain the breastfeeding relationship when an infant cannot fully feed at the breast.	❍	❍	❍	❍
Recognize techniques that help or hinder the use of an alternative feeding method.	❍	❍	❍	❍
Discuss pros and cons of alternative feeding methods in terms of ease of use, efficacy, and other factors.	❍	❍	❍	❍
Briefly describe the use of nasogastric and orogastric feeding tubes and their possible impact on breastfeeding.	❍	❍	❍	❍
Recognize stress cues an infant may exhibit while bottle-feeding.	❍	❍	❍	❍
Describe paced bottle feeding in terms of its indications, benefits, and techniques for use.	❍	❍	❍	❍
State the definition for at least five terms related to alternative feeding methods and bottle feeding.	❍	❍	❍	❍

On the next page, you will see some simple recall questions pertaining to this chapter. These are *not* the application-type questions you will find in the IBLCE exam. However, you cannot *apply* information unless you can fully *recall* that information! You should do these without looking up the answers.

When you finish with the quiz, look up the answers in the Appendix. Then, score your answers, using the Appendix. Finally, you should analyze the results of your quiz. It's not enough to just know what you got right or wrong; you must look at why you got the answers right or wrong.

Quick Quiz Chapter 14

Instructions: Circle the correct response. For a better understanding of how well you are mastering the material, try answering independently, without flipping back or looking at the source material. If you are really stuck, questions come from this workbook and from The Breastfeeding Atlas, so go back and review the appropriate material **in both sources**. *Answers are in the Appendix.*

1. The LEAST compelling reason for spoon-feeding colostrum to a newborn is that:
   A. about ½ ml of fluid stimulates the swallow reflex.
   B. expressing colostrum directly onto the spoon eliminates waste.
   C. it is the best way to preserve the breastfeeding relationship.
   D. it offers a taste and therefore a possible stimulus for waking up.

2. An alerting technique for a sleepy newborn is:
   A. initiating a quiet, rhythmic motion
   B. offering a little milk or colostrum on a spoon
   C. stroking the infant's head in the direction of hair growth
   D. using "white noise" (e.g., bathroom fan)

3. When cup feeding a term or preterm newborn, the caregiver must allow the infant to:
   A. be in a prone position
   B. lap the milk or colostrum
   C. sip the milk or colostrum
   D. swallow before offering more

4. Feeding with a commercially-available or homemade tube-feeding device would work BEST for:
   A. a medically-fragile infant with oral aversion
   B. a premature infant with a weak suck
   C. an adopted infant with a robust suck
   D. an older infant during a growth spurt

5. When using the Supplemental Nursing System™, the MOST important reason for using two tubes at the same time would be done to:
   A. increase the flow rate of the milk
   B. offer formula rather than mother's milk
   C. reduce gas-forming stomach bubbles

Analyze Your Own Quiz

- What percentage of the questions did you answer correctly?

- If you got 100% of them right, to what do you attribute your success?

- If you did not get all the questions right, can you identify your learning gap? (Example: Didn't know the information, knew the information but could not remember, knew some information but confused it with similar information, other.)

- Would you have been able to answer the questions as well if you had not read this chapter?

- What do you need to do next? (If you got them all right, what you need to do next is celebrate! Even a high-five with your child, a YESSS and a fist-pump in the air, or anything else is good! A small acknowledgement of your success is better than no acknowledgement!)

Additional Resources

1. Tender JA, Janakiram J, Arce E, et al. Reasons for in-hospital formula supplementation of breastfed infants from low-income families. *J Hum Lact.* 2009;25(1):11-17.

2. Cloherty M, Alexander J, Holloway I, Galvin K, Inch S. The cup-versus-bottle debate: a theme from an ethnographic study of the supplementation of breastfed infants in hospital in the United kingdom. *J Hum Lact.* 2005;21(2):151-162; quiz 163-156.

3. Kellams A, Harrel C, Omage S, Gregory C, Rosen-Carole C. ABM Clinical Protocol #3: Supplementary Feedings in the Healthy Term Breastfed Neonate, Revised 2017. *Breastfeed Med.* 2017;12:188-198.

4. Biancuzzo M. *Breastfeeding the Newborn: Clinical Strategies for Nurses.* St. Louis: Mosby; 2003.

5. Al-Sahab B, Feldman M, Macpherson A, Ohlsson A, Tamim H. Which method of breastfeeding supplementation is best? The beliefs and practices of paediatricians and nurses. *Paediatrics & child health.* 2010;15(7):427-431.

6. Healow LK. Finger-feeding a preemie. *Midwifery today and childbirth education.* 1995(33):9.

7. Kurokawa J. Finger-feeding a preemie. *Midwifery today and childbirth education.* 1994(29):39.

8. Oddy WH, Glenn K. Implementing the Baby Friendly Hospital Initiative: the role of finger feeding. *Breastfeed Rev.* 2003;11(1):5-10.

9. Zimmerman E, Thompson K. Clarifying nipple confusion. *J Perinatol.* 2015;35(11):895-899.

10. Wolf LS, Glass R.P. *Feeding and swallowing disorders in infancy: Assessment and management.* 2 ed: Psychological Corporation 1992.

11. Howard CR, de Blieck EA, ten Hoopen CB, Howard FM, Lanphear BP, Lawrence RA. Physiologic stability of newborns during cup- and bottle-feeding. *Pediatrics.* 1999;104(5 Pt 2):1204-1207.

12. Biancuzzo M. Breastfeeding preterm twins: a case report. *Birth.* 1994;21(2):96-100.

13. Lang S, Lawrence CJ, Orme RL. Cup feeding: an alternative method of infant feeding. *Arch Dis Child.* 1994;71(4):365-369.

14. Biancuzzo M. Creating and implementing a protocol for cup feeding. *Mother Baby Journal.* 1997;2(3):27-33.

15. McKinney CM, Glass RP, Coffey P, Rue T, Vaughn MG, Cunningham M. Feeding Neonates by Cup: A Systematic Review of the Literature. *Matern Child Health J.* 2016;20(8):1620-1633.

16. Dowling DA. Physiological responses of preterm infants to breast-feeding and bottle- feeding with the orthodontic nipple. *Nurs Res.* 1999;48(2):78-85.

17. Duarte GA, Ramos RB, Cardoso MC. Feeding methods for children with cleft lip and/or palate: a systematic review. *Brazilian journal of otorhinolaryngology.* 2016;82(5):602-609.

18. Ravi BK, Padmasani LN, Hemamalini AJ, Murthy J. Weight Gain Pattern of Infants with Orofacial Cleft on Three Types of Feeding Techniques. *Indian J Pediatr.* 2015;82(7):581-585.

19. Marofi M, Abedini F, Mohammadizadeh M, Talakoub S. Effect of palady and cup feeding on premature neonates' weight gain and reaching full oral feeding time interval. *Iranian journal of nursing and midwifery research.* 2016;21(2):202-206.

20. Malhotra N, Vishwambaran L, Sundaram KR, Narayanan I. A controlled trial of alternative methods of oral feeding in neonates. *Early Hum Dev.* 1999;54(1):29-38.

21. Aloysius A, Hickson M. Evaluation of paladai cup feeding in breast-fed preterm infants compared with bottle feeding. *Early Hum Dev.* 2007;83(9):619-621.

22. Stevens EE, Patrick TE, Pickler R. A history of infant feeding. *J Perinat Educ.* 2009;18(2):32-39.

23. Neifert M, Lawrence R, Seacat J. Nipple confusion: toward a formal definition. *J Pediatr.* 1995;126(6):S125-129.

24. Ardran GM, Kemp FH, Lind J. A cineradiographic study of breast feeding. *British Journal of Radiology.* 1958;31(363):156-162.

25. Ardran GM, Kemp FH, Lind J. A cineradiographic study of bottle feeding. *British Journal of Radiology.* 1956;31(361):11-22.

26. Pados BF, Park J, Thoyre SM, Estrem H, Nix WB. Milk flow rates from bottle nipples used after hospital discharge. *MCN The American journal of maternal child nursing.* 2016;41(4):237-243.

27. Mathew OP. Determinants of milk flow through nipple units. Role of hole size and nipple thickness. *Am J Dis Child.* 1990;144(2):222-224.

28. Gewolb IH, Vice FL, Schwietzer-Kenney EL, Taciak VL, Bosma JF. Developmental patterns of rhythmic suck and swallow in preterm infants. *Dev Med Child Neurol.* 2001;43(1):22-27.

29. McGrattan KE, Sivalingam M, Hasenstab KA, Wei L, Jadcherla SR. The physiologic coupling of sucking and swallowing coordination provides a unique process for neonatal survival. *Acta paediatrica (Oslo, Norway : 1992).* 2016;105(7):790-797.

30. Lau C, Sheena HR, Shulman RJ, Schanler RJ. Oral feeding in low birth weight infants [see comments]. *J Pediatr.* 1997;130(4):561-569.

31. Goldfield EC. A Dynamical Systems Approach to Infant Oral Feeding and Dysphagia: From Model System to Therapeutic Medical Device. *Ecological Psychology.* 2007;19(1):21-48.

32. Wilson-Clay B, Rourke JW, Bolduc MB, Stagg JD, Flatau G, Vaugh B. Learning to lobby for probreastfeeding legislation: the story of a Texas bill to create a breastfeeding-friendly physician designation. *J Hum Lact.* 2005;21(2):191-198.

33. Palmer MM, VandenBerg KA. A closer look at neonatal sucking. *Neonatal Netw.* 1998;17(2):77-79.

34. Law-Morstatt L, Judd DM, Snyder P, Baier RJ, Dhanireddy R. Pacing as a treatment technique for transitional sucking patterns. *J Perinatol.* 2003;23(6):483-488.

Chapter 15

Emergency Preparedness and Breastfeeding

If you live in the United States or another developed country, you might be wondering why the authors of *The Breastfeeding Atlas* devoted an entire chapter to breastfeeding in emergencies. But disasters can strike anywhere. We need only to think of Hurricane Katrina and the devastation it wrought on the people of New Orleans, or Hurricane Sandy and its effect on the entire Atlantic seaboard. And these aren't isolated incidents.

An emergency such as a hurricane has serious implications for a family with young children. When the floodwaters of Hurricane Agnes lapped near my sister's door years ago, she was fortunate that rescue workers came to help. But when they pound on your door at 3 AM to save you from the flood, you must move quickly. You can bring only what you can carry. For my sister, that was her children, her purse, and her diaper bag. (Luckily, she didn't need formula and its related paraphernalia!)

Hopefully, you won't ever be in the position of fleeing from disaster. But the aim of this chapter is to help you deal with a sudden emergency if it should arise, or perhaps to support your work on emergency preparedness planning in your community. Take time to read this chapter of *The Breastfeeding Atlas*. You'll find some information to help you help others—families as well as aid workers.

The purpose of this workbook is focused on photo recognition, and since there aren't any photos in chapter 15, I will confine the content here to the relevant vocabulary, and a few post-test questions based on pages 126-129 of *The Breastfeeding Atlas*. I've written some simple objectives to help you focus.

Key Words

- flash heating
- milk sharing
- milk suppression
- pasteurization
- relactation
- wet nursing

Objectives

- Identify key roles that aid workers should be trained for in order to help breastfeeding mothers in emergency situations.
- List at least three reasons why lactation consultants should participate in emergency preparedness efforts in local communities.
- List items that should be in a breastfeeding mother's emergency kit.
- Discuss wet nursing, milk sharing, relactation, milk suppression, and relief of engorgement as they relate to emergency situations.
- Give specific directives for handwashing for breastfeeding mothers and aid workers.

Recalling, Reinforcing, and Expanding Your Learning

Have you ever felt frustrated that you "learned" something, but later, can't recall it? That may be because you didn't reinforce the material you learned. And, perhaps what you originally learned isn't enough to get you through the next few decades of practice; sometimes you need to expand your learning. The exercises in this section are designed to help you recall, reinforce, and expand your learning.

What was your main motivation for reading this chapter?

❍ To study for the IBLCE exam, as a first-time candidate

❍ To review for the IBLCE exam, as a re-certificant

❍ To improve my clinical skills and clinical management

How soon do you think can use the information presented in this chapter?

❍ Immediately; within the next few days or so

❍ Soon; within the next month or so

❍ Later; sometime before I retire

Pro Tip! If you are preparing for the IBLCE exam, it would be wise to pace your studying. Set a target date for when you plan to complete the exercises, and check off them off as you go along.

Done!	Target Date	Learning Exercise
❑	____________	Learning Exercise 15-1. Terms related to breastfeeding in emergency situations.
❑	____________	Explore What You've Learned in a Journal
❑	____________	Summarize What You've Learned
❑	____________	Quick Quiz

Master Your Vocabulary

Learning Exercise 15-1. Terms related to breastfeeding in emergency situations.

Instructions: In this chapter, we'll depart from the usual matching exercise. Instead, fill in the blank. Answers are in the Appendix.

In emergency situations where some mothers are lost or somehow separated from their infants or children, the best option for feeding them might be through ________________. If so, milk can be heated briefly by bringing it to ______________, and immediately taking it off the heat. This is different than traditional Holder ______________ which is done by heating the milk to 62.5 degrees C., and holding it at that temperature for 30 minutes. Another possibility is for a willing mother to put the orphan to her own breast, an ancient practice known as ________________ .

Later, mothers and their infants or children are reunited, mothers who have "lost their milk" in the interim should be given information on ____________.

Sometimes, infants or children die in a disaster. The lactating mother will need help with __________ .

Explore What You've Learned in a Journal

- Name at least three things you learned from this chapter.

- List at least three things you still need to learn, or more fully master, in this chapter.

- Briefly describe how this information fits (or doesn't fit) with what you've seen in clinical practice, what you learned in basic or college courses, or what you've observed in your own experience breastfeeding. (In some cases, you might want to include how the information fits or doesn't fit with what "experts" say, what the media says, or whatever.)

- Describe how you will use any or all of this information. How might it be related to problems and potential solutions that occur in real life or in clinical situations?

- If you wish, include how you felt about learning this information. Were you bored? Overwhelmed? Enlightened? Worried? Something else?

Summarize What You've Learned

Instructions: Write your own summary of what you just learned in this chapter.

What are key roles that aid workers should be trained for (to help breastfeeding mothers)?	
Give three reasons why you should participate in emergency preparedness efforts in your community.	
What should be in a breastfeeding mother's emergency kit?	
In an emergency situation, what stands out in your mind about the need or management of wet nursing, milk sharing, relactation, milk suppression, and relief of engorgement?	
What would you tell mothers or aid workers about handwashing before breastfeeding or hand expressing milk?	

Self-Assessment

People often dive into a test before they have thoughtfully reflected on how well they have prepared for it. Instead, it would be helpful if they would take a few moments to give their alter-ego (their "other self") a chance to reflect on how confident they feel about mastering the stated objectives.

Instructions: Take a moment to review the chapter objectives (below). Then rate yourself. How confident are you that you have achieved each objective below?

Objective	Highly Confident	Somewhat Confident	Somewhat Unsure	Completely Unsure
Identify key roles that aid workers should be trained for in order to help breastfeeding mothers in emergency situations.	❍	❍	❍	❍
List at least three reasons why lactation consultants should participate in emergency preparedness efforts in local communities.	❍	❍	❍	❍
List what should be in a breastfeeding mother's emergency kit.	❍	❍	❍	❍
Discuss wet nursing, milk sharing, relactation, milk suppression, and relief of engorgement as they relate to emergency situations.	❍	❍	❍	❍
Give specific directives for handwashing for breastfeeding mothers and aid workers.	❍	❍	❍	❍

On the next page, you will some simple recall questions pertaining to this chapter. These are *not* the application-type questions you will find in the IBLCE exam. However, you cannot *apply* information unless you can fully *recall* that information! You should do these without looking up the answers.

When you finish with the quiz, look up the answers in the Appendix. Then, score your answers, using the Appendix. Finally, you should analyze the results of your quiz. It's not enough to just know what you got right or wrong; you must look at why you got the answers right or wrong.

Quick Quiz Chapter 15

Instructions: **Read The Breastfeeding Atlas Chapter 15**. *Circle the correct response. For a better understanding of how well you are mastering the material, try answering without looking it up. If you are review the chapter; all questions come from The Breastfeeding Atlas so go back and review the appropriate material. Answers are in the Appendix.*

1. Which of the following actions would be LEAST appropriate for an emergency worker to perform?
   - A. arranging for milk sharing
   - B. diluting powdered formula
   - C. helping a mother to hand express
   - D. doing flash heating

2. The IBCLC should participate in emergency preparedness planning in her community for all these reasons EXCEPT that it:
   - A. enables the IBCLC an opportunity to teach skills to aid workers.
   - B. helps raise community awareness of the importance of breastfeeding.
   - C. is a duty that is required by IBLCE of all lactation consultants.
   - D. is a way to include breastfeeding into the government's overall disaster plan.

3. Of the following hand hygiene practices, which is LEAST effective in reducing *E coli?*[1,2]
   - A. clipping fingernails short
   - B. drying the hands
   - C. using alcohol-based hand gels
   - D. using liquid soap
   - E. using tap water

4. If you were on a disaster planning committee in your community, which would you recommend for a breastfeeding mother's emergency kit?
   - A. 25 diapers
   - B. 50 diapers
   - C. 100 diapers
   - D. 200 diapers
   - E. 50 diaper wipes
   - F. 100 diaper wipes

5. Flash heating means:
   A. bringing the milk to a boil, then cooling it.
   B. bringing the milk to 62.5 degrees C and holding it at that temperature for 30 minutes.
   C. bringing the milk to boiling, covering it, and holding it for 30 minutes.
   D. heating the milk to 144 degrees F, then cooling it.

Analyze Your Own Quiz

- What percentage of the questions did you answer correctly?

- If you got 100% of them right, to what do you attribute your success?

- If you did not get all the questions right, can you identify your learning gap? (Example: Didn't know the information, knew the information but could not remember, knew some information but confused it with similar information, other.)

- Would you have been able to answer the questions as well if you had not read this chapter?

- What do you need to do next? (If you got them all right, what you need to do next is celebrate! Even a high-five with your child, a YESSS and a fist-pump in the air, or anything else is good! A small acknowledgement of your success is better than no acknowledgement!)

Additional Resources

1. Lin CM, Wu FM, Kim HK, Doyle MP, Michael BS, Williams LK. A comparison of hand washing techniques to remove Escherichia coli and caliciviruses under natural or artificial fingernails. *J Food Prot.* 2003;66(12):2296-2301.

2. Friedrich MN, Julian TR, Kappler A, Nhiwatiwa T, Mosler HJ. Handwashing, but how? Microbial effectiveness of existing handwashing practices in high-density suburbs of Harare, Zimbabwe. *Am J Infect Control.* 2017;45(3):228-233.

3. Shrivastav P, George K, Balasubramaniam N, Jasper MP, Thomas M, Kanagasabhapathy AS. Suppression of puerperal lactation using jasmine flowers (Jasminum sambac). *Aust N Z J Obstet Gynaecol.* 1988;28(1):68-71.

4. Oladapo OT, Fawole B. Treatments for suppression of lactation. *Cochrane Database Syst Rev.* 2009(1):CD005937.

Chapter 16
Breastfeeding the Infant with a Syndrome or Problem

Sometimes, the infant might have a condition that makes breastfeeding harder. Look to Chapter 16 of *The Breastfeeding Atlas* for what Wilson-Clay and Hoover call "special circumstances." There's nothing saying that infants with these conditions can't breastfeed, but they may need additional support to do so.

In this chapter, you'll get a glimpse of serious pathological conditions that affect an infant's health and well-being in a host of ways beyond breastfeeding. You'll begin to understand that your role in helping breastfeeding families often means venturing into highly complex situations, and your role—however limited it may seem—might be critical for helping these infants to gain a level of health they might not otherwise have.

You may find, as I have, that the "answers" for facilitating successful breastfeeding experiences for these families do not lie within these pages. Rather, the true answers come as you pay close attention to how each unique scenario unfolds, and as you allow the families and the other members of the health care team to teach you.

That being said, the excellent and unusual photos in the *Breastfeedinging Atlas (6th edition)* Chapter 16, as well as the many and varied learning exercises here, will help you to begin effective problem-solving and create individualized plans that will help the families of infants who have very complex pathologies.

I promise that after completing this chapter, you will be able to mobilize all your knowledge, skills and resources to help infants with serious physical problems to initiate and continue breastfeeding.

Key Words

- clinodactyly
- colic
- Down Syndrome
- dysphoria, dysphoric
- dysplasia
- epicanthic (epicanthal) folds
- failure to thrive
- head lag
- hydrocephalus
- hypertonia
- hypotonia
- micrognathia
- palmar crease
- reflux
- Rett Syndrome
- shunt
- syndrome
- Turner Syndrome
- turgor

Objectives

- Recognize classic physical features of infants who are affected with Down Syndrome and Turner Syndrome.
- For infants with selected structural or metabolic anomalies, recognize effects on breastfeeding (or feeding, in general) and the infant's overall health.
- Identify techniques that help to achieve optimal milk transfer in situations where the infant is affected with a temporary limitation (e.g., hypotonia) or permanent pathology (e.g., hypotonia as part of a syndrome).
- Briefly discuss what is known about dysphoric let-down in terms of its symptoms, and describe a reasonable approach to counseling a woman who experiences it.
- State the definitions of at least 10 terms that are related to selected examples of pathology.

Syndromes and Their Effects on Breastfeeding

The word *syndrome* comes from the Greek word for "concurrent." A syndrome is a collection of signs and symptoms that frequently occur concurrently, or at the same time, but without a clear cause. Some syndromes have a loosely-identified set of signs and symptoms with a vague understanding of the underlying pathology (for example, chronic fatigue syndrome). Others are caused by a chromosomal abnormality and are, therefore, present at birth. The classic signs of a syndrome may be present and obvious at birth, or they may be less obvious and go unidentified until later.

Frequently, syndromes include some type of skeletal malformation. For example, the classic sign associated with Pierre Robin Syndrome (also called Pierre Robin Sequence) is micrognathia, or an undersized jaw (**Figure 33**). Certainly, malformations affecting the face, oral cavity, head, or neck, have the most impact on feeding in general, and breastfeeding in particular. Other skeletal deformities, such as those that involve the hands, can have an impact on the self-feeding behaviors of older infants.

Sometimes, the signs of a syndrome may not be immediately evident. For example, heart or kidney malformations can impact the infant's feeding directly or create the need for treatment (such as surgery) that may affect it. When assessing the infant, it's important to keep in mind the parts we can see, as syndromes can have a multi-factorial effect on health and well-being.

Down Syndrome

Down Syndrome, also known as Trisomy 21, is a chromosomal abnormality in which two copies of chromosome 21 (one copy inherited from each parent) form one of the chromosomal pairs. In the classic form of Down Syndrome, each cell in the infant's body has three ("tri") copies of chromosome 21, rather than two.

Because syndromes are medical diagnoses, a medical doctor determines whether an infant is affected by using laboratory testing. However, it's important for other healthcare professionals to recognize the classic signs of structural malformation in infants affected with Down Syndrome, and to recognize the impact that such malformations can have on feeding in general, and especially for breastfeeding. That way, an individualized care plan can be created for the infant and the family.

Classic Signs of Skeletal Malformations

Here in the US, prenatal screening tests often identify cases of Down Syndrome during pregnancy. If such tests aren't performed, the physical traits of the newborn usually alert the primary healthcare provider to obtain a blood sample for chromosomal analysis called a karyotype test, to confirm a diagnosis of Down Syndrome. The physical traits include:

- Head and neck: low-set ears, flat bridge of the nose, almond-shaped eyes, redundant skin on the epicanthic folds (inner eyelids) (**Figure 329**). Although it is often easier to see from the back rather than the front, infants with Down Syndrome have short web-like necks.
- Hands and feet: *palmar crease* (a single transverse crease that extends across the palm of the hand) and *clinodactyly* (curvature of the fifth finger) (**Figure 331**). (Note: Not all infants affected with Down Syndrome have a palmar crease (formerly called a "Simian crease"). Conversely, some individuals with a palmar crease are not affected with Down Syndrome.)
- Generalized hypotonia: low muscle tone throughout the body, including orofacial structures.

Impact on Breastfeeding

Hypotonia (low muscle tone) throughout the body (**Figure 338**) hampers the infant's ability to position himself at the breast. If the tongue is also hypotonic, the infant will not be able to form the trough necessary to achieve good areolar compression. This affects the infant's ability to compress the tongue against the hard palate. Frequently, a weak tongue protrudes, giving the appearance that it does not "fit" within the mouth. Just as weak muscles can cause the tongue to fall forward, they also can cause it to fall to the back of the mouth, impairing the sucking motions and possibly resulting in apneic periods. Upright postures minimize the role of gravity in adding to the problem.

Creating a Plan of Care

The plan of care depends in part on when the infant is diagnosed. Some mothers may not have sought prenatal care, or they may have refused genetic testing; the birth of an infant with Down Syndrome may come as a complete surprise. Teaching and counseling should begin as soon as the diagnosis is confirmed.

Psychosocial issues are of paramount importance. Parents often grieve for the loss of the "perfect child." Mothers who had planned to breastfeed may change their minds when their initial attempts do not go well. They often assume that feeding with a bottle is easier, although this is often not the case. Parents will need much positive reinforcement. They may need to hear, many times, that infants with Down Syndrome *are* capable of breastfeeding, although this capability may not be present at birth, and parental patience is necessary for accomplishing breastfeeding goals. Parents also need many simple tips to deal with the infant's physical limitations. For milk transfer to occur, the infant must achieve an adequate seal, negative pressure, and adequate breast compression, as described in chapter 6. (**Figure 335**)

Some simple techniques can help the mother and infant to accomplish those three actions. First, it's critical to help the infant into a posture that provides optimal stability of the entire body. My go-to suggestion is the straddle position (**Figure 103**, Chapter 6.) The Dancer Hand (**Figure 333** and **334)** is also helpful for optimal seal, negative pressure, and compression. So is having the mother do deep compression of the breast (**Figure 335**).

Note that while the Dancer Hand (**Figure 333**) is helpful, the similar "U" hold (not shown here) is not. These holds differ both in terms of the placement of the hand and the purpose of the hold. With the U hold, the mother's hand is closer to her chest, to support the weight of her breast. With the Dancer Hand, the mother's hand is farther from her chest, and, although it is supportive, it forms a "shelf" for the infant's chin. This helps the hypotonic infant to latch on and stay on. However, it may not be enough. The mother may also want to compress the infant's cheeks to reduce the amount of intraoral space and thereby increase the amount of intraoral negative pressure.

Turner Syndrome

Turner Syndrome (TS) is a chromosomal condition where the second X chromosome is missing or abnormal in at least one cell line.[1] Because only the X chromosome is affected, only females have Turner Syndrome.

As the authors of *The Breastfeeding Atlas* note, Turner's Syndrome is a rare condition. One might be in clinical practice for many, many years before seeing an infant with this condition. However, this is an example of how a syndrome may have a multi-symptom impact on the infant, affecting the breastfeeding experience as well as overall growth and development.

Classic Physical Signs

Infants affected with Turner Syndrome have several structural alterations, including some that can affect breastfeeding abilities. These include:

- Orofacial malformations: a high-arched palate (**Figure 346**), micrognathia, and mandibular altered growth[2]
- Head and neck malformations: neck webbing, low-set and posteriorly rotated ears (**Figure 21** shows ears after a surgical correction with splinting), and possible hearing problems
- Other skeletal problems: several foot problems (**Figure 345**) (*The Breastfeeding Atlas* page 136 gives details)
- Cardiac disorders: coarctation of aorta, aortic stenosis, and bicuspid aortic valve require surgery, which affects breastfeeding
- Renal disorders

Other musculoskeletal problems can occur as well. For example, **Figure 347** shows an infant with Turner Syndrome who, presumably because of the associated hypotonia, developed a hip *dysplasia* (an abnormal growth or development the hip) and was fitted for a hip harness to correct it. This affected the mother's ability to find a comfortable and effective position for breastfeeding (**Figure 347**).

All or most of these structural issues can be noted at birth. However, the girl who is affected with Turner Syndrome also has metabolic problems, including

- Hormonal problems: infertility, low estrogen, hypothyroidism
- Small size for gestational age: For example, the infant in **Figure 21** and **Figure 345** was born at 38 weeks' gestation and weight 5 lb 14 oz (2665 grams).
- Preterm birth[3]
- Short stature

Rett Syndrome

Rett Syndrome is a rare genetic disorder that is characterized by small hands and feet, a deceleration of the rate of head growth (microcephaly) and other anomalies and disabilities. While infants with *Rett Syndrome* may initially seem healthy, after about six months, they tend to rapidly lose coordination, speech, and use of the hands.

Neuromuscular Problems

It would be impossible to list here all of the neuromuscular problems that can occur in a newborn. By and large, there are three main reasons for neuromuscular limitations: medications or birth trauma, prematurity, and pathological conditions.

Even full-term, healthy newborns may have been exposed to medications during labor or to trauma during delivery. (See chapter 2). These issues are often—but not always—easily identifiable, short-term, and spontaneously resolving.

Premature infants are neurologically immature, which may cause them to have neuromuscular limitations.

Other infants have true pathology, and they are affected by a brain impairment that was present in utero.

It's important to look at some specific conditions, and how they affect neuromuscular functioning and breastfeeding.

Low Tone and Feeding Problems

Hypotonia—low muscle tone—can occur in many situations. Infants who are born premature, as well as those with Down Syndrome, Rett Syndrome, hydrocephalus, and other conditions discussed in this chapter can be hypotonic. Any infant who has neurological impairment or brain impairments is likely to have hypotonia. If an infant with a history of normal muscle tone and vigorous suck suddenly has low muscle tone and a weak suck, the change could be a sign of a brain tumor, as was the case for the infant in **Figure 338**.

Generalized hypotonia of the body makes it difficult to position the infant in a way that achieves or maintains good bodily alignment while at the breast—a concept we discussed at length in Chapter 6. Hypotonia of the tongue makes it difficult for the infant to form the trough-shaped tongue necessary for breastfeeding.

Hydrocephalus

From the Greek word *hydro* (water) and *cephalus* (head), the term *hydrocephalus* is used for the condition in which there is an excessive accumulation of fluid in the brain. In lay terms, this is "water on the brain"; however, the "water" is actually cerebrospinal fluid. Infants who suffer from hydrocephalus usually have a shunt put in place (**Figure 339**) to bypass an obstruction in the fluid compartments of the brain and relieve the excess fluid buildup.

Complete Learning Exercise 16-2 Infant with hydrocephalus (Clincial Case).

The authors of the *The Breastfeeding Atlas* provide solid information about hydrocephalus. I would only add that, in my clinical experience, the disproportionately large size of the infant's head (especially before placement of the shunt) can often make positioning the affected infant extremely difficult. I distinctly remember a newborn who, from the neck down, had the appearance of a seven-pound infant. However, his actual birth weight was about 13 pounds, and his head was the size of an adult's. There's no "right" answer for how to position an infant with this condition, but the goal is for milk transfer to the infant without excessive "dragging" on the mother's nipple, as mentioned in Chapter 8.

Abnormal Posturing and Hypertonia

Unquestionably, parents and professionals alike worry about hypotonia, sometimes referred to as the "floppy baby syndrome." However, at the other end of the spectrum is *hypertonia* (**Figure 340**). Hypertonia is muscle tone that is too tense.

Chapter 3 discusses hypotonia and hypertonia.

Interestingly, page 133 describes the triggers for the infant in **Figure 340,** noting that "light touch, sudden sounds, bright lights, and motion appear to overwhelm him." Breastfeeding while exposed to such stimuli only increases his sensory defensiveness and hypertonia. Note that his reactions affect not only breastfeeding, but also his mother's perception of rejection. We don't know what happened to this infant later, but we should keep in mind that auditory and sensory overload can occur in otherwise normal children and adults, as well as in children with attention deficit disorder.

Failure to Thrive

Much has been written about failure to thrive (FTT). The authors of *The Breastfeeding Atlas* dedicate many pages to failure to thrive. Because this workbook focuses on photos, I'll show you what to look for in photos, and how to relate the information you glean to clinical management.

Definition and Description

There are many different definitions of failure to thrive (FTT); some have no relevance for the breastfed infant. The best description of failure to thrive, from Lawrence and Lawrence[4], is when the infant "continues to lose weight after 10 days of life, does not regain birth weight by three weeks of age, or gains at a rate below the 10th percentile for weight gain beyond one month of age." Lawrence and Lawrence emphasize that failure to thrive is a symptom, not a diagnosis. More importantly, FTT can be a symptom of pathology, which no amount of "better breastfeeding" can cure. For that reason, it is critically important that the primary care provider be highly involved in the management of FTT.

Feeding Management for FTT

Review these cases carefully. All infants have the same diagnosis. Begin to think about how the management was different each time, but a positive outcome was achieved.

Although it may be difficult to see on a photo, infants who have failure to thrive are usually dehydrated. One sign of dehydration is poor skin *turgor.* Skin turgor reflects tension of the fluid in the skin. If a flap of well-hydrated skin is pinched momentarily, it will snap back readily. If the skin is not well-hydrated, the skin fold persists and takes a while to return to its normal state. Often, parents and professionals alike assume they should see a sunken fontanelle if the infant is dehydrated. That is true, but *having a sunken fontanelle is a late sign of dehydration.*

Complete Learning Exercise 16-3. Infant with failure to thrive (Clinical Case).

Gastrointestinal Conditions

Infants can have any number of gastrointestinal problems. Two that have gained much attention are reflux and colic.

Reflux

Many infants spit up the fluid they take in, whether it is their mother's milk, donor milk, or artificial milk. The spit-up can be entirely normal and benign, or it can be frighteningly pathologic.

At one end of the spectrum is the infant with what could be called "passive drool." (Remember, though, that drooling is common while teething.) These infants are, according to pediatric gastroenterologists,* "happy spitters." (**Figure 11**). The parents worry, but this is unlikely to be worrisome, and will probably resolve spontaneously.

At the other end of the spectrum are infants with projectile vomiting. These infants are likely to have serious gastrointestinal pathology, and they need a complete medical evaluation by their pediatrician and/or a specialist.

Somewhere in the middle of this spectrum is reflux. It is critically important to teach parents that reflux happens to breastfed and formula-fed infants, and changing to formula doesn't improve the condition—it usually makes it worse.

Colic

Colic was first defined by Dr. Wessel's now-classic 1954 study,[5] which established the "rule of threes." Infantile colic is defined as crying for more than three hours a day, for at least three days a week, and for three weeks or longer. Although it can start or end at any time, colic usually begins at around three weeks of age, and subsides by about three months. Typically, colic-like symptoms are worse in the evening.

It's important for parents to understand that the exact cause of colic has not been identified; it's likely that several factors are involved. Although parents often want to "blame" colic on food that the mother ingests, this explanation has never been proven. In any event, like many other gastrointestinal problems, colic does not improve with formula-feeding. To the contrary, it often becomes worse with formula feeding.

A few simple interventions can help the infant who has colic. The classic "colic hold" is shown in **Figure 341.** While burping the infant, the parents should avoid holding him in a "v" position, which bends him forward and compresses the abdomen (**Figure 336**). Similarly, to avoid further compression on the abdomen, the infant may be more comfortable if he is diapered on his side (**Figure 337**), rather than lying supine.

To qualify as colic, the spit-up must be more than just a passive drool.

Other Conditions

Sometimes, surgery is needed during infancy or childhood. Certainly, any illness or surgical procedure can impact breastfeeding; some more serious than other. For example, heart surgery scar (**Figure 348).**

A little-known phenomenon is that of a dysphoric let-down. The prefix *dys-* means "difficult, bad, or abnormal," and *phoria* is from the Greek verb *fero*, meaning "to bring." If you've ever felt euphoric, you might imagine that dysphoric is the opposite feeling—a feeling that something is difficult or bad or abnormal.

There are only two case reports in the literature about dysphoric let-down.[6, 7] Wilson-Clay and Hoover also offer an interesting brief report, which was managed successfully—but differently than the other reports.

---

* Dr. Bryan Vartabedian, guest on Born to Be Breastfed.

There is no known cause for dysphoric let-down, making it difficult to know how to resolve the symptoms. Heise and colleagues[7] looked at multiple issues in hopes of identifying something that would help or hinder the symptoms: eating chocolate ice cream, smoking, drinking alcohol, taking pseudoephedrine, consuming caffeine, experiencing stress, and more. They concluded that while some substances or events might ameliorate or exacerbate the symptoms, there is no one-size-fits-all recommendation. They suggested reassuring women that they are experiencing a recognized symptom (not just a figment of the imagination) and that an alternative therapy might help.

Since dysphoric let-down is a feeling rather than a physical condition, there are no photos of it in *The Breastfeeding Atlas*. However, since it is a rather unusual condition, you should familiarize yourself with it. See page 141.

Looking Back, Looking Forward

In this chapter, we've talked about syndromes, neuromuscular problems, failure to thrive, and other conditions that affect breastfeeding.

Evidence in the education field shows that writing your own summary helps your retention. The Summarize What You've Learned exercise helps you to do this, so take just a few minutes to complete that exercise.

By now, if you have carefully viewed the images on pages 193-194 of *The Breastfeeding Atlas*, and if you've completed the written exercises here, you should feel confident able to mobilize all your knowledge, skills and resources to help infants with serious physical problems to initiate and continue breastfeeding.

Recalling, Reinforcing, and Expanding Your Learning

Have you ever felt frustrated that you "learned" something, but later, can't recall it? That may be because you didn't reinforce the material you learned. And, perhaps what you originally learned isn't enough to get you through the next few decades of practice; sometimes you need to expand your learning. The exercises in this section are designed to help you recall, reinforce, and expand your learning.

What was your main motivation for reading this chapter?

- ❍ To study for the IBLCE exam, as a first-time candidate
- ❍ To review for the IBLCE exam, as a re-certificant
- ❍ To improve my clinical skills and clinical management

How soon do you think can use the information presented in this chapter?

- ❍ Immediately; within the next few days or so
- ❍ Soon; within the next month or so
- ❍ Later; sometime before I retire

Pro Tip! If you are preparing for the IBLCE exam, it would be wise to pace your studying. Set a target date for when you plan to complete the exercises, and check off them off as you go along.

Done!	Target Date	Learning Exercise
❑	____________	Learning Exercise 16-1. Terms related to selected examples of pathological conditions.
❑	____________	Learning Exercise 16-2. Clinical Case: Infant with hydrocephalus.
❑	____________	Learning Exercise 16-3. Three clinical cases of failure to thrive (A, B, C).
❑	____________	Explore What You've Learned in a Journal
❑	____________	Summarize What You've Learned
❑	____________	Quick Quiz

Master Your Vocabulary

Unless you know a word's meaning, you cannot fully answer a question about it. There were many, many terms in this chapter; you might not need to know them all, but you never know which ones you'll need to know!

Learning Exercise 16-1. Terms related to selected examples of pathological conditions.

Instructions: Write the letter of the correct match next to each item. Answers are in the Appendix.

_____	1. clinodactyly	A.	"water on the brain"
_____	2. colic	B.	a chromosomal condition in which the second X chromosome is missing or abnormal in at least one cell line
_____	3. Down Syndrome	C.	a chromosomal condition where two copies of chromosome 21 (one copy inherited from each parent) forms one of the chromosomal pairs
_____	4. dysphoria, dysphoric	D.	a collection of signs and symptoms that frequently occur concurrently, but without a clear explanation
_____	5. dysplasia	E.	a feeling that something is bad or abnormal
_____	6. epicanthic (epicanthal) folds	F.	a rare genetic disorder characterized by small hands and feet, microcephaly and other anomalies and disabilities
_____	7. head lag	G.	a single transverse crease that extends across the palm of the hand
_____	8. hydrocephalus	H.	an abnormal growth or development
_____	9. palmar crease	I.	crying for more than three hours a day, three days a week, for three weeks or longer
_____	10. Rett Syndrome	J.	curvature of the fifth finger
_____	11. shunt	K.	device that bypasses an obstruction in the fluid compartments of the brain
_____	12. syndrome	L.	inner eyelids
_____	13. turgor	M.	tension of the skin, it reflects fluid adequacy
_____	14. Turner Syndrome	N.	weak head and neck control when being pulled up

Conquering Clinical Concepts

Learning Exercise 16-2. Clinical Case. Infant with hydrocephalus.

Instructions: Using the text on pages 132 and the accompanying photos, fill in the blanks. Answers are on page 132.

The infant in **Figure 339** was born with hydrocephalus. He willingly breastfed on both breasts until about age three months. At that time, he suddenly refused to feed on his mother's left breast.

- On which side of his head was the shunt located?

- What possible explanation might there be for his apparent contentedness in the first three months, and resistance to breastfeeding?

- During times when the infant is breastfeeding, what could you identify as the FIRST suggestion to help with his reluctance to breastfeed on the mother's left breast?

- How long did he continue breastfeeding after help from the lactation consultant?

- At age five months, what did the neurologist observe about this infant that was different from most others he had seen?

Learning Exercise 16-3. Three clinical cases of failure to thrive.

Instructions: Read the three clinical cases presented in The Breastfeeding Atlas, *pages 135-136. Begin thinking about how the cases are similar, and how they are different.*

Infant A. See Figure 342 and read the accompanying text on page 135..

- Was this infant born at term, before term, or post-term?

- How much did he weigh?

- By the time that he was 35 days old, how much did he weigh?

- A two-pronged approach was used to help him gain weight. Name the two "prongs."

- The infant was given mother's milk or formula. What else may have been considered in this case?

- He was weak, but with practice, how much fluid could he take through the tube-feeding device?

- Succinctly summarize: What was the crux of the problem in this case? How was it solved?

Infant B. (No image). See The Breastfeeding Atlas, page 135.
An infant was born weighing 6 pounds, 11 ounces (3033 grams).

- On the advice of an acquaintance, what was the mother giving the infant?

- At 18 days of age, the infant weighed 1 pound (454 grams) below his birth weight. What was his birth weight? What does he weigh now? What percentage of weight had he lost?

- The mother was advised by the health care provider to stop giving the water. Three things resulted. What were those three things?

- Succinctly summarize: What was the crux of the problem in this case? How was it solved?

Infant C. Figure 344. See text pages 135-136.

- The infant in **Figure 344** had FTT. Several factors impeded both milk production and milk transfer in this case. What were those factors?

- If you didn't know the facts and weights related to the FTT, what strong clue would suggest FTT just from looking at his photo? Is it similar to the infant in an earlier chapter (**Figure 9**)?

- Pre- and post-test weights showed that the infant had ingested _______ ml of milk during a 15-minute timeframe before becoming exhausted and falling asleep. Two goals were established: (1) to increase the mother's _______________ and (2) to increase the infant's ____________ .

- Goal #1 was accomplished by using four strategies. Name them.

- Goal #2 was accomplished by using three or four strategies. Name them.

- What laboratory data and physical assessment data were noted at the visit 36 hours later?

- What about the mother's milk supply, and her perception of her milk?

- Through telephone contact, how was it apparent that the infant's health was improving?

- Succinctly summarize: What was the crux of the problem? How was it solved?

- Above, we just worked through Case A, B, and C. What was similar about these cases? What was different?

- For you, what was the take-home message from these cases?

Summarize What You've Learned

The purpose of this chapter was to mobilize all your knowledge, skills and resources to help infants with serious physical problems to initiate and continue breastfeeding.

Sometimes, the type of information in this chapter can seem much more theoretical than clinical. Take a moment to summarize: How can you arrange the most salient points into a few bullet points? How will you use this information for individual clients in your clinical practice? How might this information be important in the bigger world of system-level changes (e.g., procedures, standing orders, etc.) or issues with populations of clients (e.g., writing patient education materials.) How might you use this information on an exam?

Main Points

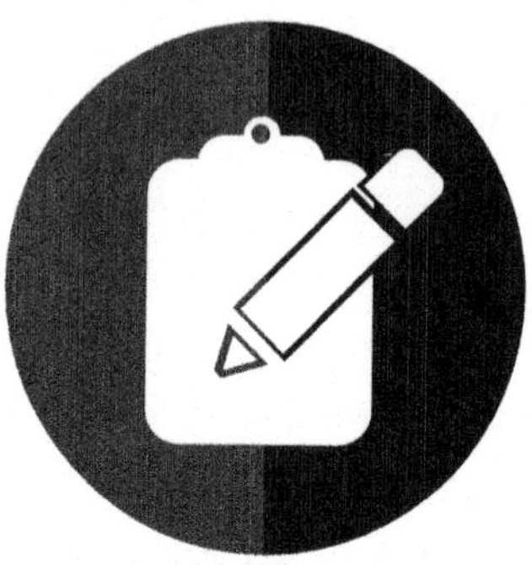

On the test

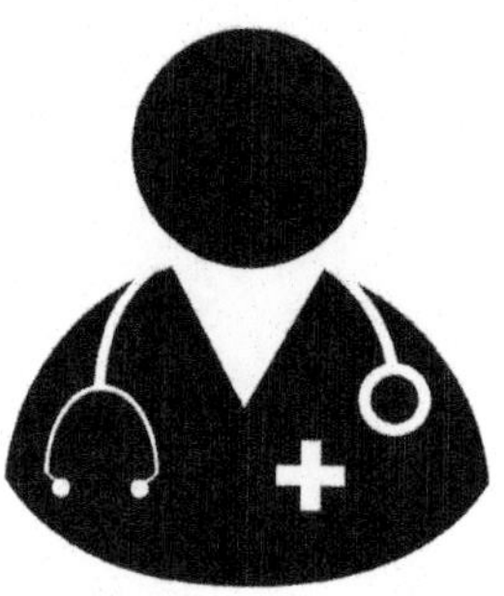

On the job

Explore What You've Learned in a Journal

Multiple studies have shown the benefits of using a learning journal. Among them are greater assimilation and integration of new information, better long-term retention of course concepts, increasing test and exam grades, and a means by which to have continuous feedback about one's own learning.

- Name at least three things you learned from this chapter.

- List at least three things you still need to learn, or more fully master, in this chapter.

- Briefly describe how this information fits (or doesn't fit) with what you've seen in clinical practice, what you learned in basic or college courses, or what you've observed in your own experience breastfeeding. (In some cases, you might want to include how the information fits or doesn't fit with what "experts" say, what the media says, or whatever.)

- Describe how you will use any or all of this information. How might it be related to problems and potential solutions that occur in real life or in clinical situations?

- If you wish, include how you felt about learning this information. Were you overwhelmed? Enlightened? Worried? Something else?

Self-Assessment

People often dive into a test before they have thoughtfully reflected on how well they have prepared for it. Instead, it would be helpful if they would take a few moments to give their alter-ego (their "other self") at chance to reflect on how confident they feel about mastering the stated objectives.

Take a moment to review the chapter objectives (below). Then, on a scale of 1 to 4, rate yourself, *in writing*. How confident are you that you have achieved each objective below?

Objective	Highly Confident	Somewhat Confident	Somewhat Unsure	Completely Unsure
Recognize classic physical features of infants who are affected with Down Syndrome and Turner Syndrome.	❍	❍	❍	❍
For infants with selected structural or metabolic anomalies, recognize effects on breastfeeding (or feeding, in general) and the infant's overall health.	❍	❍	❍	❍
Identify techniques that help to achieve optimal milk transfer in situations where the infant is affected with a temporary limitation (e.g., hypotonia) or permanent pathology (e.g., hypotonia as part of a syndrome).	❍	❍	❍	❍
Briefly discuss what is known about dysphoric let-down in terms of its symptoms, and describe a reasonable approach to counseling a woman who experiences it.	❍	❍	❍	❍
State the definitions of at least 10 terms that are related to pathology.	❍	❍	❍	❍

On the next page, you will some simple recall questions pertaining to this chapter. These are *not* the application-type questions you will find in the IBLCE exam. However, you cannot *apply* information unless you can fully *recall* that information! You should do these without looking up the answers.

When you finish with the quiz, look up the answers in the Appendix. Then, score your answers, using the Appendix. Finally, you should analyze the results of your quiz. It's not enough to just know what you got right or wrong; you must look at why you got the answers right or wrong.

Quick Quiz Chapter 16

Instructions: Circle the correct response. For a better understanding of how well you are mastering the material, try answering independently, without flipping back or looking at the source material. If you are really stuck, questions come from this workbook and from The Breastfeeding Atlas, *so go back and review the appropriate material. Answers are in the Appendix.*

1. Which of these techniques would be LEAST helpful to facilitate milk transfer in an infant with Down Syndrome?
   - A. Breast compression
   - B. Cradle hold
   - C. Dancer Hand
   - D. Upright position
2. Which of these are LEAST likely to be observed in an infant who is hypotonic?
   - A. apneic spells
   - B. constipation
   - C. inability to "cup" the breast
   - D. protruding tongue
3. The cause of dysphoric let-down is unknown, but which of these interventions is LEAST likely to alleviate the symptoms?
   - A. hypnosis or aromatherapy
   - B. increasing dietary protein
   - C. pumping after each feeding
   - D. reassurance it is a recognized phenomenon
4. Which structural problem is NOT typically associated with Turner Syndrome?
   - A. altered growth mandibular
   - B. high-arched palate
   - C. micrognathia
   - D. natal teeth

Analyze Your Own Quiz

- What percentage of the questions did you answer correctly?

- If you got 100% of them right, to what do you attribute your success?

- If you did not get all the questions right, can you identify your learning gap? (Example: Didn't know the information, knew the information but could not remember, knew some information but confused it with similar information, other.)

- Would you have been able to answer the questions as well if you had not read this chapter?

- What do you need to do next? (If you got them all right, what you need to do next is celebrate! Even a high-five with your child, a YESSS and a fist-pump in the air, or anything else is good! A small acknowledgement of your success is better than no acknowledgement!)

Additional Resources

1. Donaldson MDC, et al. Optimising management in Turner syndrome: from infancy to adult transfer. *Archives of Disease in Childhood.* 2006;91(6):513-520.
2. Simmons KE. Growth hormone and craniofacial changes: preliminary data from studies in Turner's syndrome. (0031-4005 (Print)).
3. Hagman A, et al. Women who gave birth to girls with Turner syndrome: maternal and neonatal characteristics. *Hum Reprod.* 2010;25(6):1553-1560.
4. Lawrence R, Lawrence, RM. *Breastfeeding: A guide for the medical profession.* 8 ed 2016.
5. Wessel MA, et al. Paroxysmal fussing in infancy, sometimes called colic. *Pediatrics.* 1954;14(5):421-435.
6. Cox S. A case of dysphoric milk ejection reflex (D-MER). *Breastfeed Rev.* 2010;18(1):16-18.
7. Heise AM, Wiessinger D. Dysphoric milk ejection reflex: A case report. *International Breastfeeding Journal.* 2011;6:6-6.

Chapter 17
Breastfeeding with Ankyloglossia

The law is clear: Only health care providers who are legally authorized by their state medical board to make a medical diagnosis may do so. The practice, however, is less clear: When it comes to tongue-tie, even those who are legally authorized to make a medical diagnosis may be perplexed.

In a 2013 editorial for *Breastfeeding Medicine*, Lawrence[1] explains the historical perspective of tongue-tie diagnosis and treatment, reminding us that the diagnosis is far from settled. “There is considerable controversy regarding tongue-tie as a diagnosis, the indications for treatment, and the method of treatment,” she writes. “Does the evidence support the treatment of posterior tongue-tie, and if so, how should it be performed? Who is best able to make this decision?”

If you think “controversy” is an overstatement, consider: Many health care providers disagree about such fundamental concerns as the terminology used to describe the types of tongue-tie or their characteristics! Others express concern about the reliability and validity of the tools that have been developed to determine whether surgical correction is needed.[2,3]

Although the IBLCE has made it clear that “diagnosing” is not part of the lactation consultant’s role, assessment certainly is.[4] Fortunately, the lactation consultant can avoid some of the heated controversy by keeping her cool as an expert problem-solver for suboptimal latch and milk transfer.

I promise, when you finish this chapter, you will be able to determine if or to what extent the lingual frenulum affects latch, and suggest techniques for improving it. (We will also briefly touch on lip-tie.)

This is a complicated topic. But the photos, learning exercises, case studies, and additional resources listed in this chapter will help you to learn what you need to know. You’ll also begin to get a feel for when to advocate for a medical specialist’s opinion—or even a second opinion.

Key Terms

- alveolar ridge
- ankyloglossia
- Bristol Tongue Assessment Tool (BTAT)
- frenotomy, frenulotomy, frenectomy, frenulectomy
- frenum, frenulum, frenulym, frenula
- hard/soft palate junction (HSPJ)
- Hazelbaker Assessment Tool for Lingual Frenulum Function (HATLFF)
- hypospadias
- labial
- lateralization
- lingual
- midline defects
- otolaryngologist
- range of motion
- tethered oral tissue (TOT)

Objectives

- Match key elements in tongue motion to elicitation techniques and visual examples of abnormal appearance and function.
- Recognize the signs, symptoms, and likely impact of a tongue-tied infant's ability to have full range of tongue motion.
- Predict likely consequences of dysfunctional tongue-tie for both the infant and the mother.
- Assist the parent to make an informed decision about having a frenotomy for their tongue-tied infant/child.
- Through the pictorial case reports of tongue-tied infants, identify elements of and priorities for a plan of care for the breastfeeding couplet.

Overview of Ankyloglossia

The word *ankyloglossia* comes from the Greek term *anky*, meaning "stiff, unmovable; an adhesion," and the Greek term *glossa*, meaning "tongue." It refers to the sublingual frenulum which causes a change in appearance or function of the tongue.[1]

Prevalence and Etiology

Ankylogossia has become such a hot topic over the last several years that one might wonder how common it is. Citing five studies (which used different diagnostic criteria), Segal[5] estimates the prevalence of ankyloglossia worldwide to be between 4% and 10%.

Whether tongue-ties result from genetic or environmental factors is the subject of some debate. Unquestionably, tongue-ties and lip-ties do seem to "run in families," as evidenced by the father (**Figure 352**) who requested breastfeeding help for his tongue-tied infant (not shown). Also, tongue-ties are midline defects—that is, they occur along the vertical axis of the body. Sometimes, this can signal the likelihood of other midline defects in the infant or his family. Note the infant without tongue-tie but with hypospadias (**Figure 364**), whose father and male cousin were both tongue-tied.

"Disappearing" Tongue-Ties

Some experts argue that the tongue-tie is a condition that is not subject to change, that the frenulum will not "stretch." Others tell parents that the infant's tongue-tie will "disappear" over time. Speech pathologists and other experts remind us that the tongue consists of many muscles which—like all muscles in the body—will strengthen (and therefore show better extension and retraction) with deliberate and continuous exercise. (Note the distinction between what the frenulum can do, and what the muscles can do.) So, is it possible that tongue dysfunction could improve?

Admittedly, some "tied" lingual frenula have more length and elasticity, which would presumably enable the infant to suckle better as time goes on. Some of these children, even into adulthood, may not experience much—if any—impact on speech, feeding, or dentition. There are plenty of examples of tongue-tied infants who have successfully breastfed for many months. I know these children, and authors of *The Breastfeeding Atlas* have known them—and photographed them (**Figure 374**)!

But do the tongue-ties all disappear? Are they "outgrown"? No; this language is misleading at best. The presence of a tongue-tie may be asymptomatic, or may create dysfunction, and may perhaps even be compensated for by the affected child.[6] (That's one reason why the question of whether all tongue-ties require surgical correction has been debated so hotly[7] and the evidence examined so carefully.[8]) In some cases, the infant/child is asymptomatic, or he learns to compensate. But tongue-ties can and certainly do persist into adolescence and even adulthood (**Figures 350, 351, 352, 354, 355, 358**).

Terminology, Anatomy, & Physiology

Much of the controversy and decision-making about tongue-ties is rooted in our understanding of anatomy and physiology terminology, so, let's begin by getting a clearer understanding of terms.

An infant affected with ankyloglossia has a limited range of tongue motion because of the lingual *frenulum*. From the Latin word *frenum*, meaning "bridle," this small fold of membranous tissue restrains or supports the motion of the body part to which it is attached. *Frenula* (plural of frenulum) are present throughout the body.

It appears that the terms *frenulum*, *frenum*, or *frenulym* are all correct when referring to the intraoral structures. The *lingual* frenulum connects the underside of the tongue in an anterior-posterior fashion, to the floor of the mouth. The *labial* frenulum is attached to the lips. For those frenula (plural of frenulum) that are tethered, the terms "tongue-tie" or "lip-tie" are commonly used. Less commonly, health care professionals sometimes use the phrase "tethered oral tissue" (TOT). Some contend that the term "lingual frenulum" should be used for anatomical description, and the term "tongue-tie" be reserved for a lingual frenulum associated with breastfeeding difficulties in newborns.[9] Many experts use the terms interchangeably.

Terminology for the type of tongue-tie is less clear. Many experts and authorities distinguish between frenula that are tied at the anterior, mid, or posterior part of the tongue. Hong discusses anterior and posterior frenula, and specifically describes the posterior tongue-tie as a short, thick, or fibrous cord of tissue at the base of the tongue that limits elevation.[10] Kotlow says that "all tongue-ties are posterior"[11] whereas Douglas disputes the existence of such a condition.[12] Referring to "posterior tongue-tie" as an "implausible diagnosis," she reminds us that "published studies concerning 'posterior' tongue-tie do not provide evidence that the diagnosis of 'posterior' tongue-tie has validity, or that frenotomy is effective treatment." [12 p. 504]

Indeed, when those who are legally authorized to diagnose medical conditions cannot even agree on the terminology that should be used to describe the defect, we are a long way from agreement about the options for safe and effective treatment, who should provide such treatment, or by what means it should be rendered. We are far from anything like a "one-size-fits-all" treatment.

Indicators of Ankyloglossia in Infants

Since awareness of ankyloglossia has grown in recent years, I am often asked whether a digital exam should be the default way to start a newborn exam. The answer is a resounding "No!" Your finger should be thought of as a "guest" in the infant's mouth. Starting a visit with a breastfeeding infant by launching into a digital exam makes your finger an "intruder.". You cannot expect the infant to improve his suckling "performance" under such conditions. Even adult health care recognizes that a basic principle of physical assessment is to do the poking and prying last, not first. It should not be any different for an infant.

An initial assessment should include "a nonintrusive assessment of tongue function, in addition to history, examination of the infant (and his or her oral cavity, including frenulum), and observation of a feed."[12]

Details about how to properly perform a physical assessment of the intraoral cavity is well beyond this scope of this publication. A true intraoral assessment would consider much more than just the presence or absence of a tongue-tie. As the saying goes, "the devil is in the details" and there are many details that pertain to the techniques, sequence, scope, and interpretation of conducting such an assessment—and knowing when to stop it. For more about how to perform an oral assessment when looking for tongue-tie, see a video from noted expert and author Dr. Jeanne Ballard, available on YouTube.*

My goal with this publication is to help you understand the photos in *The Breastfeeding Atlas* and, by applying some basic observations, to help you better understand real-life clinical situations. To that end, I have used some of the structural criteria identified by Hazelbaker[13] and the functional "key elements" identified in *The Breastfeeding Atlas.*

Anatomy and Physiology of the Tongue

After terminology, the next part of the controversy is the assessment and interpretation of the structure and function of the tongue.

* https://www.youtube.com/watch?v=3ty1UikV_3s

Structure: Appearance of the Tongue and Frenulum

Stories abound of infants with unusual-looking tongues, who nevertheless breastfeed successfully for many months. Other stories describe infants with normal-looking tongues who are unable to suckle effectively and are diagnosed with tongue-tie many months (or even years) later. Sometimes, tongue-ties are severe; at other times, they are almost imperceptible. As is the case when other anatomical deviations or defects are present, clinical management of breastfeeding with tongue-tie often depends on using multiple visual, tactile, and audible cues that signal what's going on.

Shape

Some tongues are round or square at the tip; others are heart-shaped) or V-shaped (**Figure 353**); others are somewhere in between. It's especially important to observe the shape of the tongue when the infant is trying to lift the tongue, since that's what he needs to do while nursing.

Elasticity

There seems to be general agreement that—just like tissue located elsewhere in the body—some lingual frenula are more elastic than others. The more elastic ones give the infant a greater ability to achieve a deep latch onto the nipple/areola.

Frenulum length

The length of the frenulum is especially important. The principle is this: A tongue-tied infant with a longer frenulum is more likely to accomplish successful milk transfer.

Attachment to tongue

This is where the anterior/posterior discussion comes in!

The lingual frenum runs vertically from the floor of the mouth to the undersurface of the tongue.

In most individuals, the frenulum is attached from the posterior aspect of the tongue to the tip (anterior portion) and moves freely. (**Figure 350**).

With all due respect to opponents of the "posterior" language, a frenulum may be tethered to the anterior or posterior part of the tongue (**Figure 36**). Those that are tethered to the posterior part of the tongue often go undiagnosed. However, in my experience, the big clue is what the palate looks like. A high-arched palate (**Figure 36**) is often indicative of a what I would call a posterior tongue-tie.

Attachment to alveolar ridge

Ideally, the frenulum is attached at the floor of the mouth, well below the lower alveolar ridge. (The ridge is where the lower tooth sockets are located.) In some cases, it might be slightly below the inferior (lower) alveolar ridge, or it might even be at the level of the alveolar ridge.

Function: Range of Motion and Key Elements of Tongue Motion in the Breastfed Infant

Successful suckling is in part dependent upon the infant's ability to compress the breast, which is best accomplished when the tongue has full range of motion.

Range of motion refers to the full distance that a body part may normally move while properly attached to another part. A restriction of range of motion means that the movement does not reach the full extent that would be possible under normal circumstances. The tongue consists of many muscles, and, like other muscles, it should move freely.

By now, it's probably no surprise to hear that opinions differ about terminology and descriptions for tongue movement. Partly, this is because some experts look at movements needed for creating optimal speech while others focus on feeding (and some focus on feeding infants or children while others specialize in feeding adults). Wilson-Clay and Hoover identify 4 elements of tongue movement in *The Breastfeeding Atlas*—lateralization, elevation, cupping, extension/retraction—required for the assessment of range of motion by a breastfeeding infant. To these, I add protrusion.

Lateralization

Lateralization means that the tongue moves to either side, horizontally (**Figure 360**).

You'll probably want to start with checking for tongue lateralization. Because this involves almost no poking and pressing of the tissue, the infant is more likely to cooperate while you check this function.

To elicit lateralization of the tongue, press lightly on the lateral aspect (side) of the tongue. Run your finger around the lower alveolar ridge, from side to side.

With normal lateralization, (**Figure 360)** the infant will move his entire tongue—the body of it, as well as the tip—and he will follow your finger from side to side. Compare the normal tongue lateralization of the girl in **Figure 358** to her sister, in **Figure 359**, who shows a limited ability to lateralize her tongue.

To improve the infant's ability to lateralize, Wilson-Clay and Hoover suggest offering the infant a gel-filled or air-filled pacifier to encourage him to use the lateral borders of his tongue.

Elevation (Lifting)

Elevation means that the tongue can lift up from the floor of the mouth (**Figure 358**).

After assessing the infant's ability to lateralize the tongue, gently and slowing pull your finger (pad side up) out of the infant's mouth while gently tickling his upper lip. This should elicit mouth-opening and tongue-elevating. Having the mouth open is important for this assessment, since the infant's mouth is open when he elevates his tongue to compress the nipple/areola against the hard palate. If he is unable to do this, he will not be able to transfer milk to himself.

In a normally functioning tongue, the entire tongue moves, with the anterior one-third of tongue elevating to contact the upper alveolar ridge (or after infancy, the upper teeth). Note that in **Figure 350** the normal tongue is attached to the floor of the mouth, and the individual can lift the anterior one-third of her tongue from the floor to the middle of her mouth. The appearance of the tongue remains unchanged. Compare this to a tongue-tied adult who tries to lift the tongue but she is unable to unable to touch the tip of her tongue to her upper gum, or upper teeth (**Figure 351**).

Now, having a better understanding of range of motion of the tongue, try to imagine what is happening inside of the infant's mouth while breastfeeding. Ideally, the infant's tongue should elevate so that the anterior one-third of the tongue—the tip—touches the superior (upper) alveolar ridge (**Figure 362**). Notice how movement in **Figure 362** differs from the movement in **Figure 361**, where the infant cannot elevate his tongue to the upper alveolar ridge, and the mother experiences nipple tissue damage.

So far, we have shown that the tongue should elevate enough to touch the superior alveolar ridge and/or the teeth, and we've explained the relationship of optimal tongue elevation to optimal milk transfer. However, while it is being elevated, the tongue should not be distorted (**Figure 357).**

Complete Learning Exercise 17-2 to compare Figure 350 and Figure 351.

17-2Cupping

Cupping is the ability of the infant's tongue to "cup" or curl around your finger during a digital assessment, or around the nipple/areolar complex while breastfeeding. Some describe it a scoop-shape or a tough-shape.

To elicit this motion, wait for the infant to "invite" your finger into his mouth; you may need to press gently on his chin (**Figure 362**) to stimulate this response. The tongue should stay in contact with your finger while he is suckling. Peristaltic movement (i.e., movement of the tongue from front to back) should be felt.

Protrusion, Extension, and Retraction

The normal tongue can protrude, extend, and retract.

When suckling the breast, a normal tongue will *extend* (stretch out) within the mouth, but it also must *protrude* (stick out) beyond the lips (**Figure 363**). This is an important distinction. Protrusion specifically means that the tongue is extended out beyond the lips, which is necessary for optimal latch-on. Regular, rhythmic cycles of extension and *retraction* (back and forth) of the tongue within the mouth propel the bolus of milk far back into the mouth so it can be swallowed. Simply stated, if the infant has difficulty extending his tongue within the mouth and beyond his lips, or if he cannot adequately cup the nipple/areola with a seal, he will not have either a good latch or good milk transfer.

To elicit this movement, lightly tickle the infant's lower lip at the midline, perhaps a few times until he opens. Alternatively, you can elicit this movement by tapping gently on the tip of the infant's tongue.

If the infant has full range of motion, he should be able to completely extend and protrude his tongue. Without full range of motion, the tongue has limited protrusion, as demonstrated by a 12-year-old girl with a tongue-tie (**Figure 355**). Limitation of movement is only part of the problem; note that trying to extend and/or protrude the tied tongue leads to distortion of the tongue's shape (**Figure 357**).

Tools for Assessment

Over the past several years, a few different tools have been developed to evaluate the need for surgical correction of a tongue-tie, including the *Hazelbaker Assessment Tool for Lingual Frenulum Function* (HATLFF), Martinelli's two-part tool, and the Bristol Tongue Assessment Tool (BTAT).

The Hazelbaker Assessment Tool for Lingual Frenulum Function (HATLFF) was designed as a means by which to make a recommendation about frenotomy (release of the frenulum) by systematically assigning a numerical score for the appearance and function of the tongue. This often-used tool has been available since 1993. Although popular, the tool is not without its critics. Some researchers have questioned whether it is valid and reliable.[2,3] Others have suggested that the level of detail it requires has made it difficult to use in clinical practice.[14,15]

Martinelli[16] has introduced a two-part tool that considers not only the structure and function of the tongue, but other factors as well. The first part addresses the infant's history, including specific questions about family history and breastfeeding. The second part addresses structure/function, but also the infant's-nutritive and nutritive sucking capabilities. Whereas other tools are more focused on the need for surgical intervention, this tool is more focused on breastfeeding capabilities and limitations.

More recently, midwives in England developed the *Bristol Tongue Assessment Tool (BTAT)*.[17] The BTAT is modeled after the HATLFF, and its outcomes have been shown to correlate closely to that tool. However, it is reportedly easier for clinicians to use. It identifies four observations, and the clinician must choose one of three descriptors7-1. Each of the four items are observed, and an overall score is assigned. (Readers are urged to look at the table in the original article[17] which is available online, and free.)

The score can be a little as 0 or as great as 8. The study says that "scores of 0-3 indicate more severe reduction of tongue function.[17 p. 345]

Consequences of Uncorrected, Dysfunctional Tongue-Tie

The problems that can result from tongue-tie in a breastfeeding infant came to the forefront about two decades ago, with Messner's now-classic article.[18] That article was followed by Hogan's excellent article.[19] Both emphasized structural and functional problems for the infant and the mother. Many experts and researchers have made similar observations since. The immediate consequences of a dysfunctional tongue-tie are twofold: inadequate milk transfer and sore nipples.

Inadequate Milk Transfer

Not all cases of inadequate milk transfer can be attributed to tongue-tie. There are any number of other possible explanations—such as that the infant is lethargic, he is recovering from birth trauma, he is being held in an awkward position—and these and other possibilities should be explored. However, a tongue-tie can indeed create sucking dysfunction when the full range of motion, as described earlier, is impeded.

Sore Nipples

Because the infant with a tongue-tie has a limited ability to draw in and/or compress the nipple/areola, the mother is highly likely to report having "sore nipples." However, as case studies demonstrate, traumatic lesions on the mothers' nipples may be extensive. In one study of twenty-four mothers, Geddes found that frenotomy solved the problem of sore nipples for all except one mother.[20]

The length of the infant's tongue may contribute to different (and even painful) sensations in the nipples. Wilson-Clay and Hoover report that the mother of this infant with an especially long tongue (**Figure 356**) reported that the painful nipples "persisted despite interventions to adjust positioning and latch." (Page 147)

Later or Ongoing Consequences

A dysfunction of the tongue is a true problem for a breastfed infant. The inability of the infant's tongue to demonstrate the full range of motion is likely to result in poor milk transfer. Inadequate milk transfer sets the stage for other problems, such as failure to thrive,[21] low milk supply, plugged ducts, mastitis, and more.

The infant's parents must decide whether to pursue surgical correction of any tongue-tie, and the decision can be a difficult one. While many experts contend that there are few short-term risks or adverse outcomes associated with a frenotomy that is done correctly,[22] others argue the procedure is sometimes ineffective in resolving breastfeeding problems and may need to be repeated a second, or even third, time. Sometimes, the resulting scar tissue can actually worsen the infant's ability to breastfeed.

Techniques to Help the Infant with Tongue-tie to Breastfeed

Before we can help an infant with tongue-tie to breastfeed, we must make sure we're working to solve the right problem. Not long ago, a mother came to me for help, reporting very "sore nipples." She was adamant that her infant's tongue was tied and needed to be clipped. After examining the infant, I felt that both the appearance and the function of his tongue was normal. I asked what her pediatrician thought, and, clearly frustrated, she told me that the pediatrician insisted the infant was "fine!" I agreed, but didn't respond. But since the tongue is only a part of breastfeeding, I did want more information.

I asked if I could observe a nursing session. Lo and behold, as soon as the mother exposed her nipples, I saw the characteristics of a severe yeast infection! No wonder she had "sore nipples"!

In short, because tongue-tie has been the topic of so much buzz, mothers who experience sore nipples are quick to self-diagnose it as the cause. As professionals, we need to be very alert for entirely different problems. After all, techniques to relieve an infant's tongue-tie won't help if the problem is something entirely different!

Basic Principles for Visual Assessment

If a tongue-tie is suspected, a visual assessment of the infant should be done when the examiner and the parent are sitting across from one another, knees touching. The knees become a "table" upon which to position the infant lying supine. [23] (Note that assessments in which the infant is not lying supine, as in **Figure 367**, are possible. However, these are not recommended.)

Visualization, while necessary, is often inadequate for identifying a "posterior" tongue-tie, as Hong[10] defines it. A "posterior" tongue-tie is often quite difficult to see (**Figure 36**); in this case, palpation is more helpful. Whereas a normal frenulum will feel like a slim, silky string, a posteriorly-tied frenum will be more likely to feel like a fibrous, knotty rope.

Feeding Observation

Visual indicators are powerful. Reviewing the four elements in the systematic assessment of infant breastfeeding[24] as described in chapter 6, some rather unusual indicators can be noted if there's a tongue-tie.

Note areolar grasp. In **Figure 365**, the presence of a wide-angle gape appears to be reassuring, but the expression on this infant's face seems to be saying, "this isn't working." Sometimes, infant gets a good grasp of the areola, but slides off shortly thereafter. In an effort to stay on, the infant may aggressively "reach" and that may be followed by—as Wilson-Clay and Hoover describe it—"flicking" their tongue as it snaps back from an extension.

Note areolar compression. Rather than smooth, long, slow, rhythmic motions of the upper and lower jaw, you may see jerky motions. This is a likely indicator of what's going on inside of the mouth. Even if an infant with a tongue-tie is suckling successfully, ultrasound studies show he is likely to have an altered suckling pattern, and position the mother's nipple further from hard/soft palate junction (HSPJ).[20,25,26] As Wilson-Clay and Hoover explain, it appears that tongue-tied infants use their tongue in a back-to-front movement (humping the posterior tongue.)

Note audible swallowing—or, more to the point—lack thereof. This cannot be overemphasized for any infant, and especially for the infant who is suspected of having an anatomic anomaly.

Other audible indicators are also important. If a clicking or clacking noise is heard while the infant is suckling, it's advisable to find the reason for it. Sometimes, such a noise is produced by an infant with normal anatomy and a poor latch.

But occasionally, this is an indicator of an anatomical defect, such as a cleft palate or a tongue-tie. In these cases, a digital exam is warranted. In some cases, this is a repeat of an earlier digital exam, and a good opportunity to bring a fresh perspective, either as the second examiner or—if you were the first examiner—by engaging someone else to be the second examiner.

Creative Infant Positioning

The value of evidence-based practice cannot be overstated, but sometimes, it seems to offer no clear alternative other than saying "goodbye and good luck!" to the struggling mother. It will be many years before we have evidence to support every suggestion we make. Without the benefit of scientific evidence, we need to try some simple, non-invasive means to help the breastfeeding dyad.

In the mid-twentieth century, tongue-ties were often noticed immediately after delivery, and clipped before the infant was wiped off and given to his mother. By about the 1970s, few practitioners seemed to address tongue-ties; science showed that tongue-tied infants could speak plainly with the help of speech therapy, so clipping the frenulum no longer seemed necessary. This, together with the fact that formula-feeding by bottle had become dominant, diminished the perception of tongue-tie as an important factor. Mothers who were motivated to breastfeed but had an infant with tongue-tie found ways to successfully breastfeed (or switched to formula).

Neither of these approaches is acceptable, but they do hold out hope for mothers who may try alternative or creative positioning.

The mother's hand may help to manipulate her breast and nipple tissue for optimal latch-on. Brief, gentle tapping or rolling of the nipple can help it to evert and increase the likelihood that it will stimulate the infant's palate. Using the teacup hold (**Figure 133** or **Figure 382)** or breast compression (**Figure 335**) may help, too. Another possibility is for the mother to hold her thumb on top and fingers below the breast, but use the thumb to gently move the nipple forward past part of the tongue restricted by the lingual frenulum. Rolling the lip out ("digital flanging") might help, too.

I like to try a prone position (**Figure 85**) with this situation. Gravity will help the tongue to fall forward, and it gives the infant the freedom to find an angle for latching that intuitively feels best for him. Again, it's not a guarantee of success, but it often helps, and it's always worth a try.

Infant Enticement

Sometimes, it can be helpful for the mother to express a little colostrum or milk for her infant to lick. If that's not possible for or acceptable to the mother, dribbling a few drops of water onto the infant's lips can be helpful. In either case, a little moisture will often cause him to lick his lips and attempt to use his tongue muscles more efficiently. Admittedly, it's no magic wand, but it might help, and it certainly won't hurt.

Equipment

Many people have asked me about the use of nipple shields for an infant who is tongue-tied. Note that Wilson-Clay and Hoover do not mention the use of this device for ankyloglossia. Was this a philosophical stance, or an oversight? (Notice that they readily suggest the use of a shield for other situations discussed in previous chapters.) The case can be made that nipple shields help to protect a mother's sore nipples. However, since nipple shields won't alter the structure or function of the tongue, there's a low likelihood that that they will improve the tongue-tied infant's latch. Rather, they might worsen the problem of low milk supply.

Finally, be sure to facilitate and check for good milk transfer in all the ways you would for an infant without a tongue-tie. We sometimes focus so much on the defect that it becomes easy to overlook the basics. For example, make sure his chin is not on his chest, that he is "changing gears" during the feeding, and that audible swallowing is heard. (Review chapter 6.)

The Infant Who Undergoes Frenotomy

Often, infants with a tongue-tie have it clipped in a procedure called a *frenotomy*, a *frenulotomy, frenectomy, or a frenulectomy.* (Technically, these terms have slightly different meanings, but are often used interchangeably.) For simplicity's sake, we will refer to this procedure as frenotomy, since *The Breastfeeding Atlas* uses this term, and it is correct, and frequently used in the scientific literature.

Pediatricians, otolaryngologists, and pediatric dentists are among those who are legally authorized to perform frenotomies. When the frenotomy is performed differs tremendously, from locale to locale. Usually, if it is done in the first 2 weeks or so, it is the pediatrician or obstetrician who performs the procedure. Thereafter, it is more likely to be the pediatric dentist or the *otolaryngologist* (ears-nose-throat or "ENT" specialist. The instrument used for frenotomy can be scissors, (**Figure 368**) scalpel, or laser.

Most frenotomies are done in the doctor's office. Generally, a young infant is placed in the mother's lap, a staff person assists by holding the infant firmly while the doctor lifts the tongue and then releases the frenulum. (An older child may be too rambunctious, and therefore may need general anesthesia.) With a gauze pad, firm pressure is applied (**Figure 369**) and some blood smudging is noted, but bleeding does not continue. Note that the infant can breastfeed almost immediately after the surgery (**Figure 370**).

Is the frenotomy effective in correcting or preventing feeding problems? I have had many conversations with literally hundreds of colleagues, and hear a general insistence that clipping an infant's tight frenulum is the ultimate solution to breastfeeding problems. These colleagues have seen so many outcomes where the infant has better latch-on, and the mother's nipple pain resolves—and they conclude that there is a cause-and-effect relationship. Like blogger Tipper Gallagher, I want to put on my "flame-retardant suit" and say that such an adamant stance seems short-sighted.[27]

Does frenotomy solve breastfeeding problems? *I*n one case (**Figure 377)** an infant was able to breastfeed successfully after the surgery, and the mother's nipples were almost healed awhile after the procedure was completed (**Figure 378**). In another case, breastfeeding problems remained unsolved. A week after the frenotomy, her tongue did not lift to touch her upper alveolar ridge (Figure 371), and problems with weight gain continued to two (**Figure 372**) and then to three (**Figure 373**) weeks later. She was given expressed hind milk in addition to nursing directly at the breast.

When it comes to published research, there is little certainty. One author even suggested that a frenotomy might be effective because of the placebo effect![22] Certainly, the results are mixed. It's difficult to evaluate the efficacy of frenotomies due to variances in methodologies and practitioners. In *The Breastfeeding Atlas*, Wilson-Clay and Hoover describe the findings from some of the studies, and the related issues. One systematic review of the literature points out that existing studies have had small sample sizes, used inconsistent methodology, looked only at short-term outcomes, and drew some questionable conclusions.[8] More recently, a Cochrane review concluded that the procedure was often successful in reducing mothers' nipple pain in the short term, but clearly stated that "no study was able to report whether frenotomy led to long-term successful breastfeeding" and emphasized that with such small samples, the certainty of the finds was limited. They concluded that "no study was able to report whether frenotomy led to long-term successful breastfeeding.[28]

Douglas raises some concerns about the possible risks of frenotomy, noting that "[t]he proliferative phase of any skin or mucosal incision is characterized by collagen deposition, granulation tissue formation, epithelialization, and wound contraction. After a deep frenotomy, which may even penetrate the decussate ligament, could the healed connective tissue prove to be less flexible than the pre-incision frenulum? Could the deep frenotomy cause substantially more pain than simple "anterior" frenotomy? Could this more invasive procedure result in subtle oral defensiveness, delaying improvement of tongue function? Could the intrusion of oral digital maneuvers postfrenotomy also contribute to subtle oral defensiveness?"[12 p. 505]

These questions are troubling, and merit careful consideration. I would also add two additional questions. First, is it possible that an especially stretchy frenulum will impair function only temporarily—if at all? Second—and perhaps more importantly— is surgery necessary? That is, is surgery the *only* strategy to resolve feeding problems in the tongue-tied infant? Speech pathologists with decades of experience have told me that, in most cases, specific exercises can help the infant's tongue to extend, retract, protrude, cup, and lateralize. Pediatric dentist Lawrence Kotlow[11] emphasizes that surgery without follow-up exercises is ineffective for sustained improvements in breastfeeding. Perhaps we should urge parents to seek input from speech pathologists, occupational therapists, and myofunctional therapists about how to resolve any tongue-tie problems.

We can and should advocate for the infant. But surgery is not always the "right" or the "only" answer, and we have a clear responsibility to help parents identify and choose from several options.

Lip Tie

A lip tie is the tethering of the labial frenum to the lip. There are several variations of normal[29] but relatively few are associated with a pathologic syndrome.[30]

Social media is full of stories about variations in the labial frenula. Thick upper labial frena ("lip ties") tend to be blamed for breastfeeding problems, but there is no substantive evidence to confirm that. To the contrary, these are likely to be normal.

The oral cavity changes dramatically during the first year of life, both in terms of form and function. [31] In young children, the frenum is generally wide and thick; during growth, it becomes thin and small."[32] Similarly, the attachment of the labial frenum moves.[29,33] Hence, it's likely that the labial frenum has many variations of normal, and these should not be presumed to be "abnormal."

Many infants with thick upper labial frena suckle well, even when the frena have an impact on appearance or other functions. Some types of labial frena can affect tooth spacing (**Figure 399**); sometimes, they can be attached to the incisive papilla. *The Breastfeeding Atlas* shows labial frena of a two-year-old child (**Figure 400**) and his grandfather (**Figure 399**), with images that clearly demonstrate that such a variation can run in families. This pair of images also demonstrates that these somewhat unusual variations can resolve with infant growth. Wilson-Clay and Hoover report that the gap in his teeth partially closed when his labial frenum migrated upward, which occurred by the age of five years" (page 159).

Complete Exercise 17-3 to work through three cases.

Looking Back, Looking Forward

In this chapter, we've talked about terminology, anatomy, physiology, and indicators of ideal function or dysfunction as related to tongue-ties. We've also described published assessment tools, as well as the visual, auditory and tactile indicators that indicate when it's time to feel reassured, and when it's time to offer help—along with some simple means to improve milk transfer, and possible consequences if the tongue-tie goes uncorrected. Finally, we've discussed the more mundane aspects of the frenotomy procedure, and wrestled with it's the very controversial discussion of its efficacy.

By now, if you have viewed the photos carefully and completed the written exercises, you should feel confident that you can determine if or to what extent the lingual frenulum affects latch, and suggest techniques for improving it.

Recalling, Reinforcing, and Expanding Your Learning

Have you ever felt frustrated that you "learned" something, but later, can't recall it? That may be because you didn't reinforce the material you learned. And, perhaps what you originally learned isn't enough to get you through the next few decades of practice; sometimes you need to expand your learning. The exercises in this section are designed to help you recall, reinforce, and expand your learning.

What was your main motivation for reading this chapter?

- ❍ To study for the IBLCE exam, as a first-time candidate
- ❍ To review for the IBLCE exam, as a re-certificant
- ❍ To improve my clinical skills and clinical management

How soon do you think can use the information presented in this chapter?

- ❍ Immediately; within the next few days or so
- ❍ Soon; within the next month or so
- ❍ Later; sometime before I retire

Pro Tip! If you are preparing for the IBLCE exam, it would be wise to pace your studying. Set a target date for when you plan to complete the exercises, and check off them off as you go along.

Done!	Target Date	Learning Exercise
❑	____________	Learning Exercise 17-1. Vocabulary words related to ankyloglossia.
❑	____________	Learning Exercise 17-2. Comparing images of tongue elevation.
❑	____________	Learning Exercise 17-3. "Lessons learned" from clinical cases.
❑	____________	Explore What You've Learned in a Journal
❑	____________	Summarize What You've Learned
❑	____________	Quick Quiz

Master Your Vocabulary

Learning Exercise 17-1. Vocabulary words related to ankyloglossia.

.Instructions: Write the letter of the correct match next to each item. Answers are in the Appendix.

_____ 1. ankyloglossia		A. relating to the lip
_____ 2. Bristol Tongue Assessment Tool (BTAT)		B. scoring tool that looks at structure and function of the lingual frenulum
_____ 3. frenotomy, a frenulotomy, frenectomy, frenulectomy.		C. ability to move the tongue from side to side in the mouth
_____ 4. frenum, frenulum, frenulym, frenula		D. hard/soft palate junction
_____ 5. HSPJ		E. commonly known as tongue-tie
_____ 6. Hazelbaker Assessment Tool for Lingual Frenulum Function (HATLFF).		F. doctor who specializes in conditions of the ears, nose and throat
_____ 7. hypospadias		G. full retraction and extension of the body part including surrounding muscles and other structures
_____ 8. labial		H. a variation on the ATLFF tool
_____ 9. lateralization		I. surgical treatment for ankyloglossia
_____ 10. lingual		J. skin flap that restricts or enables movement
_____ 11. otolaryngologist		K. relating to the tongue
_____ 12. range of motion		L. midline defect where urethra is on the underside of the penis

Conquer Clinical Concepts

Learning Exercise 17-2. Comparing images of tongue elevation

Instructions: In the table below, compare Figure 350 and Figure 351 on the following characteristics.

	Figure 350	Figure 351
How far the tongue is lifted		
Shape of the tip of the tongue when lifted		

Learning Exercise 17-3. "Lessons learned" from Clinical Cases.

Instructions: Clinical case A, B, and C are summarized below. The details of these cases are described in The Breastfeeding Atlas *on pages 148-149. Respond to each question.*

Clinical Case A. (Refer to *The Breastfeeding Atlas* page 148, and **Figures 365-373.**)

When approaching the breast, this newborn has an excellent open-wide gape (**Figure 365**), but she has a tight lingual frenulum (**Figure 366**). Note that she does not have a full range of motion for her tongue (**Figure 367**). Her parents elected for her to undergo a frenotomy, as indicated by the characteristic diamond-shaped incision/scar (**Figure 368**). After the procedure, pressure was briefly applied to the site (**Figure 369**). Ten minutes after the frenotomy, the infant was breastfeeding (**Figure 370**)! Photos show the frenotomy site at one week (**Figure 371**), two weeks (**Figure 372**), and three weeks (**Figure 373**) after having the procedure.

- At the initial assessment, list at least four infant capabilities and/or limitations.

- Briefly describe the procedure used for this frenotomy.

- What was found at the one week, two week, and three week assessments after the frenotomy? What else, if anything, would you have done? What do you see as a priority for her care?

- What did you learn from this case?

Clinical Case B. (Refer to *The Breastfeeding Atlas* page 148-149, and **Figure 374**)

Figure 374 shows an infant with the classical heart-shaped tongue that is associated with a tongue-tie. A dysfunctional suck would seem to be a likely consequence. However, as Wilson-Clay and Hoover report, this infant breastfed well and gained weight well. Also, his mother did not have sore nipples.

- Would you have performed a digital exam on this infant? Why, or why not?

- List the capabilities and limitations of the mother/infant in this situation

- What did you learn from this case?

Clinical Case C (Refer to *The Breastfeeding Atlas* page 149, and **Figures 375-378**).

The Breastfeeding Atlas shows a nine-day-old infant with a tongue-tie (**Figure 375**). As a result of his dysfunctional suckling, the mother has a damaged, infected nipple (**Figure 376**). After a frenotomy was performed, the infant was able to successfully extend, protrude and lift his tongue (**Figure 377**). Luckily, the nipple healed (**Figure 378**).

Although it is a different person, **Figure 379** shows how the tongue looks years after a frenotomy.

- If you had been the hospital nurse, what assessment data do you think you might have seen or heard in the first few days?

- What did you learn from this case?

Summarize What You've Learned

The goal of this chapter was for you to determine if or to what extent the lingual frenulum affects latch, and suggest techniques for improving it.

Instructions: Using only a few words, answer each question.

Terminology: Why is terminology a problem, and what's the controversy about?	
What signs, symptoms of either appearance or function are likely to impact the tongue-tied infant's ability to have full range of motion in his tongue?	
What are some common tools for assessment of the tongue-tie	
What are the likely consequences if the infant has a dysfunctional tongue-tie?	
How would you help the parent to make an informed decision about having a frenotomy for their tongue-tied infant?	

Explore What You've Learned With a Journal

Multiple studies have shown the benefits of using a learning journal. Among them are greater assimilation and integration of new information, better long-term retention of course concepts, increasing test and exam grades, and a means by which to have continuous feedback about one's own learning.

- Name at least three things you learned from this chapter.

- List at least three things you still need to learn, or more fully master, in this chapter.

- Briefly describe how this information fits (or doesn't fit) with what you've seen in clinical practice, what you learned in basic or college courses, or what you've observed in your own experience breastfeeding. (In some cases, you might want to include how the information fits or doesn't fit with what "experts" say, what the media says, or whatever.)

- Describe how you will use any or all of this information. How might it be related to problems and potential solutions that occur in real life or in clinical situations?

- If you wish, include how you felt about learning this information. Were you overwhelmed? Enlightened? Worried? Something else?

Self Assessment

People often dive into a test before they have thoughtfully reflected on how well they have prepared for it. Instead, it would be helpful if they would take a few moments to give their alter-ego (their "other self") a chance to reflect on how confident they feel about mastering the stated objectives.

Instructions: Take a moment to review the chapter objectives (below). Then rate yourself. How confident are you that you have achieved each objective below?

Objective	Highly Confident	Somewhat Confident	Somewhat Unsure	Completely Unsure
Match key elements in tongue motion to elicitation techniques and visual examples of abnormal appearance and function.	❍	❍	❍	❍
Recognize the signs, symptoms, and likely impact of a tongue-tied infant's ability to have full range of tongue motion.	❍	❍	❍	❍
Predict likely consequences of dysfunctional tongue-tie for both the infant and the mother.	❍	❍	❍	❍
Assist the parent to make an informed decision about having a frenotomy for their tongue-tied infant/child.	❍	❍	❍	❍
Through the pictorial case reports of tongue-tied infants, identify elements of and priorities for a plan of care for the breastfeeding couplet.	❍	❍	❍	❍

On the next page, you will see some simple recall questions pertaining to this chapter. These are *not* the application-type questions you will find in the IBLCE exam. However, you cannot *apply* information unless you can fully *recall* that information! You should do these without looking up the answers.

When you finish with the quiz, look up the answers in the Appendix. Then, score your answers, using the Appendix. Finally, you should analyze the results of your quiz. It's not enough to just know what you got right or wrong; you must look at why you got the answers right or wrong.

Quick Quiz Chapter 17

Instructions: Circle the correct response. For a better understanding of how well you are mastering the material, try answering independently, without flipping back or looking at the source material. If you are really stuck, questions come from this workbook and from The Breastfeeding Atlas, so go back and review the appropriate material. Answers are in the Appendix.

1. The most important use of the Hazelbaker Assessment Tool for Lingual Frenulum Function (HATLFF) is to:

   A. diagnose ankyloglossia

   B. document postoperative success

   C. indicate the need for frenotomy

   D. justify third-party payment for consultations

2. Parents have been told that their child's tongue-tie will "disappear." Research[6] has shown that this statement is

   A. frequently true

   B. misleading

   C. rarely discussed

3. Suction is MOST likely to be impaired when you observe that the tongue:

   A. does not seal the gap at the corners of the mouth

   B. has a heart-shaped tip

   C. is especially long

4. Of these observations, the MOST likely indicator of ankyloglossia is a tongue that is:

   A. distortion when the tongue is elevated

   B. attached at the floor of the mouth

   C. exceptionally long

   D. heart-shaped

   E. moving from front to back

5. In providing anticipatory guidance for the parent of an 18-day-old infant who will be undergoing frenotomy, which would you tell the parent is part of the procedure?

   A. admission to the hospital

   B. general anesthesia

   C. holding the infant still

   D. suturing of the wound

Analyze Your Own Quiz

- What percentage of the questions did you answer correctly?

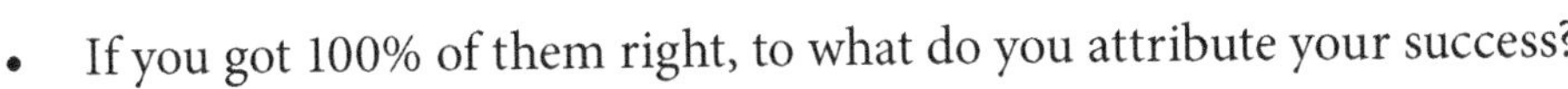

- If you got 100% of them right, to what do you attribute your success?

- If you did not get all the questions right, can you identify your learning gap? (Example: Didn't know the information, knew the information but could not remember, knew some information but confused it with similar information, other.)

- Would you have been able to answer the questions as well if you had not read this chapter?

- What do you need to do next? (If you got them all right, what you need to do next is celebrate! Even a high-five with your child, a YESSS and a fist-pump in the air, or anything else is good! A small acknowledgement of your success is better than no acknowledgement!)

Additional Resources

1. Lawrence RA. Tongue-tie-the disease du jour. *Breastfeed Med.* 2013;8(6):467-468.
2. Amir LH, James JP, Donath SM. Reliability of the Hazelbaker Assessment Tool for Lingual Frenulum Function. *International Breastfeeding Journal.* 2006;1(1):3.
3. Ricke LA, Baker NJ, Madlon-Kay DJ, DeFor TA. Newborn tongue-tie: prevalence and effect on breast-feeding. *The Journal of the American Board of Family Practice.* 2005;18(1):1-7.
4. International Board of Lactation Consultant Examiners. Advisory Opinion: Assessment, Diagnosis, and Referral. 2017. Available ***https://iblce.org/wp-content/uploads/2017/05/advisory-opinion-assessment-diagnosis-referral-english.pdf*** Accessed June 14, 2017.
5. Segal LM, Stephenson R, Dawes M, Feldman P. Prevalence, diagnosis, and treatment of ankyloglossia: methodologic review. *Can Fam Physician.* 2007;53(6):1027-1033.
6. Lalakea ML, Messner AH. Ankyloglossia: does it matter? *Pediatr Clin North Am.* 2003;50(2):381-397.
7. Ferrés-Amat E, Pastor-Vera T, Rodríguez-Alessi P, Ferrés-Amat E, Mareque-Bueno J, Ferrés-Padró E. Management of Ankyloglossia and Breastfeeding Difficulties in the Newborn: Breastfeeding Sessions, Myofunctional Therapy, and Frenotomy. *Case reports in pediatrics.* 2016;2016:3010594.
8. Francis DO, Krishnaswami S, McPheeters M. Treatment of ankyloglossia and breastfeeding outcomes: a systematic review. *Pediatrics.* 2015;135(6):e1458-1466.
9. Haham A, Marom R, Mangel L, Botzer E, Dollberg S. Prevalence of breastfeeding difficulties in newborns with a lingual frenulum: a prospective cohort series. *Breastfeed Med.* 2014;9:438-441.
10. Hong P, Lago D, Seargeant J, Pellman L, Magit AE, Pransky SM. Defining ankyloglossia: a case series of anterior and posterior tongue ties. *Int J Pediatr Otorhinolaryngol.* 2010;74(9):1003-1006.
11. Biancuzzo M. *Born to be Breastfed.* With guest, Kotlow L. Babies With Tongue and Lip Ties: What's Fact, What's False and how to overcome the Problems.
12. Douglas PS. Rethinking "posterior" tongue-tie. *Breastfeed Med.* 2013;8(6):503-506.
13. Hazelbaker A. *The Assessment Tool for Lingual Frenulum Function (HATLFF): Use in a Lactation Consultant Private Practice.* Pasadena, CA, Pacific Oaks College; 1993.
14. Madlon-Kay DJ, Ricke LA, Baker NJ, DeFor TA. Case series of 148 tongue-tied newborn babies evaluated with the assessment tool for lingual frenulum function. *Midwifery.* 2008;24(3):353-357.

15. Ngerncham S, Laohapensang M, Wongvisutdhi T, et al. Lingual frenulum and effect on breastfeeding in Thai newborn infants. *Paediatrics and international child health.* 2013;33(2):86-90.

16. Martinelli RL, Marchesan IQ, Berretin-Felix G. Lingual frenulum protocol with scores for infants. *The International journal of orofacial myology : official publication of the International Association of Orofacial Myology.* 2012;38:104-112.

17. Ingram J, Johnson D, Copeland M, Churchill C, Taylor H, Emond A. The development of a tongue assessment tool to assist with tongue-tie identification. *Arch Dis Child Fetal Neonatal Ed.* 2015;100(4):F344-348.

18. Messner AH, Lalakea ML, Aby J, Macmahon J, Bair E. Ankyloglossia: incidence and associated feeding difficulties. *Arch Otolaryngol Head Neck Surg.* 2000;126(1):36-39.

19. Hogan M, Westcott C, Griffiths M. Randomized, controlled trial of division of tongue-tie in infants with feeding problems. *J Paediatr Child Health.* 2005;41(5-6):246-250.

20. Geddes DT, Langton DB, Gollow I, Jacobs LA, Hartmann PE, Simmer K. Frenulotomy for breastfeeding infants with ankyloglossia: effect on milk removal and sucking mechanism as imaged by ultrasound. *Pediatrics.* 2008;122(1):e188-194.

21. Forlenza GP, Paradise Black NM, McNamara EG, Sullivan SE. Ankyloglossia, exclusive breastfeeding, and failure to thrive. *Pediatrics.* 2010;125(6):e1500-1504.

22. Power RF, Murphy JF. Tongue-tie and frenotomy in infants with breastfeeding difficulties: achieving a balance. *Arch Dis Child.* 2015;100(5):489-494.

23. Academy of Breastfeeding Medicine. Protocol #11: Guidelines for the evaluation and management of neonatal ankyloglossia and its complications in the breastfeeding dyad. 2004; .Available at ***http://www.bfmed.org/Media/Files/Protocols/ankyloglossia.pdf***

24. Shrago L, Bocar D. The infant's contribution to breastfeeding. *J Obstet Gynecol Neonatal Nurs.* 1990;19(3):209-215.

25. Geddes DT, Kent JC, Mitoulas LR, Hartmann PE. Tongue movement and intra-oral vacuum in breastfeeding infants. *Early Hum Dev.* 2008;84(7):471-477.

26. Geddes DT, Kent JC, McClellan HL, Garbin CP, Chadwick LM, Hartmann PE. Sucking characteristics of successfully breastfeeding infants with ankyloglossia: a case series. *Acta Paediatr.* 2010;99(2):301-303.

27. Gallagher T. Tongue tie: One IBCLC's moderate approach. September, 12, 2016; ***http://www.theboobgeek.com/blog/tongue-tie.html*** June 20, 2017.

28. O'Shea JE, Foster JP, O'Donnell CP, et al. Frenotomy for tongue-tie in newborn infants. *Cochrane Database Syst Rev.* 2017;3:Cd011065.

29. Townsend JA, Brannon RB, Cheramie T, Hagan J. Prevalence and variations of the median maxillary labial frenum in children, adolescents, and adults in a diverse population. *General dentistry.* 2013;61(2):57-60; quiz 61.

30. Priyanka M, Sruthi R, Ramakrishnan T, Emmadi P, Ambalavanan N. An overview of frenal attachments. *Journal of Indian Society of Periodontology.* 2013;17(1):12-15.

31. Ranly DM. Early orofacial development. *J Clin Pediatr Dent.* 1998;22(4):267-275.

32. Khursheed D, Zorab, S. S., Zardawi, F. M., Talabani, R. M. Prevalence of Labial Frenum Attachment and its Relation to Diastemia and Black Hole in Kurdish Young Population. *IOSR Journal of Dental and Medical Sciences.* 2015;14(9):97-100.

33. Boutsi EA, Tatakis DN. Maxillary labial frenum attachment in children. *Int J Paediatr Dent.* 2011;21(4):284-288.

Chapter 18

Breastfeeding With Cleft Lip and Palate

A young man in his late teens stepped aside to let me move through a crowded aisle. My nurse brain—which is always switched on—noticed an almost invisible scar on his lip. I found myself wondering how bad the cleft had been, but feeling certain that his friends and acquaintances might never have guessed he was born with a cleft lip. Moments later, the crowd shifted, and I noticed that the young man was apparently part of a sports team, and his last name was printed on the back of his jacket. The clues all lined up—an unusual last name, his age, and being in the neighborhood where his family had lived many years ago. I instantly knew who he was. His mother had wanted desperately to breastfeed him. I had felt woefully inadequate to help them. He was born with clefts of the lip and both palates, and had undergone five surgeries.

If you ever have an opportunity to work with a family whose child has a cleft, you will never forget them, or their circumstances. While writing this chapter, I realized that I am as intrigued now as I was decades ago by all that there is to know about—and how much can be done to facilitate —breastfeeding for infants who are affected with a cleft.

Reading this chapter won't make you an expert. But with the excellent photos on pages 197-198 of *The Breastfeeding Atlas*, and the learning exercises that are provided in this workbook, you should be able to complete the post-test in a matter of minutes. As for helping families to have a successful breastfeeding experience? Well, that will take a little longer!

I promise that when we finish this chapter, you will be able to recognize various types of orofacial clefts, their impact on breastfeeding, and strategies to initiate and continue successful milk transfer.

Key Words

- alveolar ridge
- bifid uvula
- bowel malrotation
- cleft lip
- cleft palate
- complete palatal cleft
- endotracheal (ET) tube
- grooved palate
- intubation
- incomplete palatal cleft
- isolated clefts
- nasogastric (NG) tube
- Pierre Robin Syndrome (Sequence)
- Pigeon feeder
- primary palate
- orotracheal
- secondary palate
- SpecialNeeds® feeder
- submucous cleft
- Van der Woude Syndrome
- velum

Objectives

- Name orofacial clefts using widely-accepted terminology and classifications.
- Recognize a submucous cleft through visualization and palpation techniques, along with its management implications.
- Recognize conditions that are associated with, overlooked, or mistaken for orofacial clefts.
- Discuss at least four aspects of feeding difficulties that the infant with a cleft is likely to encounter.
- Provide anticipatory guidance for infants who will undergo surgery for orofacial cleft defects.
- Depending on the extent of the lesion, choose the technique that is most likely to help the infant with a cleft to achieve an adequate seal, negative pressure, and mandibular compression.

Overview of Cleft Lips and Cleft Palates

Cleft lip and cleft palate, relatively common congenital defects, are likely to have a serious effect on breastfeeding. A cleft changes the orofacial structure in a manner that makes it difficult for the infant to get a good seal, create adequate negative pressure, and compress the lactiferous ducts enough to facilitate optimal milk transfer. (See Chapter 6.)

By definition, a cleft is a type of lesion. More specifically, the cleft is a gap in the tissue that results from failure of anatomical parts to fuse during embryonic development. This chapter is devoted to orofacial clefts. A cleft lip usually develops at around five weeks of gestation; a cleft palate occurs later, at around seven weeks.

The reasons for a cleft defect are complex, but most are attributed to environmental or genetic factors.[1] For example, many studies have looked at the relationship between folic acid and orofacial defect, although a cause-and-effect relationship is unclear.[2] Unquestionably, cleft defects do run in families (**Figure 352**), and statistics show that having a family member with a cleft increases the likelihood that an infant will also be affected. However, family history is not entirely explainable by a gene theory only. After all, family members tend to be exposed to the same environmental factors.

Isolated clefts are those that are not associated with any recognizable anomalies; non-isolated clefts occur with other known anomalies. For example, a cleft palate rarely occurs without a cleft lip.[3] Many times, orofacial clefts are part of a syndrome, such as Van der Woude Syndrome, Pierre Robin sequence (as shown in the "receding" chin in **Figure 398**), velocardiofacial syndrome, or median facial dysplasia.[4]

The LAPAL Classifications

Cleft defects were first identified in 1923.[5] For many years, the most popular classification system for such conditions was the classification developed by Kernahan and Stark in 1958.[6] Since then, several modifications have been suggested by others. Currently, the Cleft Foundation uses the LAPAL classification.[7] This approach addresses the location and extent of the clefting through a right-to-left description of the affected structure: (**L**) right side of the Lip, (**A**) right Alveolar ridge and primary palate, (**P**) secondary Palate, (**A**) left Alveolar ridge and primary palate, and (**L**) left side of the Lip.

Cleft Lips

A cleft lip is seen in **Figure 380** and **Figure 381**. These images show cleft lips with very small gaps; often, the gap can be much wider, even without involvement of the alveolar ridge or the palate.

Cleft Palates

There are two parts to the human palate: the primary palate and the secondary palate. The primary palate includes the alveolar arch, while the secondary palate includes the hard and soft palate. The *alveolar ridge* (also called alveolar margin) is a separate structure; the inferior alveolar ridge is part of the mandible, and the superior alveolar ridge is part of the maxilla where the tooth sockets are located. Kosowski and colleagues[8] explain that the hard palate "is formed by the palatine processes of the maxillae and by the horizontal lamina of the palatine bones. It is covered by oral and nasal mucosa."[8 p. 165] The soft palate is also called the *velum*.

Certainly, a cleft is a gap—a discontinuation of the normal tissue. However, orofacial clefts differ substantially. A cleft palate may be either unilateral (one-sided) or bilateral (both sides). It may or may not involve the alveolar ridge. It may be either complete or incomplete.

According to Kosowski,[8] an incomplete cleft involves only the secondary palate. A *complete cleft* is one that affects the alveolar arch and the entire length of the secondary palate. The infant in **Figure 389** has a cleft of the alveolar ridge, the alveolar arch, and the entire length of the secondary palate.

A cleft of a soft palate is seen in **Figure 383** and **Figure 384**.

A cleft may be immediately apparent when the infant is born. (Sometimes, it can be seen during an ultrasound, prenatally.) Other times, it is only apparent during a careful examination of the infant; often, they are identified during a thorough physical exam by a primary care provider before hospital discharge. However, small clefts are sometimes missed.

Sometimes, an infant has a *submucous cleft*. This means that the cleft is covered by a mucous membrane in either the soft or the hard palate Because of this covering, the submucous cleft can be difficult to see; often such clefts go undiagnosed even into adulthood.[9] Shining a light onto the palate will greatly aid in visualizing the defect (**Figure 383**). Palpation, rather than visualization, is probably more effective in identifying such clefts.

If a submucous cleft is located within the soft palate, there will be a lack of muscular tissue and incorrect positioning of the muscles that make up the palate. If the submucous cleft is located within the hard palate, it is midline, and feels like a notch or a depression. Often,[10] a submucous cleft palate is associated with a *bifid uvula* (**Figure 385**). (The term *bifid* is from the Latin from *bi-* meaning 'doubly', and *fidus* and *findere* which means 'to split'.)

A submucous cleft can affect speech[10] and feeding capabilities. Swallowing is most likely to be affected due to the incorrect positioning of the muscles. Such a cleft is likely to cause chronic otitis media as well. Usually, ear infections need to be treated medically or surgically, but speech and feeding problems are less apparent and more easily resolved. Parents may inquire about the possibility of surgery for the submucous cleft, but should be informed that the condition may not warrant surgery.

A submucous cleft should not be repaired on the presumption that it will impair feeding or speech function. In a group of 130 adult clients, 44% of submucous clefts "remained asymptomatic into adulthood, and none required surgical intervention."[11]

Grooved Palate

People often look at a photo of a "grooved" palate (**Figure 390**) and ask, "How can you tell that it isn't a cleft palate?" No one would benefit from my initial inclination to reply, "Because it doesn't look like a cleft! A groove doesn't look like a gap!" But let's back up a little.

A grooved palate may occur naturally, such as with Down Syndrome (**Figure 391**) or Turner Syndrome (**Figure 346**) and many other syndromes, including Pierre Robin Syndrome (Sequence), (not shown here). But the condition is highly likely to result from the placement of an endotracheal (ET) tube. An ET tube is placed into the trachea to provide respiratory support (or, perhaps, medication). This procedure is referred to as *intubation*. (Note: The term *intubation* applies only to placement of a tube into the trachea, and should not be confused with the placement of a feeding tube into the stomach.)

Look for the grooved palate to reflect the size and shape of the ET tube. In **Figure 390**, try to visualize the very narrow, straight, smooth, firm ET tube that was pressed into the infant's soft tissue for a period of time. Palatal grooving can occur in as few as 12 hours after insertion of the ET tube, and when the infant has been intubated for 15 days or more, more than 87% have a grooved palate. The size used for successful intubation varies substantially, based on the newborn's gestational age and/or any congenital defects, but for an infant born at less than 37 weeks, an ET tube of 3.5 mm in diameter, or smaller would be likely. (To provide some perspective, a standard #2 pencil is 7 mm in diameter on the outside.)

A full discussion of grooved palates is beyond the scope of this publication, but it is important to be aware that such a condition exists because it's highly likely you will see them in clinical practice, and you will want to be able to recognize them. In a review article covering 12 studies of palatal and areolar grooves, Hohoff and colleagues[12] provide many details and insights, such as that those two types of grooves never co-occur. Interestingly, only three of the twelve studies define the "grooved" palate, and each of those definitions differ from the other. Perhaps the most useful definition was that it presents as "*an architectural deformity of the palate caused by external pressure from the orotracheal tube.*" (The prefix *endo-* means "within," and *orotracheal* simply means that the tube is advanced into the trachea through the mouth.)

Hohoff and colleagues[12] point to studies showing that intubation "does not invariably lead to grooving" but the incidence of palatal grooving in premature infants is about 90% among those who are intubated. Premature newborns are at high risk for breathing difficulties, and are therefore more likely to be intubated. However, any newborn—including those born at term—may have difficulty breathing and be intubated. The grooved palates that result can persist for many years, as is seen in a 12-year-old (**Figure 391**). It may pose no problem to infant feeding.

Breastfeeding Goals and Anticipatory Guidance

I am often asked whether a baby with a cleft defect can breastfeed exclusively. The answer is an emphatic "maybe." Clarren's seminal research[13] shows that some can and some cannot, and this fits with both my clinical observations and case reports in *The Breastfeeding Atlas*! The more severe the cleft, the less likely the infant will be able to suckle well enough to get all his nourishment at the breast.

Most breastfeeding advocates are eager to help a mother achieve her breastfeeding goals. I am eager to affirm that many infants with cleft defects can successfully breastfeed.[14] However, the infant in **Figure 392** is unlikely to be able to accomplish *exclusive* breastfeeding. He has a complete cleft of the lip and palate, and a cleft of the alveolar ridge. He was not supplemented in the hospital, and he began losing significant amounts of weight. By Day 4, he had dark, scant urine output and few small dark stools (**Figure 393**). (Note that, as explained in Chapter 4, the lack of a yellow stool on Day 4 is worrisome.) Meanwhile, bilirubin levels rose. With expert guidance from Wilson-Clay, he was repositioned three times, but he still was unable to transfer milk to himself, as evidenced by pre-test and post-test weighing.

Because of the mother's commitment to exclusive breastfeeding, the hospital nurse was probably reluctant to introduce supplementation. However, given the extent of the lesions, even when the infant had his mouth on the breast and his jaws moving, he wasn't transferring milk. Wilson-Clay immediately realized this.

Sometimes, when faced with a clinical situation such as a severe cleft, we need to help parents modify their goals. This infant will have many needs: He will likely need several surgeries, treatments for recurrent otitis media, and much more. Hence, the parents should be reminded of the protective components of human milk, the efficacy of frequent skin-to-skin contact, and the need to protect the mother's milk supply so that feedings may be given by an alternative method (**Figure 395**). Exclusive, direct breastfeeding may be possible later, but not at the moment.

The psychological impact of an infant's serious facial defect on his parents cannot be overstated. Often, the only time the infant looks "normal" is when he is suckling at breast; so, for a number of physical and psychological reasons, this should be encouraged. Just as importantly, the parents should be reassured that surgical reconstruction is almost always highly successful. Note the dramatic improvement in appearance of this infant only days after his reconstructive surgery (**Figure 396**). Seeing before-and-after photos of other infants—or better yet, seeing and talking with adults who have had cleft repairs—can help parents have realistic high hopes for their children.

Clinical Management Strategies

As discussed in Chapter 3, any and all feeding strategies should aim to help the infant with achieving and maintaining 1) seal of the lips, (2) negative intraoral pressure, and (3) mandibular (jaw) compression of the nipple. **Focusing on these three cornerstones is critical for the infant with a cleft.** In addition, an infant with a cleft palate will need to transfer milk without excessive gagging. For an infant affected with a cleft lip and/or a cleft palate, some simple techniques and specialized equipment can be helpful.

Helpful Techniques

It's helpful to remind the parents that the goal of any first feeding is for the newborn to become acquainted with the breast. Optimal latch and milk transfer is of less importance. Some do better during the colostral phase, when they don't have a large volume of milk to cope with. Others do better after the mother's full and elastic breast/nipple fills the gap in oral tissue.

It is critical to give appropriate anticipatory guidance to the parents before the infant attempts a feeding in which an abundance of milk is likely to be released. Let them know that, especially for the infant who has a cleft palate, suckling the milk may cause gagging, spitting, and pulling away from the breast. Emphasize that, unlike artificial baby milk (i.e., formula), human milk is physiologic and is not harmful if aspirated.[15]

Have a bulb syringe handy, but suggest an upright feeding position (**Figure 394**) to minimize the possibility of aspiration. It may not have been reasonably possible with this particular dyad (**Figure 394**), but my go-to position for an infant with a cleft defect is the seated straddle position (**Figure 103**), because it provides so much stability, but any upright or semi-upright position is good. If bottle-feeding, a semi-upright position and holding the bottle horizontally, as explained in chapter 14, is helpful. In **Figure 387**, the infant was exhibiting feeding aversion. Flexing the hips can help to avoid or minimize hyperextension (**Figure 386**) of the body.

The teacup hold (**Figure 382**) is one means by which to plug the gap of a cleft lip and achieve a good seal. Take time to carefully review **Figure 133** in Chapter 7, which shows the teacup hold without the infant attached. Here, in **Figure 382**, notice that the mother correctly uses the teacup hold with her fingers off-center from the nipple/areolar and the infant's mouth.

Another way to fill the gap of the cleft is by having the mother use her thumb to fill the cleft. The "sandwich" hold might even work; it very much depends on the width and shape of the cleft in the lip. I'm a fan of the Dancer hand (**Figure 333**) for achieving a good seal or creating a smaller intraoral space and therefore greater negative pressure. However, this will not work with every dyad. Each lesion is different, each breast is different, and each infant behaves or reacts differently. I can even think of instances where the cleft was more of a small notch than a large gap, so I did not suggest any special technique at all, and yet milk was successfully transferred for months! As the authors of *The Breastfeeding Atlas* so aptly remind us, sometimes we need to use some experimentation and common sense.

Note that achieving good negative pressure is usually much more difficult with a cleft palate than with a cleft lip. Ideally, with a malleable breast, the infant can occlude the cleft in the palate. If the cleft is particularly large, however, that might not be possible. Meanwhile, since it's not a "closed system," negative pressure is low or nonexistent.

Achieving optimal compression is unlikely to occur without some special techniques, such as the mother compressing her breast while the infant suckles (**Figure 394**).

Helpful Equipment

In most cases, a regular bottle with a regular nipple doesn't work well at all. The authors of *The Breastfeeding Atlas* show the usefulness of a SpecialNeeds® Feeder (**Figure 395**) (also known as the Haberman® feeder), a Pigeon Feeder® (**Figure 397**), and a spoon. (Note that, like the Pigeon Feeder, Dr. Brown's Specialty Feeding System also has a one-way valve.) I heartily agree that these can work well. I have also used a syringe, or a syringe attached to a length of pediatric catheter tubing, or a #5 French feeding tube. All are good alternatives for some infants, and less effective for others. Trial and error is key to finding out what works.

In my experience, different plastic surgeons and cleft teams have different preferences for how to give oral feedings after surgery. When possible, find out such preferences ahead of time, and teach the parents to use that method from the start. This streamlines infant feeding education, supports the parents and infant in growing comfortable with the method, and reduces the likelihood of "feeding aversion" after surgery. (In the past, I have found that what some providers called an infant's postoperative "feeding aversion" was actually an aversion to an unfamiliar method or technique. See Chapter 16 for a discussion of feeding aversion.)

Looking at *The Breastfeeding Atlas*' **Figure 388,** you might be surprised to see an infant with a cleft who was fed through a *nasogastric tube* (NG). A closer reading shows that this infant has some rather unusual feeding behaviors and conditions, including a *bowel malrotation*—a condition where the intestines have been twisted in a way that can cause an obstruction. This is an excellent example of how easy it is to assume that a problem such as inadequate intake is due to the visible problem—in this case, the cleft. In fact, inadequate intake and subsequent poor weight gain can be due to other problems—invisible problems such as a bowel malrotation—or other pathology.

To me, the most helpful "equipment" in feeding an infant with cleft is the mother's hand. Mentioned only rarely in the professional literature[16]—but well-known among those who have worked in resource-poor countries—hand expressing milk directly into the infant's mouth is a popular method for successfully feeding infants affected by orofacial clefts. Here in the United States, where multiple pieces of equipment are available, the approach is undervalued. It is often not even considered in this situation.

Surgery and Postoperative Care

Parents have many questions about the repair of their infant's cleft defect. It's imperative that they make contact with their child's cleft repair team as soon as possible after birth. An orofacial cleft represents multi-factorial physical and emotional issues, and a multi-disciplinary cleft team is equipped to optimize care and health outcomes for the infant.

The parents that I've encountered ask many who-what-where-when-how questions. In my experience—and borne out by the professional research, as well as the case scenarios in *The Breastfeeding Atlas*— the answers vary greatly. Answers often depend on the preferences of the surgeon and the cleft team, but more importantly, on the extent of the clefting, and the general health status of the infant, including whether the clefting is isolated or part of a syndrome. To some degree, even the distance from the family's home to the hospital where the surgery is performed will affect the answers. If you are preparing for a certification exam, here are some short answers that might serve as general guidelines.

Who

Usually, the surgery is performed by a plastic surgeon who has subspecialized in reconstruction of pediatric and/or craniofacial defects. I would venture to say that relatively few have treated breastfeeding infants, and this is one reason why it's important for a lactation specialist to become part of the cleft team. On page 155, *The Breastfeeding Atlas* mentions a surgeon who witnessed a post-operative infant's lengthy attempt at breastfeeding; the astute mother quoted the surgeon as saying quietly, "You know, I guess I've never seen a breastfed baby."

Where

In no case will the local community hospital be equipped for this type of surgery. Some families can have their infant's cleft repair at a craniofacial center, such as the one in Atlanta.* For those without a craniofacial center nearby, this option may be completely out of the question—especially if the infant needs multiple surgeries. Instead, a regional referral center is likely to offer specialists, subspecialists, and equipment for the surgery their infant needs.

The location of their child's treatment center can affect the parents in many ways, including the amount of time, absence from their jobs, and the expenses and hassles of travel—not to mention the fatigue and the worry of being away from any other children, and more. These factors can create stressors that may make it difficult for the mother to produce and express her milk. (I am reminded of one infant who had multiple surgeries—as is often the case—to repair his cleft lip and cleft palates; his parents lived in a rural locale about 100 miles from the regional referral center, and they had other small children at home.)

* ***https://www.choa.org/medical-services/craniofacial-disorders*** Accessed August 4, 2017.

What

How will the surgery affect the child's appearance, and his oral functions? What factors related to preoperative fasting, medications, and sleep could affect breastfeeding? What is the average stay in the hospital? What follow-up visits will be needed? Parents should be fully informed, and instructed about the postoperative course.

When

Parents often are eager to know how soon the repair will be scheduled, but this is not an answer we can anticipate. Sometimes, surgery is performed early.[17] Other times, the surgeon's preference or the infant's condition warrants a much longer wait. Further, surgery for cleft palate defects is often a two-step process, since research has shown better outcomes.

Historically, an informal metric to assess fitness for surgery was the 10-10-10 rule: 10 weeks of age, 10 pounds of weight, and 10 g/dL of hemoglobin. The other unwritten "rule" seemed to forbid breastfeeding until 10 days after the surgery, because of the fear that sucking would damage the suture line. To my knowledge, there is no evidence that this is a real risk for a breastfed infant. To the contrary, studies by Darzi[18] and, much earlier, Weatherly-White[19] showed that early breastfeeding in the first several hours after surgery was beneficial, and appeared to have no adverse effects for the baby or the suture line.

Looking Back, Looking Forward

In this chapter, we've talked about terminology and classifications of clefts, submucous clefts as they relate to feeding issues, conditions that associated with, overlooked, or mistaken for orofacial clefts, the feeding difficulties that an infant with a cleft is likely to encounter, and some ideas for how to provide anticipatory guidance to the parents of a breastfed infant affected with a cleft. Finally, we addressed techniques that are most likely to help the infant with a cleft to achieve an adequate seal, adequate negative pressure, and adequate compression.

Evidence in the education field shows that writing your own summary helps your retention. The Summarize What You've Learned exercise helps you to do this, so take just a few minutes to complete that exercise now.

By now, if you have viewed the photos carefully, and if you've completed the written exercises, you should feel confident that you can recognize various types of orofacial clefts, their impact on breastfeeding, and strategies to initiate and continue successful milk transfer.

Recalling, Reinforcing, and Expanding Your Learning

Have you ever felt frustrated that you "learned" something, but later, can't recall it? That may be because you didn't reinforce the material you learned. And, perhaps what you originally learned isn't enough to get you through the next few decades of practice; sometimes you need to expand your learning. The exercises in this section are designed to help you recall, reinforce, and expand your learning.

What was your main motivation for reading this chapter?

- ❍ To study for the IBLCE exam, as a first-time candidate
- ❍ To review for the IBLCE exam, as a re-certificant
- ❍ To improve my clinical skills and clinical management

How soon do you think can use the information presented in this chapter?

- ❍ Immediately; within the next few days or so
- ❍ Soon; within the next month or so
- ❍ Later; sometime before I retire

Pro Tip! If you are preparing for the IBLCE exam, it would be wise to pace your studying. Set a target date for when you plan to complete the exercises, and check off them off as you go along.

Done!	Target Date	Learning Exercise
❑	____________	Learning Exercise 18-1. Vocabulary related to cleft lip and palate.
❑	____________	Learning Exercise 18-2. Case study of infant with cleft.
❑	____________	Explore What You've Learned in a Journal
❑	____________	Summarize What You've Learned
❑	____________	Quick Quiz

Master Your Vocabulary

Learning Exercise 18-1. Vocabulary related to cleft lip and palate.

Instructions: Write the letter of the correct match next to each item. Answers are in the Appendix.

_____	1. bifid	A.	cleft covered by mucous membrane
_____	2. bowel malrotation	B.	twisted intestines that become obstructed
_____	3. bilateral	C.	cleft not associated with a syndrome
_____	4. complete cleft of the palate	D.	split
_____	5. endotracheal (ET)	E.	syndrome most commonly associated with cleft defect
_____	6. grooved palate	F.	tube within the trachea to support respiration
_____	7. incomplete cleft palate	G.	placement of a tube into the trachea
_____	8. intubation	H.	includes the palatal arch
_____	9. isolated cleft	I.	typically includes a cleft palate and micrognathia
_____	10. nasogastric (NG)	J.	squeezable bottle with nipple
_____	11. orotracheal	K.	both sides
_____	12. palatal arch	L.	involves the entire hard and soft palate
_____	13. Pierre Robin Syndrome	M.	feeding tube inserted through the nose
_____	14. Pigeon feeder	N.	ET tube is inserted through the mouth
_____	15. primary palate	O.	bottle with 1-way valve, variable flow and long teat
_____	16. secondary palate	P.	soft palate
_____	17. SpecialNeeds feeder	Q.	includes the hard and soft palate
_____	18. submucous cleft	R.	involves only the secondary palate
_____	19. Van der Woude Syndrome	S.	depression in palatal tissue, either naturally or from ET tube
_____	20. velum	T.	bony arch at the roof of the mouth

Conquer Clinical Concepts

Learning Exercise 18-2. Case study of infant with cleft.

Instructions: This study refers to the infant shown in Figures 392-296. The details of this case are described in The Breastfeeding Atlas on pages 157-158 Fill in the blanks.

The nurse at the hospital thought she heard the infant swallowing. Wilson-Clay thought she heard swallowing, too. By Day 4, there were several good indicators:

- The mother achieved good ________________
- The mother demonstrated excellent ________________
- The baby sounded as if he was ______________________

But also by Day 4, there were several worrisome indicators:

- discharge ____________, using an accurate scale, was undocumented
- lack of an adequate number of ____________
- urine was _____________ (color) and ___________ (amount)
- ___________ levels were rising
- weight _______ was continuing

Wilson-Clay zeroed in on the indicators that were happening on Day 4; she knew the story didn't add up. If the infant was truly swallowing, the clinical picture would have looked differently. Presumably, she realized two other important factors: (1) infants who have neurological or structural defects can sometimes "sound" like they are swallowing but in fact, they are not, and (2) the likelihood of this successful milk transfer with such a severe defect was unlikely.

She knew that the most critical information was lacking: results of pre- and post- __________ . When she did this, she had proof of _______________. Her first few recommendations included:

- having the mother _______________________
- offering the baby ________________________

However, as is often the case with infants who have severe clefting, the infant was unable to _____________ his sucking. Hence, the lactation consultant and the mother decided to try using a ____________________________.

After the repair of the cleft, the mother had difficulty maintaining an adequate milk supply. She took _____________, some unnamed _________________, pumped at __________________ and used a _______________at the breast.

Milk production was not the only problem, however. She also had trouble with milk ____________ .

Problems continued even after the surgery of the ________________. The infant had trouble getting milk through any method that required substantial __________________. He was frustrated, and the mother ended up feeling ____ and _______. Shortly thereafter, both the infant and her toddler came down with a virus. Despite good social and professional support, the mother decided to wean.

In cases like these, it's best to:________ the mother's efforts, assist with __________________ and address the possibility of ________________________

Questions to ponder:

- As the old saying goes, we all have 20/20 vision with hindsight. But without the benefit of hindsight, if you had been the hospital nurse, would you have wondered if it was okay for this infant to get all of his nutrition at the breast?

- Have you ever thought, on first impression, that a newborn was swallowing, only to later discover that, in fact, he was not?

- Would you have been wondering what was written on this newborn's hospital discharge plan?

- If you had been in a position to write the discharge plan, what would you have picked out as a priority, or priorities?

Explore What You've Learned in a Journal

Multiple studies have shown the benefits of using a learning journal. Among them are greater assimilation and integration of new information, better long-term retention of course concepts, increasing test and exam grades, and a means by which to have continuous feedback about one's own learning.

- Name at least three things you learned from this chapter.

- List at least three things you still need to learn, or more fully master, in this chapter.

- Briefly describe how this information fits (or doesn't fit) with what you've seen in clinical practice, what you learned in basic or college courses, or what you've observed in your own experience breastfeeding. (In some cases, you might want to include how the information fits or doesn't fit with what "experts" say, what the media says, or whatever.)

- Describe how you will use any or all of this information. How might it be related to problems and potential solutions that occur in real life or in clinical situations?

- If you wish, include how you felt about learning this information. Were you overwhelmed? Enlightened? Worried? Something else?

Summarize What You've Learned

The purpose of this chapter is to help you recognize various types of orofacial clefts, their impact on breastfeeding, and strategies to initiate and continue successful milk transfer.

Sometimes, the type of information in this chapter can seem much more theoretical than clinical. Take a moment to summarize: How can you arrange the most salient points into a few bullet points? How will you use this information for individual clients in your clinical practice? How might this information be important in the bigger world of system-level changes (e.g., procedures, standing orders, etc.) or issues with populations of clients (e.g., writing patient education materials.)

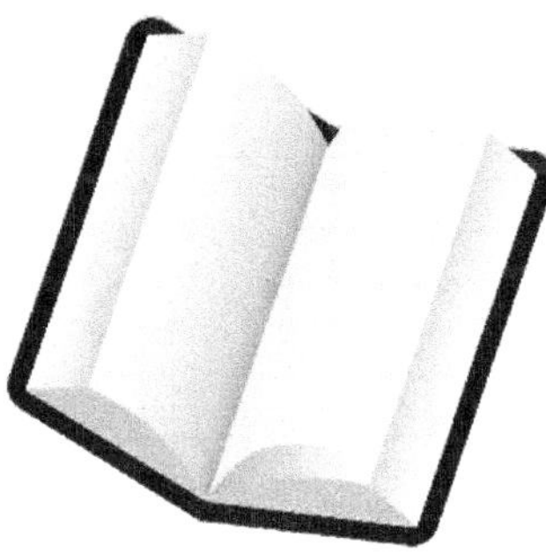

Main Points

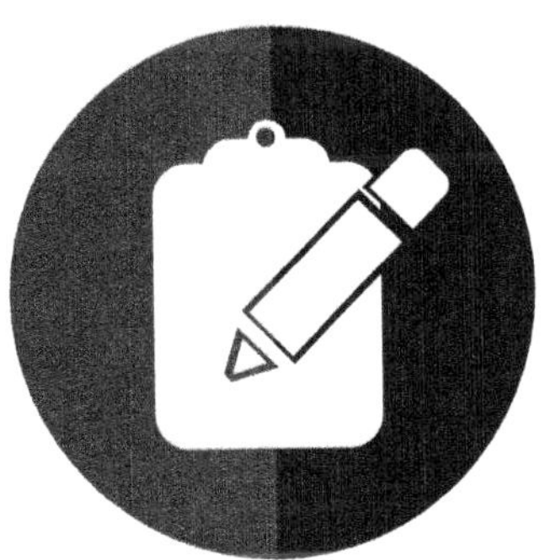

On the test

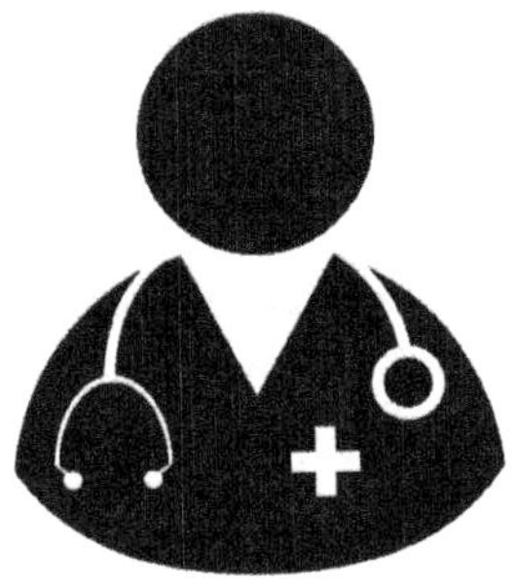

On the job

Self-Assessment

People often dive into a test before they have thoughtfully reflected on how well they have prepared for it. Instead, it would be helpful if they would take a few moments to give their alter-ego (their "other self") a chance to reflect on how confident they feel about mastering the stated objectives.

Instructions: Take a moment to review the chapter objectives (below). Then rate yourself. How confident are you that you have achieved each objective below?

Objective	Highly Confident	Somewhat Confident	Somewhat Unsure	Completely Unsure
Name orofacial clefts using widely-accepted terminology and classifications.	❍	❍	❍	❍
Recognize a submucous cleft through visualization and palpation techniques., along its management implications.	❍	❍	❍	❍
Recognize conditions that are associated with, overlooked, or mistaken for orofacial clefts.	❍	❍	❍	❍
Discuss at least four aspects of feeding difficulties that the infant with a cleft is likely to encounter.	❍	❍	❍	❍
Provide anticipatory guidance for infants who will undergo surgery for orofacial cleft defects.	❍	❍	❍	❍
Depending on the extent of the lesion, choose the techniques that is most likely to help the infant with a cleft to achieve an adequate seal, negative pressure, and mandibular compression.	❍	❍	❍	❍

On the next page, you will see some simple recall questions pertaining to this chapter. These are not the application-type questions you will find in the IBLCE exam. However, you cannot apply information unless you can fully recall that information! You should do these without looking up the answers.

When you finish with the quiz, look up the answers in the Appendix. Then, score your answers, using the Appendix. Finally, you should analyze the results of your quiz. It's not enough to just know what you got right or wrong; you must look at why you got the answers right or wrong.

Quick Quiz Chapter 18

Instructions: Circle the correct response. For a better understanding of how well you are mastering the material, try answering without looking it up. If you are really stuck, questions come from this workbook and from *The Breastfeeding Atlas* so go back and review the appropriate material. Answers are in the appendix.

1. Baby Bethel was born at 32 weeks' gestation. During morning report, a new lactation consultant says Bethel has a cleft palate. This diagnosis does not appear in her medical record. Her medical record is MOST likely to show that she was:

   A. abused while still in utero

   B. exposed to an unusual virus

   C. intubated for several days

   D. resuscitated immediately after birth

2. Whether an infant or child affected with an orofacial cleft defect can accomplish exclusive breastfeeding is MOST often predicted by:

   A. the extent of his cleft.

   B. the lactation consultant's skill.

   C. his mother's past experience.

   D. a supportive NICU environment.

3. Most times, a cleft lip and/or a cleft palate is:

   A. caused by maternal alcoholism.

   B. inherited from the parent.

   C. isolated (nonsyndromic).

   D. repaired at a community hospital.

4. A submucous cleft is often:

   A. a serious impediment.

   B. asymptomatic.

   C. repaired within the week.

   D. repaired within the year.

5. A cleft that runs the length of the primary and secondary palate is called a:

   A. bilateral cleft.

   B. complete cleft.

   C. incomplete cleft.

   D. unilateral cleft.

Analyze Your Own Quiz

- What percentage of the questions did you answer correctly?

- If you got 100% of them right, to what do you attribute your success?

- If you did not get all the questions right, can you identify your learning gap? (Example: Didn't know the information, knew the information but could not remember, knew some information but confused it with similar information, other.)

- Would you have been able answer the questions as well if you had not read this chapter?

- What do you need to do next? (If you got them all right, what you need to do next is celebrate! Even a high-five with your child, a YESSS and a fist-pump in the air, or anything else is good! A small acknowledgement of your success is better than no acknowledgement!)

Additional Resources

1. Shkoukani MA, et al. Cleft palate: a clinical review. *Birth defects research. Part C, Embryo today : reviews.* 2014;102(4):333-342.

2. Wehby GL, Murray JC. Folic acid and orofacial clefts: a review of the evidence. *Oral diseases.* 2010;16(1):11-19.

3. Watkins SE, et al. Classification, epidemiology, and genetics of orofacial clefts. *Clinics in plastic surgery.* 2014;41(2):149-163.

4. Venkatesh R. Syndromes and anomalies associated with cleft. *Indian journal of plastic surgery : official publication of the Association of Plastic Surgeons of India.* 2009;42 Suppl:S51-55.

5. Allori AC, et al. Classification of Cleft Lip/Palate: Then and Now. *Cleft Palate Craniofac J.* 2017;54(2):175-188.

6. Kernahan DA, Stark RB. A new classification for cleft lip and cleft palate. *Plastic and reconstructive surgery and the transplantation bulletin.* 1958;22(5):435-441.

7. Liu Q, et al. A simple and precise classification for cleft lip and palate: a five-digit numerical recording system. *Cleft Palate Craniofac J.* 2007;44(5):465-468.

8. Kosowski TR, et al. Cleft Palate. *Seminars in Plastic Surgery.* 2012;26(4):164-169.

9. Ha KM, et al. Submucous cleft palate: an often-missed diagnosis. *J Craniofac Surg.* 2013;24(3):878-885.

10. Oji T, et al. A 25-year review of cases with submucous cleft palate. *Int J Pediatr Otorhinolaryngol.* 2013;77(7):1183-1185.

11. McWilliams BJ. Submucous clefts of the palate: how likely are they to be symptomatic? *Cleft Palate Craniofac J.* 1991;28(3):247-249; discussion 250-241.

12. Hohoff A, et al. Palatal development of preterm and low birthweight infants compared to term infants – What do we know? Part 2: The palate of the preterm/ low birthweight infant. *Head & Face Medicine.* 2005;1:9-9.

13. Clarren SK, et al. Feeding infants with cleft lip, cleft palate, or cleft lip and palate. *Cleft Palate J.* 1987;24(3):244-249.

14. Biancuzzo M. Clinical focus on clefts. Yes! Infants with clefts can breastfeed. *AWHONN Lifelines.* 1998;2(4):45-49.

15. Lawence RA, Lawrence R. M. *Breastfeeding: A guide for the medical profession.* 8 ed.

16. Pathumwiwatana P, et al. The promotion of exclusive breastfeeding in infants with complete cleft lip and palate during the first 6 months after childbirth at Srinagarind Hospital, Khon Kaen Province, Thailand. *J Med Assoc Thai.* 2010;93 Suppl 4:S71-77.

17. Jiri B, et al. Successful early neonatal repair of cleft lip within first 8 days of life. *Int J Pediatr Otorhinolaryngol.* 2012;76(11):1616-1626.

18. Darzi MA, et al. Breast feeding or spoon feeding after cleft lip repair: a prospective, randomised study. *Br J Plast Surg.* 1996;49(1):24-26.

19. Weatherley White RC, et al. Early repair and breast-feeding for infants with cleft lip. *Plast-Reconstr-Surg.* 1987;79(6):879-887.

Appendix

Answers by Chapter

Chapter 1
Introduction

Aha! There are no exercises in Chapter 1! But I did offer you a challenge! I asked you to dive in, and take a learning approach that you may never have experienced before.

Take just a moment to think about how it went.

The aim of this workbook is to help you to:

- accurately distinguish between similar but different conditions shown in the photos
- use written exercises to recall and apply knowledge of typical features
- provide detailed context and clarification of terms as they may relate to items on the IBLCE exam

Do you feel that you have accomplished that?

Let me know!

Chapter 2
Infant States and General Appearance

Master Your Vocabulary

Learning Exercise 2-1. Terms describing normal and variations of normal well-being in newborns.

1	N	10	M
2	Q	11	G
3	H	12	I
4	E	13	P
5	K	14	D
6	J	15	F
7	O	16	B
8	C	17	L
9	A		

Conquer Clinical Concepts

Learning Exercise 2-2. Comparing four observations that are clues to sleep states.

	Deep Sleep	Light Sleep	Drowsy	Quiet Alert	Active Alert ("Fussy")	Crying
Bodily Movement	Nearly still	Some	Variable	Minimal	Variable; smooth movements	Increased, with motor activity, ruddy color
Eye Movement	No	yes, lightly, beneath the lids	Occasional	Open, and bright	Open, but dull	Tightly closed or open
Facial Movements or Expression	No	Perhaps, briefly	Perhaps, some	Attentive	Little or none	Grimaces
Breathing	Smooth, regular	Irregular	Irregular	Regular	Irregular	Irregular
Responsiveness	Low	Possible	Often easy to awaken infant, or help him to return to sleeping	High, to positive stimuli	Present but may be delayed	Highly reactive to noxious stimuli
Other observations, comments	(Up to you…)	(Up to you…)	(Up to you…)	(Up to you…)	(Up to you…)	(Up to you…)

Learning Exercise 2-3. Common examples of birth trauma. (Wordfind)

```
C E A T B J S T B Z R L W A N Y I Z R N
A E X T H B E N M J R C K A E R G J U S
P C F N A R A T C L I B V R N U I T C O
U A R N O U A N H Q L E X A S J B Q H X
T M N S F I R N G N I E Z R D N C G S Y
S O C D D S D N B A V U J L G I V N I G
U T R L C I F A C I A L P A L S Y E C E
C A I C B N R S J N I U E I L U I N H N
C M I U I G L L O E O D Q N C X F R I D
E E I D Y Q A C T E X A H E U E O C U E
D H A P E U E D A L O P A I A L T A A P
A O A B R A S I O N S X E D D P Y I O R
N L O S W C U U F N C M H S C L W E B I
E A Y R K E I A Y L T H E F A A K C O V
U H F R A C T U R E D C L A V I C L E A
M P C C V A I N W S M G O I P H O E T T
H E O R X X O D K E T B E O U C Y A T I
E C R M Z D O P R A N F S O B A V C D O
D L T H G E C S V I N S E T M R X A N N
G A B G E E V S X A S Y T T H B I R N T
```

Learning Exercise 2-4. Technology and issues related to traumatic birth

1.	E	5.	B
2.	H	6.	A
3.	G	7.	D
4.	F	8.	C

Learning Exercise 2-5. Differences between cephalohematoma and caput succedaneum.

	Cephalohematoma	Caput succedaneum
Collection of...	Blood	Fluid
Cross sutures	No	Yes (almost always)
Location	Beneath the scalp	Within the scalp
Result of...	Birth trauma, including use of assistive devices	Pressure on the head
Possible complications	Jaundice, or more serious problems, discomfort	Pointy "cone head", discomfort
Breastfeeding issue or implications...	Positioning to reduce pressure on the head Colostrum is a priority, "early and often," to help reduce likelihood of hyperbilirubinemia	Positioning to reduce pressure on the head
Resolves...	Within a few months	Within several days

Quick Quiz Chapter 2

1. C
2. B
3. B
4. C
5. B

Chapter 3
Infant Orofacial Assessment and Feeding Reflexes

Master Your Vocabulary

Learning Exercise 3-1. Terms related to data-gathering, assessment for skin and orofacial structures and function.

1. N
2. B
3. K
4. I
5. D
6. R
7. G
8. P
9. C
10. J
11. S
12. L
13. Q
14. A
15. T
16. E
17. H
18. M
19. F
20. O

Conquer Clinical Concepts

Learning Exercise 3-2. Recognizing normal and alterations in normal lip tone.

Lip Tone

Indicators

· Visual

Tight (pursed) lips indicate excessive tone

· Palpable

Normally, some resistance should be felt

· Auditory

Audible swallowing is reassuring

Clicking or smacking is nonreassuring

A&P Connections

· Structure:
Name of Main Muscle

Orbicularis oris

· Function:
Muscle's Main Function

Creates seal around nipple and areola, which results in negative pressure

Ideally, lips should be flagged around the breast

Clinical

· Reasons

general hypotonia
traumatic birth
neuromuscular deficit

· Consequences

Low tone impairs:
negative pressure
adequate seal
Infant often falls asleep

Non-Muscle Problems of Lip

tight labial frenum or any structure that restricts movement

"lip retraction" ("lip bunching")

Learning Exercise 3-3. Comparison of major differences between craniosynostosis and plagiocephaly

	Craniosynostosis	Plagiocephaly
fusion of the skull?	Yes, one (or more) of the sutures in the infant's skull closes early	skull sutures are not fused.
how common	1 out of every 2500 births	half of children in the United States have some degree of plagiocephaly
effects	asymmetry of the skull	head is misshapen, typically at the back
usual intervention	serious medical condition that often requires surgery	reduce "tummy time"
treatment practitioner?	surgeon (specialist)	primary care provider

Learning Exercise 3-4. Comparison of Mongolian slate blue spots and indicators of bruising related to physical abuse

	Mongolian spot	Bruising
Color	blue, blue-gray	blue in the beginning
Color changes	fade to a lighter blue over the years	change to different colors, typically in this order: red, blue or purple, green, yellow, brown over several days
Location	usually buttocks; may be back, legs, shoulders, upper arms, and scalp.	Anywhere. Note that infants/children **seldom** have a bruise on the buttocks from an accidental injury
Flat or raised?	flat; normal skin texture	raised
Size	2-8 cm (1-3 inches)	any
Shape	irregular	more regular; depends on weapon (or hand) used
Onset/resolution	present at birth, or shortly thereafter; usually resolves within several years	present any time; resolves within about 2 weeks
Other characteristics?	non-tender to the touch	tender to the touch

Learning Exercise 3-5. Comparison of three types of vascular nevi.

	Stork bite	Hemangioma	Port wine stain
Other names	angel kisses salmon patches	strawberry mark	---
How common?	extremely common	Somewhat; about 5-10% of newborns	Uncommon; about 3 in 1000 infants
Color, shape, size	smooth flat with the skin's surface	Superficial are bright red or purple (Figure 60). Deep hemangiomas, colors are more muted; they may even be skin color. Most are mixed—both superficial and deep	smooth, flat. shape can change into a pebbly texture. not bright red. Pink at birth, then grow darker. Typically, they are a muted maroon color.
Most likely location	forehead nose eyelids back of neck can be elsewhere	face scalp back chest can be anywhere	face scalp back chest can be anywhere
Onset, progression, resolution	not necessarily present at birth may rapidly and dramatically develop a few weeks later almost all lighten and fade completely	may appear several weeks after birth. All hemangiomas are visible by the time the infant is 6 months old.	can be treated (or masked with makeup) never disappear spontaneously
Implication for care?	Frequently mistaken for erythema or bruising	Can be treated, but parents usually forego treatment because most of them fade.	Sometimes associated with some pathology Usually, they are harmless

Quick Quiz Chapter3

1. A
2. E
3. F
4. D
5 A

Chapter 4
Infant Stools and Urine Output

Master Your Vocabulary

Learning Exercise 4-1. Matching terms related to infant output.

1. A
2. F
3. B
4. D
5. C
6. E
7. G

Conquer Clinical Concepts

Learning Exercise 4-2. Comparison of meconium, transitional, and milk stools.

	Meconium	Transitional Stool	Milk Stool
Color	dark-green or a tarry-black	olive green, or greenish-brown	bright yellow and watery yellow and yogurt-like
Consistency	sticky and even a little shiny	slippery, slimy	Loose, unformed stools are common in the first month or so. "mustard-like seeds" of milk stools are very common
Frequency/ Timing	within the first 24 hours	Meconium stools give way to transitional stools within a day or two	Ideally, onset is no later than Day 4.
Number	at least one meconium stool	At *least* 2 stools on Day 2, and at *least* 3 stools by Day 3.	Day 1 at least one stool Day 2 at least two stools Day 3 at least three stools Day 4 at least three to four through the first month.
Volume	Every newborn is different	Minimum: at least the size of a US quarter or it doesn't "count." Maximum: don't worry too much.	Minimum: at least the size of a US quarter or it doesn't "count." Maximum: don't worry too much.

Learning Exercise 4-3 Recognizing and correctly documenting types of infant output.

Question	Answer
How will you recognize various clues to determine if stool or urine output is normal, a variation of normal, or a worrisome condition that requires medical follow-up?	Five worrisome signs that require immediate medical follow-up by the primary healthcare provider: • Color: The infant's stool is white, black, or contains streaks of bright red. • Infant's reaction: The infant screams out in pain or bleeds while defecating. • Mucous: The presence of mucous, with or without blood, could indicate an infection or a food intolerance. • Changes: Dramatic changes in stool after introducing a new food or medication may indicate an allergy. • Consistency: Stool that has a more yogurt-like consistency at around age 1, or more than 5 runny stools a day after age 1. Urine output: • At least 1 wet diaper within the first 24 hours of life. Day 2 At least 2 wet diapers by Day 2 • Day 3, at least 3 wet diapers • Day 4, at least 4 wet diapers • Day 5, and thereafter: at least 6-8 wet diapers, assuming newborn has been taking in milk (including colostrum) since birth. • Urine should always be light yellow, or straw-colored.
Name factors that affect whether stool is normal.	• the age of the infant • timing of the mother's milk "coming in" • infant's overall behavior during suckling and at other times • the mother's intake (food, fluids, or medications) • the extent to which the infant is breastfed (exclusively, partially, or not at all)
How can you distinguish stool/urine output in the diaper from other observations (e.g., oozing from circumcision, pseudo-menses, other)?	• consistency • time of appearance/disappearance • amount • texture • location

Quick Quiz Chapter 4

1. D
2. C
3. B
4. D

Chapter 5
Appearance of Human Milk

Master Your Vocabulary

Learning Exercise 5-1. Basic terms related to mothers and milk-making.

1. L
2. H
3. A
4. B
5. F
6. E
7. I
8. J
9. C
10. G
11 D
12. K

Conquer Clinical Concepts

Learning Exercise 5-2 Comparisons of Lactogenesis I, II, and III.

	Lactogenesis I	Lactogenesis II	Lactogenesis III
Also called...	(Does not apply)	Onset of copious milk secretion	lactation or galactopoesis
Onset	middle of pregnancy	Around 3-4 days postpartum	as long as milk is removed from the gland on a regular basis.
Typical volume per 24 hours	drops during pregnancy average 30 ml might be as little as a few drops	Day 2, about 175 ml Day 7, about 600 ml; less if stimulation was delayed or infant did not suckle	By 1 month, about 750-800 ml/24 hrs
Color	Usually yellow	More white	Bluish white
Consistency	Thick, sticky	Fluid	Fluid
Primary control is through...	Hormones	Primarily endocrine (hormonal) and some autocrine control	Primarily autocrine control as time goes on, and secondarily through endocrine control
Other comments	Higher in protein, lower in fat	Physiologic engorgement	Some consistency in patterns

Quick Quiz Chapter 5

1. A
2. B
3. E
4. B
5. D

Chapter 6
Positioning and Latch Techniques

Master Your Vocabulary

Learning Exercise 6-1. Matching anatomical terms of movement and direction.

1. I
2. D
3. A
4. J
5. H
6. K
7. F
8. B
9. C
10. G
11. E

Learning Exercise 6-2. Stick figures to show the meaning of directional terms.

Everyone draws their understanding in a little different way! You might want to see these "actions" in videos if you are having trouble drawing them.

There are many videos available that describe these terms. Most are long, and more specific than you might want or need. Here are a few that will give you the information you need to draw your own stick figures.

A little corny, but this gives clear descriptions!!
https://www.youtube.com/watch?v=DuxCiNdOtD8

Woman and man, fairly good: *https://www.youtube.com/watch?v=vdScqySvcxc*

Supination, pronation, adduction, abduction, rotation
https://www.pinterest.com/pin/247979523206875511/

Flexion, extension, hyperflexion, hyperextension supination, pronation

https://www.pinterest.com/pin/247979523206875511/

https://www.youtube.com/watch?v=DuxCiNdOtD8

woman and men, pretty good: *https://www.youtube.com/watch?v=vdScqySvcxc*

Conquer Clinical Concepts

Learning Exercise 6-3. Recognizing reasons to use or avoid positions, and their common pitfalls.

	Best reasons to use, and/or advantages	Least likely reasons to use	Pitfalls to avoid
Cradle hold	Older infant who supports himself.	newborns, small infants hypotonic infants	Optimal latch-on may not occur in infants who need substantial support.
Cross-cradle (transitional) hold	infants who are hypotonic or small. mother who feels a little unsure of herself and wants to have a firmer grip. mother can move the infant from one side using the cross-cradle to the other side using the football hold.	Any situation where the mother's hand or wrist or arm is stressed by supporting the infant's head. Many new mothers have an IV in their hand or wrist the first few days; others have a problem that lasts much longer, for example, carpal tunnel syndrome.	Mother may inadvertently push on the infant's head and hyperflex his neck
Football hold	cesarean surgery, large breasts, obese mothers (maybe)	Any situation where the mother's hand or wrist or arm is stressed by supporting the infant's head	A vigorously kicking infant may reflexively push his feet against the bed or chair. (Techniques to minimize this are discussed in the chapter)
Side-lying hold	Nighttime feedings, cesarean delivery, sore episiotomy painful hemorrhoids	Small breasts	infant may slide off chest-to-chest or tummy-to-mummy position. If the mother falls asleep during breastfeeding, this could increase the infant's risk for suffocation
Straddle hold	Hypotonic infants with orofacial structural defects.	If the newborn is especially small, and/or if the mother is obese.	Discomfort or awkwardness

Learning Exercise 6-4 Matching specific positions and holds to their descriptions.

1. E
2. I (or G)
3. F
4. C
5. G
6. D
7. A
8. B
9. H

Quick Quiz Chapter 6

1. C
2. B
3. A
4. D
5. C

Chapter 7
Nipple Inversion, Eversion, & Elasticity

Master Your Vocabulary

Learning Exercise 7-1. Vocabulary for everted, inverted, and short nipples.

1.	B	7.	D
2.	J	8.	C
3.	L	9.	E
4.	H	10.	A
5.	K	11.	F
6.	I	12.	G

Conquer Clinical Concepts

Learning Exercise 7-2 Using shells and shields.

1. A nipple shell could be worn either during pregnancy or after delivery. However, it can only be worn between feedings.

2. If a mother's nipple has little or no elasticity, it is unlikely to provide adequate stimulation to the infant's palate.

3. Although infants can initially "accommodate" a large-diameter shield, it is difficult for them to sustain an adequate seal around it.

Learning Exercise 7-3. Determining if the infant using a shield is well latched.

	Infant is latched well	Infant is poorly latched
Mouth, gape	big gape; open-wide mouth	small gape
Where will the lips be?	on the "body" of the shield	on the shaft of the shield
Rhythmic sucking?	rhythmic suckling audible swallowing	non-rhythmic suckling little or no audible swallowing
Milk inside the shield's teat?	presence of milk in the teat	milk not inside the teat
Weight Gain	steady weight gain	weight loss, or inadequate weight gain

Quick Quiz Chapter 7

1. C
2 B
3. A
4. A
5. B

Chapter 8
Nipple Lesions

Learning Exercise 8-1. Matching common skin lesions to their description.

1.	Q	11.	L
2.	T	12.	C
3.	F	13.	N
4.	B	14.	I
5.	O	15.	D
6.	S	16.	G
7.	R	17.	K
8.	P	18.	E
9.	J	19.	H
10.	M	20.	A

Learning Exercise 8-2 Recognizing common prefixes, roots, and words.

Prefix/Suffix	Meaning	Word in this chapter
-ema, emia	blood	erythema
-it is	inflammation	folliculitis, dermatitis, mastitis
-osis	condition or disease	diagnosis, prognosis, candidosis, ecchymosis
-phasic	having phases	biphasic, triphasic
a-	not; without	atopic, asymptomatic, amastia, atypical
ab-	away from	abnormal
aller-	Denoting something as different	allergy allergen
anti-	against	antibiotic, antifungal, antiviral
bi-	twice; double	biphasic, bifid
cya-	blue color	cyanotic
cutane-	skin (Latin)	subcutaneous
derm-	skin (Greek)	epidermis, dermis, subdermis
ec(t)-	out, away	telectasia
epi-	on; upon	epidermis
erythr(o)-	redness or being flushed	erythemia
hist-	tissue	histamine
hyper	above	hyperpigmentation
hypo	beneath	hypodermis, hypopigmentation
necr(o)-	death	necrotic
ser-, sero-	watery; fluid	serous
tri	three	triphasic
-ule	small, diminutive	nodule, pustule, ductule, lobule
urt-	herbaceous plant with jagged leaves and stinging hairs	urticaria
vas(o)-	duct; blood vessel	vasoconstriction, vasodilation
-ema, emia	blood	erythema

Learning Exercise 8-3. Identifying those "white spots" on nipples

1. It is round in shape. White plaque caused by yeast is more likely to follow the skin crevices. This is the biggest clue.

2. It does not appear to be raised off the skin (Admittedly, a little hard to tell in a photo.)

3. The texture does not appear "velvety." (Again, it's a little hard to tell in a photo.)

Learning Exercise 8-4. Comparison of herpes and impetigo lesions.

	Herpes	Impetigo
Lesion type (appearance)	clustered vesicles	clustered vesicles, followed by honey-colored crusts
Lesion distribution	lips, nose, face	lips, nose, face, breasts
Lesion size	< 1 cm	< 1 cm
Associated sensation	tingling, itchy, painful	itchy, painless
Causative pathogen	Viral: Herpes simplex	Bacterial: Strep or Staph
Effectively resolved with…	antiretroviral treatment	antibiotic treatment
Recurrent?	Signs/symptoms recur	Unlikely
Contagious?	Highly	Highly
Transmission?	Direct contact: sexual or oral contact Droplet Autotransmission	Direct contact (touching) Indirect contact: inanimate objects, surfaces, etc.

Learning Exercise 8-5. Conditions associated with skin lesions.

1. G
2. F
3. A
4. C
5. D
6. E
7. H
8. B

Quick Quiz Chapter 8

1. D
2. C
3. D
4. A
5. C

Chapter 9
Congenital and Acquired Variations of the Breasts and Nipples

Master Your Vocabulary

Learning Exercise 9-1. Vocabulary for selected anatomical variation

1. F
2. H
3. E
4. B
5. D
6. I
7. C
8. L
9. J.
10. A
11. G
12. K

Learning Exercise 9-2. Matching terms to their graphic image.

Everyone draws a little differently! Your drawing should depict these characteristics.

- **amastia** means that a mammary gland and possibly the nipple are absent
- **amazia** (also *amasia*) is a condition in which the breast is absent but the nipple is present
- **athelia** means lack of a nipple
- **hyperadenia** or **hypermastia** means extra mammary glands; this is an observable characteristic
- **hyperplasia, hyperplastic** means growth of cells within the ducts and/or lobules; this is *internal* and cannot be observed so the breasts look normal
- **hypomastia** means hypoplasia that affects the *mammary* gland, specifically
- **hypoplasia, hypoplastic** refers to *any* gland that is lacking in normal amount of tissue
- **macromastia** means large breasts with normal glandular tissue
- **mammoplasty** means the woman has had either an augmentation or a reduction; this is a surgical procedure that changes the size of the breast
- **micromastia** means small breasts with adequate glandular tissue
- **symmastia** means a web-like appearance

Learning Exercise 9-3. Impact of congenital variations on lactation

Likelihood of Exclusive Breastfeeding

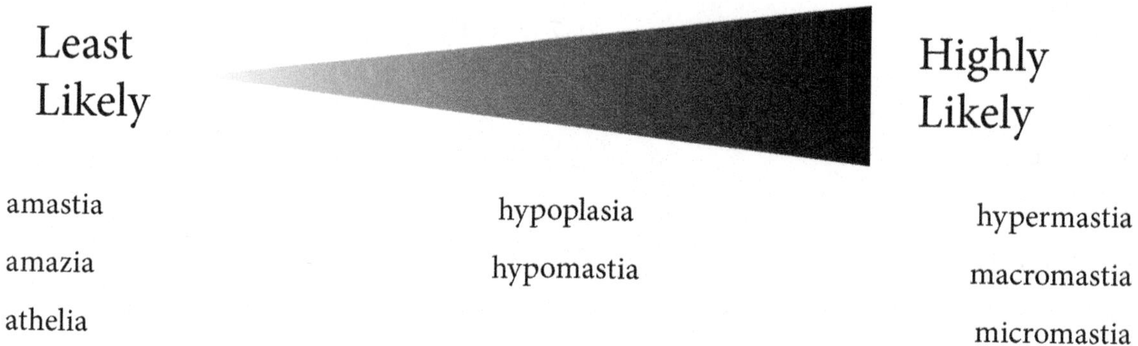

Quick Quiz Chapter 9

1. E
2. B
3. B
4. A
5. A

Chapter 10
Impact of Breast/Nipple Anatomy on Clinical Management

Master Your Vocabulary

Learning Exercise 10-1. Recognizing photos of nipple and flange issues.

1. E
2. B
3. C
4. I
4. A
6. G
7. D
8. J
9. F
10. H

Learning Exercise 10-2. Using correct terminology for parts of a pump.

1. E
2. F
3. B
4. A
5. D
6. C

Conquer Clinical Concepts

Learning Exercise 10-3. Recognizing and labeling parts of a flange.

1. The rim is at A
2. The flare is at B; the entire shaded part
3. The shaft (tunnel) is at C
4. The connector is at D

Learning Exercise 10-4. Nipple length and diameter and their clinical indicators and implications.

Nipple length: What are possible consequences of an especially long nipple?	infant gagging poor milk transfer dwindling milk supply skin damage to the nipple dehydration failure to thrive skin infection.
Nipple diameter: What are three ways that nipple diameter be measured, or estimated?	calipers circle template ruler coins
Nipple diameter: What is considered the diameter of most nipples?	About 15 mm or 16 mm. Range is about 23-40 mm
Nipple diameter: What 5 or 6 factors affect nipple size and diameter?	changes in pregnancy engorgement (especially during the postpartum period) location (the right is usually larger)3 activity (at rest vs. feeding or pumping) ethnicity duration of lactation
Nipple diameter: How do large-diameter nipples impact latch?	disproportion between the infant's mouth and the mother's nipple can make it difficult for the infant to accommodate her nipple.
What indicators suggest that the flange size is incorrect, and how can you tell for sure?	Discomfort redness cracks at the base of the nipple abrasions (more)
Compare nipples at rest to nipples during a pumping session. What happens?	While pumping, the nipple can increase in length—sometimes substantially.

Quick Quiz Chapter 10

1. D
2. B
3. A
4. C
5. A

Chapter 11
Engorgement, Oversupply, and Mastitis

Learning Exercise 11-1. Terms related to milk stasis and milk overproduction.

1. E
2. D
3. L
4. B
5. M
6. O
7. F
8. K
9. G
10. I
11. A
12. N
13. C
14. H
15. J

Learning Exercise 11-2. Terms related to lactational mastitis.

1. E
2. M
3. I
4. B
5. L
6. F
7. K
8. H
9. D
10. G
11. J
12. C
13. A

Conquer Clinical Concepts

Exercise 11-3. Comparison of physiologic and pathologic engorgement.

	Physiologic Engorgement	Pathologic Engorgement
Likely maternal perception	Tender, uncomfortable	Painful; very painful
Breast is soft, firm or hard?	Firm; about as firm as your chin	Hard; about as hard as your forehead
Appearance of skin	Veins visible, but skin normal color	Shiny; taut Redness, or red streaking
Other?	Resolves spontaneously, sooner or later.	Usually progresses to a plugged duct and/or mastitis.

Quick Quiz Chapter 11

1. D
2. A
3. C
4. B
5. D

Chapter 12
Breast Cancer and Issues for Lactation

Master Your Vocabulary

Learning Exercise 12-1. Terms related to breast cancer diagnosis and treatments.

1. P
2. K
3. O
4. H
5. Q
6. L
7. J
8. G
9. A
10. C
11. M
12. D
13. F
14. E
15. N
16. B
17. I

Conquer Clinical Concepts

Learning Exercise 12-2. Comparing lactation observations that may be precancerous.

Observation	Commonly-observed in lactating mothers	Suspicious observations
Breast size	Enlarged bilaterally with milk; breast may be fuller than the other	Enlargement that is not explainable by milk supply, and accompanied by other concerning observations
Breast symmetry	Approximately equal	Unequal, and not explainable by difference in milk supply
Color	Normal skin color, or reddened area can be easily explained.	Reddened in one area, and other observations are concerning.
Edema	Present especially in the early days after epidural anesthesia; less likely thereafter	Edema accompanied by heat and redness that cannot be explained by mastitis.
Induration	Possible in the presence of an abscess	No abscess present
Peau d'orange	Possible if abscess is present	Possible
Discharge	A little blood, usually bilateral, most notable after a feeding and explainable by a poor latch; becomes better with optimal latch or "resting"	Copious, spontaneous bloody or clear unilateral discharge that persists over many days or weeks.
Mastitis	May recur in the same place but is treatable with appropriate antibiotic therapy.	Mastitis-like symptoms that do not respond to antibiotic therapy.
Lumps	Decrease or disappear within a few or several days, lumps are fluid-filled and regularly shaped. Lumps in the breast feel similar to one another.	Persist for more than 2 weeks; lumps are solid, irregularly shaped. Lump is solitary, or feels different from other lumps in the breast

Learning Exercise 12-3. Venn diagram to show similarities and differences between ultrasounds and mammograms.

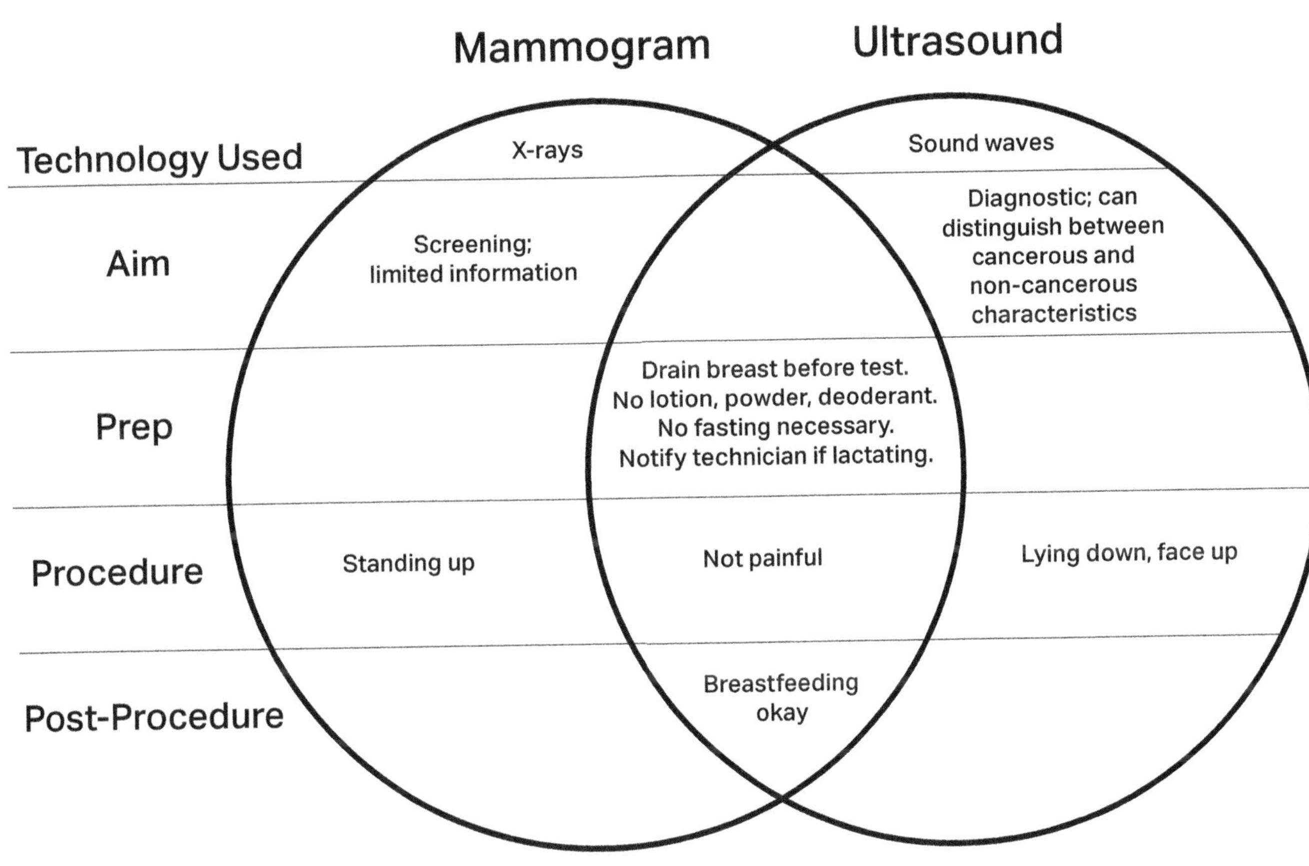

Learning Exercise 12-4. Case Study A (Figure 273-275)

- Answers are on page 104 of *The Breastfeeding Atlas.*
- The woman in the case has scars from two incisions A **circumareolar** incision was made from the biopsy made during her childbearing years. This fairly short thin line is faintly visible at the areola edge; the lesion was benign.
- After her childbearing years were over, the more recent **curvilinear incision** was used to perform a lumpectomy to remove a cancerous lesion; the scar is seen in the photo. (A radial incision, not seen in the photos but shown in the diagram below, is generally avoided in a younger woman, to lessen the cosmetic impact of the surgery.) A lumpectomy is performed to remove a cancerous lesion, and to **create clean margins**.
- **Yes**, it is okay to wash radiation-bronzed skin; see *The Breastfeeding Atlas* page 104 for details.

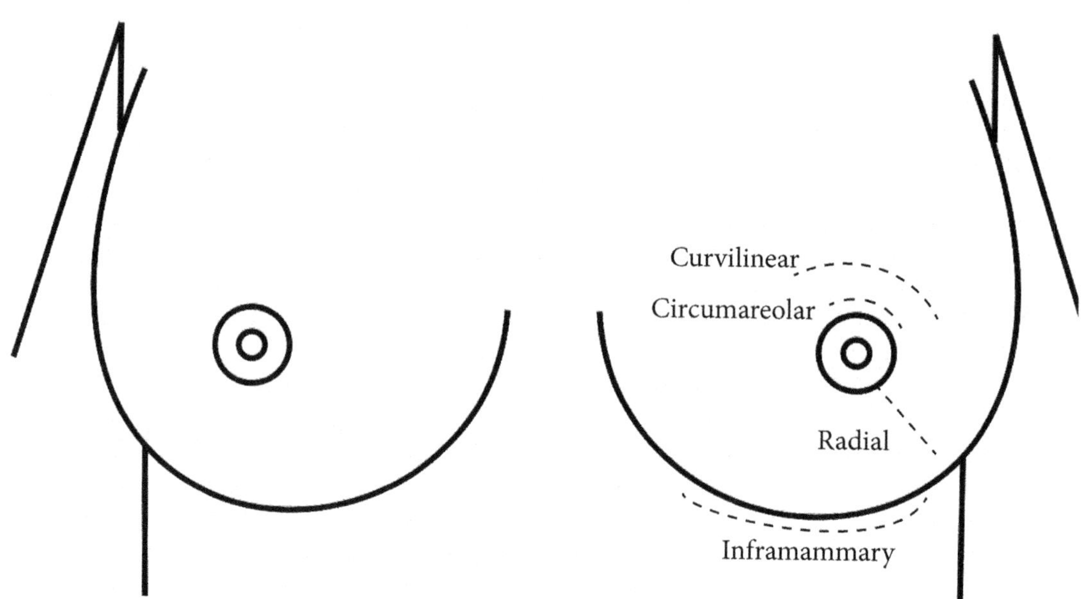

Reprinted with permission from Marie Biancuzzo's Comprehensive Lactation Course.

Learning Exercise 12-5. Case Study B (Figure 277)

- Each professional must form his or her own philosophy about these sorts of things. Mine might be different from yours, or from the authors of *The Breastfeeding Atlas* or any other professional or any other publication. Sometimes, "resting" make sense if it will give the woman some relief. If she suggests an ultimatum, ("If I can't rest my nipples…I'll quit!) then definitely, agree to the "rest" strategy! Returning to nursing after having had a bottle for five days is likely to present little or no problem.
- It was unrelated. Read the details in *The Breastfeeding Atlas.*

Learning Exercise 12-6. Case Study C (Figures 278-280)

- Emergency weaning was initiated because the mother was about to begin chemotherapy, which would be considered incompatible with breastfeeding.
- The woman gave birth to a healthy child (Page 105)
- Two likely causes would be cancer, or possibly abscess.
- She breastfed the infant for five months (Page 105)

Learning Exercise 12-7. Case Study D (Figures 281-283)

Answers are in *The Breastfeeding Atlas.*

The take-home message for the lactation professional is: Be an advocate for the mother, and help her to advocate for herself!

Quick Quiz Chapter 12

1. A
2. D
3. A
4. B
5. A

Chapter 13
Twins, Triplets and Tandem Nursing

Learning Exercise 13-1. Basic vocabulary related to twins, triplets and tandem nursing

1. B
2. E
3. F
4. G
5. A
6. D
7. C

Learning Exercise 13-2. Recognizing feeding strategies in photos.

1. B
2. E
3. D
4. C
5. A

Conquer Clinical Concepts

Learning Exercise 13-3. Techniques for sequential or simultaneous feedings.

Sequential	• Works well in the first month or more when newborns need more support (and mothers are still learning how to provide it.) **Figure 287** is an example • Works well for those who choose to do sequential feedings indefinitely.
Simultaneous	• Most mothers do not have the coordination to achieve simultaneous feeds (until they are more comfortable handling their twins.) • Works well when mother has mastered the skill of handling both infants at once. In the early days, few can manage it. It may take a month of more. • Works better when developmental changes occur during the first months of the twins' life—such as being able to hold their own heads up, sit up assisted, or sit up independently.
Cradle/Cradle	• Does not work well for good alignment because newborns, especially preterm newborns, need substantial postural support that a double cradle-hold in a "V" (**Figure 288**) cannot reliably provide. • Works better after infants have better muscle tone.
Football/ Football	• Works well when mothers want to begin simultaneous feedings of twins (**Figure 290**). • Works well to provide good head, neck, and shoulder support for each twin while keeping both in the *en face* position.
Side-lying	• Works better for older infants. • Might work fine for sequential feeding, if the infant does not need much support.
Standing	• Works well for toddlers who are on the go!
Use of pillows	• Works well to help with positioning, especially in the early days.

Learning Exercise 13-4. Recognizing key indicators of positioning.

Figure 289. Indicators for postural/positional changes needed.

- Mother's hand is on the back of the infant's neck
- Mother appears to be slouched
- Both infants are on a pillow, but mother's arms are unsupported
- Mother is not supporting her breast

Figure 290. Two indicators that should help to achieve good milk transfer.

- Good visualization
- Mother is supporting each twin's head, neck, and shoulders

Figure 297. If you were counseling the mother shown in this photo, you might want to praise her for doing such a good job, but offer her a gentle caution to interrupt breastfeeding and seek help if she experiences contractions.

Quick Quiz Chapter 13

1. C
2. A
3. C
4. D
5. D

Chapter 14
Alternative Feeding Methods

Master Your Vocabulary

Learning Exercise 14-1. Vocabulary related to alternative feeding methods.

1. B
2. G
3. F
4. D
5. H
6. E
7. I
8. A
9. C

Conquer Clinical Concepts

Learning Exercise 14-2. Comparison of the standard positioning and reverse positioning techniques.

	Standard Positioning Techniques	Reverse Positioning Techniques
What is a likely reason for using the technique?	to deliver fluid to an infant	to deliver fluid to an infant who is showing resistance to the tube
How is the tube entering and contacting the tongue?	enters mouth centered along palate and tube is in contact with upper lip	lower lip and tongue are in contact with the tube (**Figure 320**).
Where is the tube positioned in relation to the breast/nipple?	*above* the nipple	at the side of the breast
How far should the tube extend beyond the nipple?	about ¼ inch beyond the nipple	touches, but does not extend past the nipple (**Figure 319**)

Learning Exercise 14-3. Recalling pertinent details on techniques for alternative feeding methods.

1. When cup feeding, it is critical to wait for the infant to **swallow** before offering more milk.
2. Paced feeding can be used with **any** alternative feeding method.
3. When pacing the feeding, the caregiver should pause if the infant does not spontaneously breath after **3** to **5** sucks.
4. In paced feeding, the fluid is held **horizontal** to the infant's lips.
5. Trying to completely withdraw the bottle from the infant's mouth may result in him exerting more **negative** pressure on the nipple.
6. There is no need have milk **fill** the teat when bottle-feeding an infant.
7. Finger-feeding should be done with the caregiver's finger pad-side **up**.
8. The purpose of paced feeding is to help the infant avoid coping with **excessive milk volume** (or fast flow).
9. Feeding with a syringe is best accomplished when the syringe is **combined with finger feeding**.
10. An infant is not a candidate for using a nursing supplementer unless he can **compress the mother's nipple and the tube**.

Learning Exercise 14-4. Indications and contraindications for alternative feeding devices when supplementation is medically indicated.

Device	Indication(s)	Contraindication(s)
Bottle	To deliver fluid with a familiar device	Any medical contraindication to oral feedings, as determined by the physician.
Spoon feeding	To deliver fluid, especially when mother has colostrum. To help rouse a sleepy baby	Any medical contraindication to oral feedings, as determined by the physician.
Finger feeding	To deliver fluid to an infant who cannot get some or all of his feeding at the breast	Any medical contraindication to oral feedings, as determined by the physician
Cup feeding	To deliver fluid to an infant who cannot get some or all of his feeding at the breast.	Any medical contraindication to oral feedings, as determined by the physician
Nursing supplementer	To deliver fluid to an infant who cannot suckle well enough to get all of his feeding at the breast.	Any infant who cannot compress with breast well enough to obtain fluid from the device. Any medical contraindication to oral feedings, as determined by the physician
Paladai	To deliver fluid to an infant who cannot suckle well enough to get all of his feeding at the breast.	Any medical contraindication to oral feedings, as determined by the physician

Learning Exercise 14-5. Advantages and disadvantages of alternative feeding devices.

Device	Advantage(s) over other alternative methods	Disadvantages compared to other alternative methods
Bottle	Familiar to parents and professionals Easily available	often blamed for so-called "nipple confusion" infant may reject a rubber nipple
Spoon feeding	can be held next to the nipple no waste; no need to transfer milk to or from another device can be used to easily help rouse the infant	offers no opportunity for sucking
Finger feeding	offers the opportunity to suck feels, tastes, and smells similar to skin on the breast	some infants may resist tube some parents may not like doing it
Cup feeding	easily available; *any* cup is acceptable easy to clean; preferred by World Health Organization has had much research to show ease and efficacy	offers no opportunity for sucking critics say milk spills or it's difficult to learn/teach
Nursing supplementer	Keeps the infant "practicing" feeding at the breast while delivering fluid and calories provides breast stimulation but *cannot be used as sole source of stimulation* to the breast	may be awkward for mother to use cannot be used for infant who has poor ability to compress breast and tube *traditional* positioning does not work well for infant with aversion to tubes
Paladai	infants with clefts took more milk with paladai than with cups or spoons maximum volume in the least amount of time lightweight, portable, easy to clean.	may not be easily available

Quick Quiz Chapter 14

1. C
2. B
3. D
4. C
5. A

Chapter 15
Emergency Preparedness and Breastfeeding

Master Your Vocabulary

Learning exercise 15-1. Terms related to breastfeeding in emergency situations.

In emergency situations where some mothers are lost or somehow separated from their infants or children, the best option for feeding them might be through **milk sharing**. If so, milk can be heated briefly by bringing it to **boiling point (or 100° C, 212° F)** and immediately taking it off the heat. This is different than traditional Holder **pasteurization** which done by heating the milk to 62.5 degrees C., and holding it at that temperature for 30 minutes. Another possibility is for a willing mother to put the orphan to her own breast, an ancient practice known as **wet nursing**.

Later, mothers and their infants or children are reunited, mothers who have "lost their milk" in the interim should be given information on **relactation**.

Sometimes, infants or children die in a disaster. The lactating mother will need help with **suppression.**

Quick Quiz Chapter 15

1. B
2. C
3. C
4. C
5. A

Chapter 16
Breastfeeding with a Syndrome or Problem

Master Your Vocabulary

Learning Exercise 16-1. Terms related to selected examples of pathological conditions.

1. J
2. I
3. C
4. E
5. H
6. L
7. N
8. A
9. G
10. F
11. K
12. D
13. M
14. B

Conquer Clinical Concepts

Learning Exercise 16-2. Infant with hydrocephalus.

- The shunt was located on the left side of his head
- It's entirely possible that the infant either perceives pain in a way that he did not previously, or that he has the wherewithal to realize that he now can avoid such pain.
- The FIRST suggestion should be to change posture/positioning.
- He continued to be exclusively breastfed for six months, and partially breastfed for four years!
- At age five months, the neurologist observed that this infant had more favorable brain development than what he typically saw.

Learning Exercise 16-3. Three clinical cases of failure to thrive.

Answers are in *The Breastfeeding Atlas*, page 135-136.

Quick Quiz Chapter 16

1. B
2. B
3. C
4. D

Chapter 17
Breastfeeding With Ankyloglossia

Master Your Vocabulary

Exercise 17-1. Vocabulary words related to ankyloglossia

1. E
2. H
3. I
4. J
5. D
6. B
7. L
8. A
9. C
10. K
11. F
12. G

Conquer Clinical Concepts

Exercise 17-2. Comparing images of tongue elevation

	Figure 350	Figure 351
How far the tongue is lifted	can touch upper teeth	cannot touch upper teeth
Shape of the tip of the tongue when lifted	same as at rest	heart-shaped

Learning Exercise 17-3. "Lessons learned" from clinical cases.

Case A

At the initial assessment, the infant demonstrates several capabilities and limitations

- tight, fleshy lingual frenum
- flat tongue; difficulty forming a central groove
- struggled with bottle-feeding and cup feeding; spilled milk
- behavior agitated during feeding

Procedure used

- performed by ENT
- seated on mother's lap
- mother and nurse held firmly
- snipped with scissors

Observations at one week post-frenotomy

- a small, white lesion present on the underside of the tongue
- infant still having trouble gaining weight
- tongue tip does not lift past midline plane

Observations at two weeks' post-frenotomy

- incision is completely healed
- tongue can achieve cup shape

Observations at three weeks' post-frenotomy

- better able to coordinate and swallow fluids
- stamina improved; longer and more effective feeding
- improved but slow weight gain

Clinical Case B

Each professional must determine how to practice within his or her scope of practice and personal philosophy. I feel very clear about my role, responsibilities, scope of practice, and personal philosophy. I do not stick my fingers in infants' mouths unless I have a reason to. (Similarly, when I am in the role of labor and delivery nurse, I do not perform a vaginal exam on a woman unless I have a reason to!) Taking a line from my close friend Debi Bocar, RN PhD IBCLC, I consider my finger a "guest" in the infant's mouth.

Here, the authors tell us that this infant demonstrated effective feeding skills, was gaining weight, and his mother did not experience sore nipples. I do not see a reason for a digital exam in this case. (Doing a baseline digital exam shortly after birth is a good reason to do a digital exam; the reason is to establish a baseline.)

Clinical Case C

In the first day or so in the hospital, clicking or smacking may have been noted during the feeding. It's highly likely that the mother's nipples were "sore" during those days, but likely as not, there was no routine inspection of the mother's nipples or breasts. It would be interesting to see what risk factors for yeast were present.

Quick Quiz Chapter 17

1. C
2. B
3. A
4. D
5. C

Chapter 18
Breastfeeding With Cleft Lip and Palate

Master Your Vocabulary

1. D
2. B
3. K
4. L
5. F
6. S
7. R
8. G
9. C
10. M
11. N
12. T
13. I
14. J
15. H
16. Q
17. O
18. A
19. E
20. P

Conquer Clinical Concepts

Answers are on page 157-158 of The Breastfeeding Atlas

Quick Quiz Chapter 18

1. C
2. A
3. C
4. B
5. B

About Marie

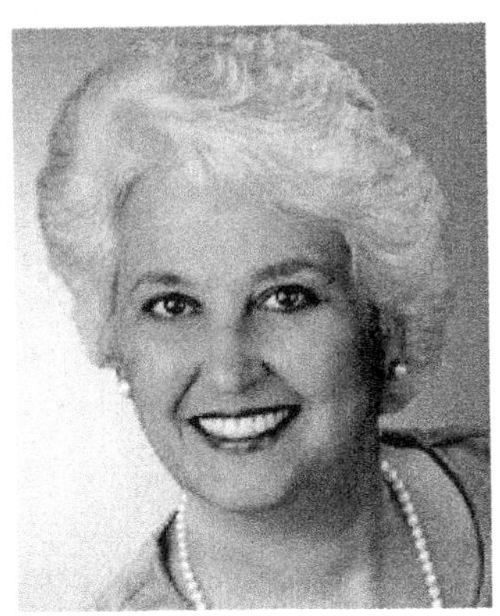

Marie Biancuzzo, RN MS CCL IBCLC, is an internationally-recognized expert in breastfeeding and the founder of Breastfeeding Outlook. As the company's educational director, Marie has taught more than one-quarter of the current IBCLCs in the US and helped them to meet their goals. Marie has more than 30 years of clinical expertise with breastfeeding management, and her company has been recognized by the International Board of Lactation Consultant Examiners and the American Nurses Association as a long-term provider of continuing education. Marie is the author of *Breastfeeding the Newborn: Clinical Strategies for Nurses*, many independent study modules and peer-reviewed articles, as well as the host of *Born to be Breastfed*, a weekly online radio show.

Other Books by Marie

How to Pass the IBLCE Exam This Time: Making the Sure-Footed Climb to Success After Failure (Gold Standard Publishing, 2017)

Test-Taking Strategies: A Guide to Taking and Passing the IBLCE Exam, 4th ed. (Gold Standard Publishing, 2015)

Breastfeeding the Newborn: Clinical Strategies for Nurses, 2nd ed. (Gold Standard Publishing, 2002)

Sore Nipples: Prevention and Problem Solving, 3rd ed. (Gold Standard Publishing, 2016)

Additional Resources from Marie

Born to be Breastfed (VoiceAmerica, 2013-current). Weekly online radio podcasts.

Comprehensive Lactation Course: Cornerstones of Clinical Care & Exam Success (Four-day seminar plus 60 hours online learning, locations vary)

Marie Biancuzzo's Lactation Exam Review (Two-day seminar, locations vary)

Picture Perfect: Finding the Clues, Getting the Answers, and Passing the IBLCE Exam (One-day seminar, locations vary)

Lactation flash cards (Gold Standard Publishing, 2016). Available on the Apple App Store or Google Play

Online learning programs (Topics vary but include Baby-Friendly or Ten Steps training, colic, common breast problems, engorgement, ethics, galactagogues, tandem breastfeeding, nipple shields, postpartum depression, mastitis, and more. See BreastfeedingOutlook.com for details.)

Radio Shows

All of Marie's *Born to be Breastfed* radio shows are recorded and available at ***http://borntobebreastfed.com*** or ***https://www.voiceamerica.com/show/2248/born-to-be-breastfed.***

They are also available as podcasts, which you may subscribe to, via **iTunes** or **Stitcher** on portable devices.

Here are shows that are most relevant to the topics in this workbook.

Babies With Tongue and Lip Ties: What's Fact, What's False and How to Overcome the Problems
Guest: Lawrence Kotlow
Air Date: August 29, 2016
https://www.voiceamerica.com/episode/93984/babies-with-tongue-and-lip-ties-whats-fact-whats-false-and-how-to-overcome-the-problems

Cleft Lip or Palate: Smart Strategies to help you breastfeed your baby
Guest: Leslie Turner
Air Date: July 25, 2016
https://www.voiceamerica.com/episode/93287/cleft-lip-or-palate-smart-strategies-to-help-you-breastfeed-your-baby

How Biological Nurturing is Key to Relaxed, Joyful Nursing for Mother and Newborn
Guest: Susan Colson
Air Date: January 16, 2017
https://www.voiceamerica.com/episode/96805/how-biological-nurturing-is-key-to-relaxed-joyful-nursing-for-mother-and-newborn

The Number 1 Guide to Looking at Your Breastfed Baby's Number Two
Guest: Bryan Vartabedian
Air Date: July 3, 2017
https://www.voiceamerica.com/episode/99744/the-number-1-guide-to-looking-at-your-breastfed-babys-number-two

Breastfeeding Twins, Triplets, and More!
Guest: Karen Gromada
Air Date: November 11, 2013
https://www.voiceamerica.com/episode/73969/breastfeeding-twins-tripletsor-more

Tongue and Lip Ties: New science challenges the status quo
Guest: Pamela Douglas
Air Date: October 16. 2017
https://www.voiceamerica.com/episode/102970/tongue-and-lip-ties-new-science-challenges-the-status-quo

Your guilt-free quick guide to a positive experience of mother-led weaning
Guest: Ariadne Brill
Air Date: August 14, 2017
https://www.voiceamerica.com/episode/100723/your-guilt-free-quick-guide-to-a-positive-experience-of-mother-le

You CAN Understand Your Baby! Find Out How
Guest: Di Bustamante
Air Date: January 23, 2017
https://www.voiceamerica.com/episode/97020/you-can-understand-your-baby-find-out-how

Don't Fear Baby's Tears: Keys to Aware Parenting
Guest: Aletha Solter
Air Date: April 24, 2017
https://www.voiceamerica.com/episode/98595/dont-fear-babys-tears-keys-to-aware-parenting

What Your Mother Never Told You About the Love Hormone!
Guest: Wendy Jones
Air Date: July 17, 2017
https://www.voiceamerica.com/episode/99967/what-your-mother-never-told-you-about-the-love-hormone

The Intergenerational Secret Service Inside You--and Your Baby
Guest: Toni Harman
Air Date: November 28, 2016
https://www.voiceamerica.com/episode/95830/the-intergenerational-secret-service-inside-you-and-your-baby

Epige-WHAT? Why it Matters for Your Milk and Your Baby
Guest: Jenny Thomas
Air Date: January 25, 2016
https://www.voiceamerica.com/episode/90090/epige-what-why-it-matters-for-your-milk-and-your-baby

Breastfeeding a Baby Affected With Down Syndrome: You Can Do It!
Guest: Doris Stevick
Air Date: August 21, 2017
https://www.voiceamerica.com/episode/100881/breastfeeding-a-baby-affected-with-down-syndrome-you-can-do-it

CPSIA information can be obtained
at www.ICGtesting.com
Printed in the USA
BVOW09s1354010318
509335BV00007B/139/P

9 781931 048576